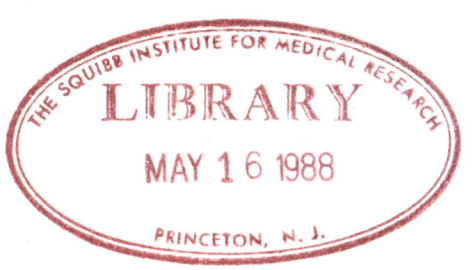

NEW CONCEPTS IN ALZHEIMER'S DISEASE

Pierre Fabre Monograph Series

Series Editors:

M. BRILEY, J. P. COUZINIER, P. LENOBLE and
J. TISNE-VERSAILLES
Centre de Recherche Pierre Fabre
Avenue Jean Moulin 17
81100 Castres Cédex
France

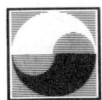

PIERRE FABRE MONOGRAPH SERIES
VOLUME 1

NEW CONCEPTS IN ALZHEIMER'S DISEASE

Edited by

M. BRILEY

Département de Pharmacologie Biochimique
Centre de Recherche Pierre Fabre
Avenue Jean Moulin 17
81100 Castres Cédex
France

A. KATO

Département de Pharmacologie
Centre Médical Universitaire
1211 Geneva
Switzerland

M. WEBER

Laboratoire de Pharmacologie et de Toxicologie Fondamentales
Route de Narbonne 205
31400 Toulouse
France

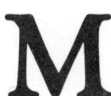

First published 1986

Published by
THE MACMILLAN PRESS LTD
Houndmills, Basingstoke, Hampshire RG21 2XS
and London
Companies and representatives
throughout the world

Printed in Great Britain by
Camelot Press Ltd,
Southampton

British Library Cataloguing in Publication Data
New concepts in Alzheimer's disease.—(Pierre
Fabre monograph series; v. 1)
1. Alzheimer's disease
I. Briley, M.   II. Kato, A. C.   III. Weber, M.
IV. Series
618.97'68983   RC523
ISSN 0269-7866
ISBN 0-333-41356-3

Contents

The Contributors

Amato, S.
   Department of Pharmacology
   University Medical Centre, University of Geneva
   1211 Geneva 4
   Switzerland

Anderton, B. H.
   Department of Immunology
   St George's Hospital Medical School
   Cranmer Terrace
   London SW17 0RE
   UK

Baron, J. C.
   Service Hospitalier Frédéric Joliot
   CEA, Département de Biologie
   91406 Orsay
   France

Birdsall, N. J. M.
   Division of Physical Biochemistry
   National Institute for Medical Research
   The Ridgeway, Mill Hill
   London NW7 1AA
   UK

Blusztajn, J. K.
   Laboratory of Neuroendocrine Regulation
   Department of Nutrition and Food Sciences
   Massachusetts Institute of Technology
   26245 Cambridge
   MA 02139
   USA

Bouras, C.
   Division of Morphological Psychopathology
   Institutions Universitaires de Psychiatrie
   1225 Chêne-Bourg
   Geneva
   Switzerland

Bowen, D. M.
    Department of Neurochemistry
    Institute of Neurology
    33 John's Mews
    London WC1N 2NS
    UK

Briley, M.
    Department of Biochemical Pharmacology
    Centre de Recherche Pierre Fabre
    17, avenue Jean Moulin
    81100 Castres Cédex
    France

Brion, J.-P.
    Laboratoire d'Anatomie Pathologique et de Microscopie Electronique
    Université Libre de Bruxelles
    Route de Lennik 808
    1070 Brussels
    Belgium

Brown, M.
    Department of Biochemical Pharmacology
    Centre de Recherche Pierre Fabre
    17, avenue Jean Moulin
    81100 Castres Cédex
    France

Bruni, A. C.
    Servizio di Neurologia dell'Ospedale Civile
    Regione Calabria
    USL no. 17
    Lamezia Terme
    Italy

Casamenti, F.
    Department of Pharmacology and Toxicology
    University of Florence
    Viale Morgagni 65
    50134 Florence
    Italy

Chopin, P.
    Department of Biochemical Pharmacology
    Centre de Recherche Pierre Fabre
    17, avenue Jean Moulin
    81100 Castres Cédex
    France

Choulli, K.
    Laboratoire de Psychobiologie des Comportements Adaptatifs
    INSERM – U. 259
    Domaine de Carreire
    Rue Camille-St-Saëns
    33077 Bordeaux Cédex
    France

Conneally, P. M.
  Indiana University Medical Center
  Indianapolis
  Indiana
  USA

Constantinidis, J.
  Division of Morphological Psychopathology
  Institutions Universitaires de Psychiatrie
  1225 Chêne-Bourg
  Geneva
  Switzerland

Davison, A. N.
  Department of Neurochemistry
  Institute of Neurology
  National Hospital
  Queen Square
  London WC1N 3BG
  UK

Delteil, C.
  Laboratoire de Pharmacologie et de Toxicologie Fondamentales
  205, route de Narbonne
  31400 Toulouse
  France

Diana, G.
  Department of Neuroscience
  University of Rome
  Citta Universitaria
  00186 Rome
  Italy

Eckenstein, F. P.
  Department of Neurobiology
  Harvard Medical School
  25 Shattuck Street
  Boston
  MA 02115
  USA

Eder-Colli, L.
  Department of Pharmacology
  Centre Médical Universitaire, Université de Genève
  1211 Geneva 4
  Switzerland

Erkman, L.
  Department of Pharmacology
  Centre Médical Universitaire, Université de Genève
  1211 Geneva 4
  Switzerland

Flament-Durand, J.
Laboratoire d'Anatomie Pathologique et de Microscopie Electronique
Université Libre de Bruxelles
Route de Lennik 808
1070 Brussels
Belgium

Foncin, J.-F.
Laboratoire de Neurohistologie de l'École Pratique des Hautes Études
Division Montyon Hôpital de la Salpétrière
47, boulevard de l'Hôpital
75651 Paris Cédex 13
France

Froment, Y.
Department of Pharmacology
Centre Médical Universitaire, Université de Genève
1211 Geneva 4
Switzerland

Geffard, M.
IBCN – CNRS
Rue Camille-St-Saëns
33077 Bordeaux
France

Gibbons, K.
Neurogenetics Laboratory
Massachusetts General Hospital
32 Fruit Street
Boston
MA 02114
USA

Giess, M. C.
Laboratoire de Pharmacologie et de Toxicologie Fondamentales
205, route de Narbonne
31400 Toulouse
France

Gussela, J. F.
Neurogenetics Laboratory
Massachussets General Hospital
32 Fruit Street
Boston
MA 02114
USA

Haines, J.
Indiana University Medical Centre
Indianapolis
Indiana
USA

Haugh, M. C.
Department of Immunology
St George's Hospital Medical School
Cranmer Terrace
London SW17 0RE
UK

Hefti, F.
Department of Neurology
University of Miami
Miami
FL33101
USA

Henderson, C. E.
Neurobiologie Moléculaire
Institut Pasteur
25, rue du Docteur-Roux
75724 Paris Cédex 15
France

Heral, X.
Department of Biochemical Pharmacology
Centre de Recherche Pierre Fabre
17, avenue Jean Moulin
81100 Castres Cédex
France

Herman, J. P.
Laboratoire de Psychobiologie des Comportements Adaptatifs
INSERM – U. 259
Domaine de Carreire
Rue Camille-St-Saëns
33077 Bordeaux Cédex
France

Hobbs, W.
Neurogenetics Laboratory
Massachusetts General Hospital
32 Fruit Street
Boston
MA 02114
USA

Hulme, E. C.
Division of Physical Biochemistry
National Institute for Medical Research
The Ridgeway, Mill Hill
London NW7 1AA
UK

Kahn, J.
Department of Neuropathology
Institute of Psychiatry
University of London
De Crespigny Park
Denmark Hill
London SE5 8AF
UK

Kato, A. C.
   Department of Pharmacology
   Centre Médical Universitaire
   Université de Genève
   1211 Geneva 4
   Switzerland

Kromer, W.
   Zentrum Pharmakologie
   Medizinishe Hochschule
   Hanover
   FRG

Lerner-Natoli, M.
   Laboratoire de Neurobiologie du Développement
   INSERM – U.249 et EPHE
   Institut de Biologie
   Boulevard Henri IV
   34060 Montpellier Cédex
   France

Maire, J.-C.
   Laboratory of Neuroendocrine Regulation
   Department of Nutrition and Food Sciences
   Massachusetts Institute of Technology
   26245 Cambridge
   MA 02139
   USA

Mansour, H.
   Laboratoire de Neurobiologie du Développement
   INSERM – U.249 et EPHE
   Institut de Biologie
   Boulevard Henri IV
   34060 Montpellier Cédex
   France

Martinou, J. C.
   Laboratoire de Pharmacologie et de Toxicologie Fondamentales
   205, route de Narbonne
   31400 Toulouse
   France

Middlemiss, D. N.
   Merrell-Dow Research Institute
   Strasbourg Center
   16, rue d'Ankara
   67084 Strasbourg
   France

   Present address:
   Continental Pharma
   Parc Scientifique de Louvain-la-Nueve
   Rue Grabonpré 11
   1348 Mont-Saint-Guibert
   Belgium

Miller, C. C. J.
   Department of Immunology
   St George's Hospital Medical School
   Cranmer Terrace
   London SW17 0RE
   UK

Le Moal, M.
   Laboratoire de Psychobiologie des Comportements Adaptatifs
   INSERM – U.259
   Domaine de Carreire
   Rue Camille-St-Saëns
   33077 Bordeaux Cédex
   France

Moret, C.
   Department of Biochemical Pharmacology
   Centre de Recherche Pierre Fabre
   17, avenue Jean Moulin
   81100 Castres Cédex
   France

Nadaud, D.
   Laboratoire de Psychobiologie des Comportements Adaptatifs
   INSERM – U.259
   Domaine de Carreire
   Rue Camille-St-Saëns
   33077 Bordeaux Cédex
   France

Nee, L.
   National Institutes of Health
   Bethesda,
   Maryland
   USA

Oberlé, I.
   Laboratoire de Génétique Moléculaire des Eucaryotes du CNRS
   Unité 184 de Biologie Moléculaire et de Génie Génétique de L'INSERM
   Faculté de Médecine
   11, rue Humann
   67085 Strasbourg Cédex
   France

Orzi, F.
   Department of Neuroscience
   University of Rome
   Citta Universitaria
   00186 Rome
   Italy

Palmer, A. M.
   Department of Neurochemistry
   Institute of Neurology
   33 John's Mews
   London WC1N 2NS
   UK

Palumbo, E.
   Department of Neuroscience
   University of Rome
   Citta Universitaria
   00186 Rome
   Italy

Peck, B. S.
   Division of Physical Biochemistry
   National Institute for Medical Research
   The Ridgeway, Mill Hill
   London NW7 1AA
   UK

Pedata, F.
   Department of Pharmacology and Toxicology
   University of Florence
   Viale Morgagni 65
   50134 Florence
   Italy

Pepeu, G.
   Department of Pharmacology and Toxicology
   University of Florence
   Viale Morgagni 65
   50134 Florence
   Italy

Polinsky, R.
   National Institutes of Health
   Bethesda
   Maryland
   USA

Privat, A.
   Laboratoire de Neurobiologie du Développement
   INSERM – U.249 et EPHE
   Institut de Biologie
   Boulevard Henri IV
   34060 Montpellier Cédex
   France

Probst, A.
   Neuropathology Division
   Institute of Pathology
   University of Basle
   Schonbeinstrasse 40
   4056 Basle
   Switzerland

Raynaud, B.
   Laboratoire de Pharmacologie et de Toxicologie Fondamentales
   205, route de Narbonne
   31400 Toulouse
   France

St George-Hyslop, P. H.
  Neurogenetics Laboratory
  Massachusetts General Hospital
  32 Fruit Street
  Boston
  MA 02114
  USA

De St Hilaire-Kafi, S.
  Division of Morphological Psychopathology
  Institutions Universitaires de Psychiatrie
  1225 Chêne-Bourg
  Geneva
  Switzerland

Salmon, D.
  CNRS
  Laboratoire d'Anthropologie Physique du Collège de France
  Paris
  France

Simon, H.
  Laboratoire de Psychobiologie des Comportements Adaptatifs
  INSERM – U.259
  Domain de Carreire
  Rue Camille-St-Saëns
  33077 Bordeaux Cédex
  France

Soreq, H.
  Department of Neurobiology
  The Weizmann Institute of Science
  Rehovot 76100
  Israel

Stockton, J. M.
  Division of Physical Biochemistry
  National Institute for Medical Research
  The Ridgeway, Mill Hill
  London NW7 1AA
  UK

Taghzouti, K.
  Laboratoire de Psychobiologie des Comportements Adaptatifs
  INSERM – U.259
  Domaine de Carreire
  Rue Camille-St-Saëns
  33077 Bordeaux Cédex
  France

Taguchi, T.
  Neurobiologie Moléculaire
  Institut Pasteur
  25, rue du Docteur-Roux
  75724 Paris
  France

Tanzi, R.
Neurogenetics Laboratory
Massachusetts General Hospital
32 Fruit Street
Boston
MA 02114
USA

Touzeau, G.
Department of Pharmacology
Centre Médical Universitaire
Université de Genève
1211 Geneva 4
Switzerland

Ulrich, J.
Neuropathology Division
Institute of Pathology
University of Basle
Schonbeinstrasse 40
4056 Basle
Switzerland

Le Van Thai, A.
Laboratoire de Pharmacologie et de Toxicologie Fondamentales
205, route de Narbonne
31400 Toulouse
France

Vidal, S.
Laboratoire de Pharmacologie et de Toxicologie Fondamentales
205, route de Narbonne
31400 Toulouse
France

Weber, M.
Laboratoire de Pharmacologie et de Toxicologie Fondamentales
205, route de Narbonne
31400 Toulouse
France

Wurtman, R. J.
Laboratory of Neuroendocrine Regulation
Department of Nutrition and Food Sciences
Massachusetts Institute of Technology
26245 Cambridge
MA 02139
USA

Zakut, H.
Department of Obstetrics and Gynecology
Edith Wolfson Hospital
The Sackler Faculty of Medicine
Tel-Aviv University
Holon
Israel

Zigmond, M. J.
  Department of Biological Sciences
  University of Pittsburgh
  Pittsburg
  USA

Preface to the series

Created in 1961, the Pierre Fabre Group is one of Europe's youngest research-based ethical pharmaceutical and beauty-care groups. From its base in Castres in south-west France, the group has expanded in the last 25 years to become one of the major privately owned French companies in its field.

The Pierre Fabre Research Centre, which has existed in its present form for about 10 years, has adopted a basic strategy of encouraging collaboration between its own research centre in Castres and academic research scientists throughout the world. The creation of the Pierre Fabre Monograph Series is a further development of this strategy. Certain monographs in this series will be based on international symposia organised or sponsored by the Pierre Fabre Research Centre. Others will group together chapters from acknowledged international experts and dynamic young scientists destined to become tomorrow's experts. In all cases, the subjects of these monographs will be those presenting a major challenge to therapeutic medicine.

The Editorial Board:
M. Briley
J. P. Couzinier
P. Lenoble
J. Tisne-Versailles

Preface

In the early twentieth century, Alzheimer's disease would have been described as a minority disease. Demographic changes that have occurred in all developed countries, coupled with major medical advances in other areas, have made Alzheimer's disease one of the commonest problems in old age and a major health problem for the end of this century.

The realisation of these facts in the last few years by public health authorities, grant-giving bodies and the pharmaceutical industry has led to an explosion of interest in widely differing areas touching on Alzheimer's disease. This multidisciplinary approach is essential for a disease which is obviously more complex than a deficit in a single neurotransmitter system. The danger is, however, that different specialists, each concentrating on one part of the problem, may not be sufficiently aware of progress in other areas.

The editors of this first volume in the Pierre Fabre Monograph Series thus set themselves the task of bringing together chapters describing work in areas extending from animal behaviour to molecular genetics and from positron emission tomography to immunology; some chapters relating specifically to Alzheimer's disease, others describing techniques which may soon be applied to this problem. It is hoped that in this way, the book may make a small contribution to our knowledge of Alzheimer's disease.

The symposium on which this book is based was held in Castres in south-west France in October 1985. It was sponsored by the Centre de Recherche Pierre Fabre (CRPF) and the Centre National de la Recherche Scientifique (CNRS) with generous contributions from the Conseil Général de Midi-Pyrénées and The Macmillan Press.

We would like to thank everyone from the CRPF who helped with the symposium, especially the members of the Biochemical Pharmacology Department who undertook the local organisation. Special thanks are due to Martine Dehaye for her most efficient and charming handling of the secretariat for both the symposium and this book. Our thanks also to Elisabeth Carilla for her invaluable help as editorial assistant.

Castres, Geneva and Toulouse, 1986   M. B.
                                                                                      A. K.
                                                                                      M. W.

1

New Concepts in the Pathophysiology of Alzheimer's Disease

A. N. Davison

1.1 Normal Ageing

It is generally accepted that intellectual functioning decreases slowly from the third decade of life to the sixth and more abruptly thereafter. General intelligence, as evaluated by environmental criteria, appears to be maintained over a much greater period of adult life and to decline at a much slower rate than does mental ability as assessed in certain types of intelligence tests. There are exceptional individuals who retain remarkable intellectual powers throughout their lives. Their brains are presumably free of gross pathology, indeed plaques and tangles are not invariably present in the brains of all elderly individuals. Thus it is not mandatory for ageing to be associated with cognitive loss accompanied by neuropathological changes. In the opinion of Wisniewski and Merz (1984) measurable and visible variation from normal brain structure function is, by definition, pathological. If by reason of their number and location, these pathological changes elicit a clinical expression, they are defined as disease. Although gerontologists seem to avoid discussion of illness, Wisniewski and Merz (1984) argue that 'normal aging' may simply be a stage of pathology without clinical expression.

In contrast, in relatively rare occurrences, elderly persons with no apparent clinical cognitive impairment may have considerable brain atrophy, even exceeding that found in some demented patients. Tomlinson (1980) quotes two cases of intellectually well-preserved old people in whom plaque formation was heavy throughout all areas of the cerebral cortex, in a concentration similar to that which occurs in Alzheimer's disease.

In the great majority of apparently normal old subjects, however, a small number of plaques and tangles are found. The plaques in normal subjects are identical at both light and electron microscopic level with those of Alzheimer's disease. Most of the morphological changes are found in the outer cortical layers, in the depths of sulci and in the structures of the anterior temporal lobes, particularly the amygdaloid nucleus and overlying cortex and in the hippocampus and hippocampal gyrus. As in Alzheimer's disease, however, there is a tendency for all the senile changes to be more concentrated in the anterior temporal lobes than in any other part of the brain. Thus the difference between normal and Alzheimer-diseased subjects of the pre-senile period becomes largely quantitative (Tomlinson, 1980).

1.1.1 Brain Atrophy and Nerve Cell Loss

Progressive decline in brain weight begins at about 45–50 years of age and reaches its lowest value after the age of 86 years, by which time the mean brain weight has decreased by about 11 % relative to that in young adults (DeKaban, 1978). Loss in brain weight suggests fall-out or shrinkage of neurons, to which could be attributed the behavioural changes seen in the elderly. Brody (1955) has reported a steady loss of cerebral cortical neurons from mature to elderly individuals and thus it has been calculated that 'every day of our adult life more than 100,000 neurons die'. However, loss of neurons does not occur throughout the brain. Konigsmark and Murphy (1970) found no change in the number of neurons with age in the human ventral cochlear nucleus and these authors emphasised that there is still no conclusive evidence that loss of brain weight, volume or even function in the later decades of life can be ascribed to neuronal loss. In the human inferior olive there is also only a small loss of nerve cells between the ages of 20 and 80 years (Monagle and Brody, 1971). However, Tomlinson et al. (1981) found gradual loss of the pigmented cells of the locus coeruleus from early middle to old age. Some subjects of 80-90 years of age possess only 30-40 % of the neurons found in the most populated younger person's brain. In the basal forebrain (substantia innominata region) nerve cells of the nucleus basalis of Meynert are reduced in number by 30 % in elderly subjects (Mann et al., 1984).

1.1.1.1 Changes in the Cortex

Due to the difficulties of making quantitative measurements on cortical neuronal populations there has been considerable controversy on the subject. Even allowing for shrinkage and other artefacts it does seem that extensive loss of large cortical neurons occurs throughout normal life. Henderson et al. (1980) report some loss of cells in different regions of the cortex. The greatest loss found was in large neurons, where the mean reduction over the period from 20 to 90 years of age was between 40 and 60 %, while loss of small nerve cells and glia was between 12 and 43 %. This was confirmed by Anderson *et al.* (1983), who found neuronal loss of about 1 % per year from the neocortex and medial hippocampus. Ball (1977) has measured the number of cortical neurons in the hippocampal cortex. In normal ageing between the ages of 45 and 90 years, there was a linear decrease in neuronal density to 20 % of the total original density. The elderly person may therefore be more susceptible to neuronal dysfunction compared with the younger subject with his full complement of healthy nerve cells.

1.1.2 Alterations in the Neuropil

In some regions of the ageing brain, examination by the Golgi method shows that there is loss of dendritic processes and synaptic contacts (Schiebel and Tomiyasu, 1978). In their study Buell and Coleman (1979) saw grossly atrophic dendritic arborisation, although the intensity of such change was no different in adult (mean age 51.2 years) than in elderly (mean age 79.6 years) subjects. In the normal ageing human parahippocampal gyrus, Buell and Coleman (1979) found continued growth of dendritic arborisation. Indeed, the net length of individual terminal segments of the average apical tree increased by 0.21 μm/year from 44 to 92 years of age. This suggests unexpected plasticity within the ageing brain; possibly this reactive synaptogenesis (Cotman & Scheff, 1979) is in response to neuronal loss.

The data then available suggested to Buell and Coleman (1979) a model in which there are two populations of neurons in the normal ageing cortex: one a group of dying neurons with shrinking dendritic trees; the other a larger group of surviving neurons with expanding dendritic trees. They postulated that, with increasing age, there is a shift of individual neurons from the surviving to the dying population. The rate at which this shift takes place may be a function of genetic and non-genetic or extrinsic (toxicological, behavioural, infectious) factors. Even aged neurons have the capacity to grow new synapses following partial denervation, although the extent and rate of growth is diminished with increased age. Cotman and Scheff (1979) unilaterally removed the entorhinal cortical input and examined septohippocampal afferents. At 12 days post-lesion, younger (three-month-old) rats demonstrated a 22 % increase in out-growth of the fibre plexus on the lesioned side, compared with a 10–11 % increase in 28-month-old animals. Sixty days post-lesion, synaptic profiles were nearly normal in young animals, but the increase in the aged animals was significantly less than normal bouton density. Similarly, neuronotrophic activity induced by injury occurs at a slower rate in adults than in neonates (Nieto-Sampedro *et al.*, 1983). Axonal transport of glycoproteins is significantly slowed in the septo-hippocampal pathway of the 25-month-old, compared to that of three-month-old animal (Geinisman *et al.*, 1977). It is possible that, with ageing, loss of synapses may be due to insufficient axonal transport or, alternatively, that a decrease in the number of neurons in the medial septal nucleus (or simply loss of axons) may account for the 35 % decrease in glycoprotein transport.

1.1.3 Neurotransmitters

In man, small declines in the brain catecholamine concentration are seen with age. Unexpectedly, monoamine oxidase (a mitochondrial enzyme) activity is increased in the ageing brain. The major alterations found are loss in dopamine and noradrenaline transmitter systems (loss of 50 % throughout life (Winblad et al., 1978)), possibly correlated with altered sleeping habits, depressive illness and dyskinesia. Although there is some disagreement it appears that the cholinergic system is less affected by age (White et al., 1977).

1.2 The Pathophysiology of Alzheimer's Disease

There are many neurological, general medical and psychiatric conditions which can lead to a possible diagnosis of a primary dementing illness. Dementia, as defined by McKhann et al. (1984), is the decline of memory and other cognitive functions, in comparison with the patient's previous level of function, as determined by a history of decline in performance and by abnormalities noted from clinical examination and neuropsychological tests. A diagnosis of dementia cannot be made when consciousness is impaired by delirium, drowsiness, stupor, or coma or when other clinical abnormalities prevent adequate evaluation of mental status. Dementia is a diagnosis based on behaviour and cannot be determined by computerised tomography, electroencephalography, or by other laboratory methods, although specific causes of dementia may be identified by these means. The commonest example of dementia is Alzheimer's disease. This condition is typified by an acquired progressive decline in memory with global cognitive impairment. Ultimate diagnosis depends on neuropathological assessment of a defined density of plaques and tangles in the brain. Clinical and pathological criteria have led to identification of groups in which diffuse or focal degenerative changes occur (e.g. Pick's disease and dementia accompanying Huntington's chorea). In the case of multiinfarct dementia the step-wise decline in cognitive ability is associated with multiple areas of ischaemia. The cause of the disease is vascular (Hachinski, 1983), and is clearly associated with strokes, which produce signs of focal neurological damage. In Sourander and Sjogren's (1970) study of 258 cases of dementia only 72 were considered to have cerebrovascular disease, while more than half had Alzheimer's disease. In epidemiological studies (e.g. Barclay et al., 1985) family histories of dementia have been demonstrated in about a third of cases. Female relatives are twice as likely to be demented as male relatives. This suggests that an autosomal dominant sex-linked genetic factor may be involved in the aetiology of Alzheimer's disease. Nuclear defects are indicated by the demonstrated changes in nucleolar volume seen in neurons from patients with Alzheimer's disease (Mann et al., 1985). Of particular interest, therefore, are the observations of Bradley and his colleagues (Robison et al., 1985). They found that when fibroblasts and lymphoblasts are grown in tissue culture they have increased chromosomal aberrations when exposed to various types of DNA-damaging agents (e.g. methylmethane sulphonate, but not u.v.). Damaged DNA from the fibroblasts of Alzheimer patients fails to repair in comparison to controls. This mechanism may be important in the amitotic neuron since some loss of bases occurs naturally with age, and defective DNA could lead to faulty transcription. Similarly, in cases of familial Alzheimer's disease repair of strand breaks in fibroblast DNA were found (Li and Kaminskas, 1985) to be slower than in age-matched controls. Damage induced by bleomycin was repaired at an equal rate in both Alzheimer and control fibroblasts.

1.2.1 Brain Atrophy in Alzheimer's Disease

Atrophy of the brain is a common finding in Alzheimer's disease, particularly in the cerebral cortex, with frontal and temporal lobes being most involved. The hippocampus and amygdaloid are usually considerably shrunken (Perry, 1984). Regional variation in brain atrophy was examined by Hubbard and Anderson (1981). They found (Table 1.1), in comparison to age-matched controls, that there was a marked reduction in cranial capacity in the relatively younger group of Alzheimer patients. Marked atrophy was present only in the temporal cortex of the 85-year-old brains. In this series the mean volume of cerebral white matter was found to be reduced by 12 % and this presumably accounts for the dilated ventricles frequently found in dementia (quantitative computed tomographic analysis of ventricular volume is significant in about 84% of demented patients (Damasio et al., 1983)).

1.2.2 Nerve Cell Loss

1.2.2.1 The Subcortex and Brain Stem

In 1981 Rossor proposed that Alzheimer's disease was an example of degenerative disorder in which there was loss or dysfunction of nerve cells of the iso-dendritic core. Thus cells from the locus coeruleus, substantia nigra, substantia innominata and septal nuclei share a non-specialised isodendritic pattern corresponding to the reticular formation. Loss of other cell groups could be due to trans-synaptic degeneration after the loss of ascending input.

An example is the apparent loss of large cells (diameter above 30 μm) from the basal nucleus of Meynert (Whitehouse et al., 1982) which is the principal source of cholinergic fibres to the neocortex. However Pearson et al. (1983a) have evidence that shrinkage of nerve cells rather than cell death may have occurred, because a similar disappearance of large cells from the basal nucleus is seen in human and monkey brain after lesions in the cortex (Pearson et al., 1983b; Sofroniew et al., 1983). Alternatively, Perry et al. (1982) conclude that loss of cholinergic neurons may be a secondary rather than primary change in

Table 1.1 Regional variation in brain atrophy in Alzheimer's disease

| | Cranial Capacity | | | | | |
| | Younger group (mean age 73) | | | Elderly group (mean age 85) | | |
	Controls	Alzheimer's disease	Difference (%)	Controls	Alzheimer's disease	Difference (%)
Number of patients	12	7		6	8	
Fronto-parietal cortex	19.9	17.3	−13	18.5	18.0	n.s.
Temporal cortex	6.8	5.6	−18	7.0	5.5	−21
Temporal white matter	3.4	2.5	−26	2.9	2.4	n.s.
Cerebral ventricles	1.8	2.8	+53	2.4	2.6	n.s.

Data after Hubbard and Anderson (1981)

Alzheimer's disease. The reduction in choline acetyltransferase (ChAT) activity could be ascribed to 'down regulation' in enzyme synthesis, possibly brought about by the absence of trophic factor.

1.2.2.2 Changes in the Cortex

Hubbard and Anderson (1985) have examined cerebral cortical neuronal populations in Alzheimer's disease using a stereological procedure utilising cortical and cellular volume measurements to correct for shrinkage. Loss of large neurons was 26 % in the frontal cortex and 33 % in the temporal cortex in Alzheimer patients of mean age 86 years as compared to controls of mean age 84 years. No significant change was seen in the population of small neurons or glial cells.

Extensive pyramidal cell loss was seen by Mann et al. (1985) in the temporal cortex and hippocampus (Table 1.2). These results are in broad agreement with previous findings of Terry et al. (1981) and Mountjoy et al. (1983). Neuropil

Table 1.2   Loss of neurons in different brain regions in Alzheimer's disease

	Nerve cell number (Number of neurons per mm^3)		Percentage loss
	Controls	Alzheimer's	
Temporal cortex layer III	14,743 ± 198	6123 ± 335	58*
Temporal cortex layer V	19,500 ± 216	7695 ± 457	60*
Nucleus basalis of Meynert	327 ± 17	168 ± 13	49*
Neurons per section			
Dorsal tegmental nucleus of raphe	37 ± 1	33 ± 1	12*
Substantia nigra	465 ± 17	430 ± 10	7.5

Mean cell number ± SEM are shown
*Significant differences
From Mann et al. (1985)

density (Hubbard and Anderson, 1986) was reduced by between 12 and 17 % in both elderly (over 80 years old) and younger Alzheimer patients. Tangles are found predominantly in the large pyramidal neurons of layers three and five (see also Pearson et al., 1985). Damage to or loss of large cortical neurons could be associated with the findings of reduced uptake of deoxyglucose in different regions of the association cortex (Foster et al., 1983).

1.2.3 Histopathological Features

Neuritic plaques and filamentous tangles are the most widespread neuropathological changes seen in Alzheimer's disease. There are also granulovacuolar degeneration in the hippocampus, Hirano body formation and perivascular congiophilic amyloid deposition.

Plaques are widely distributed in the neocortex. The hippocampus amygdaloid and hippocampal gyrus are usually heavily affected. Plaques are rarely found in the cerebellar cortex and never in the spinal cord (Brun, 1983). The typical plaque is spherical with in amyloid plaque core diameter of about 13 μm, although the total plaque is somewhat larger. The rim of the neuritic plaque consists of nerve cell processes or neurites filled with intracellular paired helical filaments, dense bodies and mitochondria. Some of the neurites contain balloon-like swellings suggesting attempted regeneration of dystrophic processes. Glial cells and their processes and lipofuscin aggregates may be found. The centre of the plaque contains amyloid and aluminosilicates (Candy et al., 1986). Both neurofibrillary tangles and the dystrophic neurites that comprise senile plaques contain abundant pairs of helically wound, 10 nm filaments and some straight filaments with diameters of 10–20 nm. Many senile plaques contain deposits of extracellular, 8–10 nm amyloid filaments. Selkoe et al. (1985) have developed a novel method for high-grade purification of these amyloid cores by fluorescence-activated cell sorting, although recoveries by this method are low. Amino acid analysis of the amyloid reveals a high content of glycine and other non-polar residues and a composition similar to that of PHF fractions. Moreover, claims that tangle-specific antibodies react intensely with purified amyloid cores have not yet been confirmed in formalin-fixed paraffin-embedded samples. Thus, Masters and his colleagues (Masters et al., 1985a) propose that in Alzheimer's disease there is a progressive accumulation of highly insoluble, modified fibrous proteins with unique antigenic characteristics in neuronal perikarya and neurites. The subunit proteins (A–4) are the building blocks of neurofibrillary tangles, amyloid plaque cores and, ultimately, amyloid congophilic angiopathy. Depending on the environment in which they are assembled or polymerised, either twisted or straight filaments result. Amyloid plaques are also present in the brain of certain strains of mice infected with the scrapie agent but these structures differ from those seen in Alzheimer's disease.

The tangles which are intracellular inclusions found in the neuronal cell body form a second important feature of Alzheimer's disease. They are usually seen in the cerebral cortex, especially in the hippocampus and in some parts of the subcortex but not in the cerebellum, spinal cord or peripheral nervous system. Biochemical analyses indicate that both paired helical filaments and 15 nm straight filaments are highly insoluble, rigid protein polymers which resist chemical or enzymatic breakdown. Selkoe and his colleagues at Harvard (Selkoe et al., 1985a, 1985b) have used their insolubility to enrich for tangles in the presence of strong detergents. Evidence of a similar inertness in vivo comes from the observation that these fibres (tangle ghosts) are sometimes seen extracellularly following neuronal death. Immunochemical studies indicate that paired helical filaments contain epitopes shared with normal neurofilaments (Anderton *et al.*, 1982), but also contain unique or novel epitopes distinct from neurofilaments and other normal brain proteins. There is evidence that phosphorylated neuro-filament (200 kD), normally in axons and terminals, accumulates within the perikayra. Selko *et al.* (1985) have recently found that certain epitopes of the microtubule-associated protein-2 are also associated with paired helical fila-ments. Studies by Masters and his colleagues (Masters *et al.*, 1985b) have shown homology between some amino acid sequences of paired helical filament and human amyloid protein. Antibodies directed against isolated neurofilament rods crossreact with human neurites and amyloid (plaques and vascular). There are several striking similarities between the A–4 proteins of Alzheimer's disease and the filaments and polypeptides associated with the unconventional virus disease sheep scrapie. There are morphological resemblances between the filaments and a similarity in amino acid compositionof the A–4 monomer and the 7 kD deglycosylated scrapie-associated protein, but no sequence homology (Masters *et al.*, 1985b).

1.2.4 Neurotransmitters

The major change in neurotransmitter activity is in the cholinergic activity of the amygdala, the hippocampus, the basal forebrain (nucleus basalis) and the neo-cortex. Loss of choline acetyltransferase activity in the cortex has been ascribed to reduction in presynaptic terminals originating in projections from the basal forebrain. This conclusion is based on concomitant (Table 1.3) reduction in acetylcholine (ACh) synthesis, choline uptake and ChAT activity in tissue prisms from biopsy samples of Alzheimer patients (Sims *et al.*, 1983). There is a highly significant correlation between cognitive impairment and reduction in acetyl-choline synthesis by fresh brain tissue (Francis *et al.*, 1985). However, post-synaptic muscarinic receptors largely remain unaltered. Fine *et al.* (1985) have described experiments on rats with lesions in the nucleus basalis. One group of rats received transplants of cholinergic-rich tissue from the ventral forebrain of embryos. Controls had transplants of non-cholinergic hippocampal cells. Six months after surgery the animals show significant impairment in passive avoid-ance tests. Those animals with cholinergic cell transplants showed substantial improvement in retention in a passive avoidance performance test. These experi-ments are of relevance to treatment with cholinergic agonists and indicate theoretical bases for replacement therapy.

Amongst other transmitters affected are 5-hydroxytryptamine (5-HT) and 5-HT-receptor concentration, which is reduced. Bowen and Davison (1985) suggest that these 5-HT receptors may be localised on the tangle-forming gluta-mergic neurons of the cortex. 5-HT concentration is reduced in the more severely affected samples of temporal cortex and in the limbic areas. It is possible that

Table 1.3   Comparison of values for different presynaptic cholinergic markers in Alzheimer's disease and control fresh biopsy tissue. Neurosurgical samples were taken for diagnostic purposes and were histologically assessed

	Stimulated choline uptake (pmol/min/mg protein)	Stimulated acetylcholine synthesis (d.p.m./min/mg protein)	ChAT activity (pmol/min/mg protein)
Controls	3.04 ± 0.33 (6)	6.6 ± 1.2 (22)	86 ± 21 (11)
Alzheimer disease	1.72 ± 0.58 (6)	3.9 ± 1.2 (6)	37 ± 25 (6)
Other non-Alzheimer	2.71	4.9	70
Dements	2.73	8.5	74

Data from Sims *et al.* (1983)

reduction in 5-HT concentration is due to loss or dysfunction of cells in the raphe nucleus (Ishii, 1966). While depolarisation-induced release of 5-HT is reduced in fresh tissue-prisms in Alzheimer patients, catecholamine release is unchanged.

In the cerebral cortex, where large neurons are lost or are affected by the presence of neurofibrillary tangles, it is likely that glutamate is the neurotransmitter involved (Pearce *et al.*, 1984). Glutamate concentration in the CSF of Alzheimer patients but not in that of other amino acids correlates with measures of cognitive impairment (Smith *et al.*, 1985). Sasaki *et al.* (1985) have found a reduction in glutamate content in the cortex and basal ganglia of Alzheimer patients. Specific binding of radioactive L-glutamate to caudate nucleus membranes (Pearce *et al.*, 1984) and its distribution as determined by an autoradiography in the neocortex (Greenamyre *et al.*, 1985) provide some evidence of reduced glutamergic innervation and receptor concentration (Table 1.4). Further work will show the extent to which this cortical transmitter system is affected in dementia and if this is a primary event in the pathological process.

Table 1.4   Binding of different ligands to receptors in the cortex

	$[^3H]$ quinuclidinyl benzylate	L-$[^3H]$ glutamate
		Cortex
Control (5)	1.73 ± 0.21	2.17 ± 0.07
Alzheimer's disease (6)	1.55 ± 0.17	$1.17 \pm 0.18*$

After Greenamyre *et al.* (1985)
Binding to receptors was determined autoradiographically.
No significant differences were seen in glutamate binding to the caudate, putamen or nucleus basalis or in muscimol and flunitrazepan binding.
* = significant difference.

1.2.5 Mechanisms of Cell Loss and Dysfunction

Like other cells, those of the nervous system are affected throughout life by the process of 'wear and tear'. Accumulating evidence now indicates that the sum of the deleterious free radical reactions continuously going on throughout the cells and tissues constitutes the ageing process or is a major contributor to it. Lost neurons are not replaceable and plasticity is decreased in the elderly brain. Some groups of neurons such as those of the substantia nigra, the hippocampus, amygdala, locus coeruleus or the nucleus basalis of Meynert are particularly susceptible to ageing and disease, whereas other neurons (especially small nerve cells) are less vulnerable. In mammalian systems the free radical reactions are largely those involving oxygen (Harman, 1981). Since large neurons (e.g. cortical pyramidal or Purkinje cells) with high metabolic activity seem to be especially affected it is likely that their rate of oxygen utilisation leads to toxic superoxide radical formation. The age-increased activity of monoamine oxidase also leads to peroxide formation. As a result, lipid peroxidation products (e.g. lipofuscin) may accumulate. Changes in DNA, including strand breakage and base modification, may now be attributed to free radical (e.g. hydroxyl radical) action; and impaired repair mechanisms (Robison *et al.*, 1985) explain defects in protein synthesis (Mann *et al.*, 1981; Sajdel-Sulkowska and Marotta, 1984). Similarly, impaired genetic control mechanisms may affect synthesis of trophic factors in a particular region of the CNS. Survival and sprouting of nerve cells in culture has been shown to be stin.ulated by muscle extracts and their derived growth factors. Thus, co-cultivation of septal and hippocampal explant results in enhanced growth and cholinergic activity in comparison to that of the separate tissues (Appel, 1981). Recent work suggests that nerve growth factor (NFG) might play a similar role in forebrain cholinergic neurons to that seen in peripheral adrenergic neurons. Schwab *et al.* (1979) found that NGF injected into the hippocampus of the rat is specifically taken up by nerve terminals. The protein is retrogradely transported to cholinergic neurons of the medial septal nucleus and those of the diagonal band of Broca. In a detailed study by Pearson *et al.* (1985) of the distribution of plaques and tangles, areas of the association cortex were found to be severely involved but the motor, somatic, sensory and primary visual areas were virtually unaffected. The neurofibrillary tangles were in clusters with a laminar distribution suggesting that the disease follows interconnected pathways. Pearson and his colleagues (Pearson *et al.*, 1985) make the interesting suggestion that the olfactory system is involved in the pathogenesis. The disease would be thought to spread via cortico-cortical association fibres so that changes in the basal nucleus would be secondary to cortical pathology. A possibility is that a virus, e.g. herpes (Tomlinson and Esiri, 1983), could infect the olfactory system. Persistent virus may lead to eventual cell death or to a defect in host expression. An example is neuroblastoma cells infected with lymphocytic choriomeningitis virus, which (despite normal morphology, growth rates and protein synthesis) show reduced synthesis of acetylcholine, ChAT and AChE (Oldstone *et al.*, 1977). Another example is herpes simplex virus (type 1) infection of a cloned rat pheochromatocytoma cell line maintained in tissue culture (Rubenstein and Price, 1984). Reduction in ChAT and AChE activities is seen well before cell death. The possibilities of latent herpes infection and entry of the virus into the limbic system via the trigeminal ganglia has been discussed by Ball (1982). Despite these interesting suggestions viral genomic material has not so far been identified in Alzheimer's disease nor have primates been infected by innoculation of post-mortem brain preparations.

1.3 Summary

Even in non-familial cases of dementia there is some evidence of a genetic factor. This may be linked to defective expression of neurofilament protein. In this respect there is a link with accumulation of tangles and amyloid which have some degree of homology. It may be speculated that neurons containing tangles or undergoing granulo-vacular degeneration would not be able to release trophic factors and that trans-neuronal degeneration would result. However, the environmental or aetiological factors associated with Alzheimer's disease are not known.

Although there has been a failure to transmit Alzheimer's disease to primates it is possible that, as in Parkinson's disease, a virus may be implicated at some stage in the pathogenesis. Finally, free-radical formation has been considered as an alternative mechanism for death of large neurons within the CNS. Although tangles are found in several other dementing conditions (e.g. dementia pugilistica, Parkinson-dementia complex of Guam) Alzheimer-type plaques and tangles are not invariably found. For example, in dementia of Parkinson's disease there is a low neuritic plaque count and a normal population of tangles (Perry *et al.*, 1985). In addition, memory loss is not necessarily associated with defects in the cholinergic system and/or loss of nucleus basalis nerve cells. We have proposed (Bowen and Davison, 1985) that damage to or loss of cortical cells may be a more general finding in dementing illness.

References

Anderson, J. M., Hubbard, B. M., Coghill, G. R., and Slidders, W. (1983). The effect of advanced old age on the neurone content of the cerebral cortex – observations with an automatic image analyser point counting method. *J. Neurol. Sci.*, **58**, 235–46.

Anderton, B. H., Breinburg, D., Downes, M. J., Green, P. J., Tomlinson, B. E., Ulrich, J., Wood, J. N., and Kahn, J. (1982). Monoclonal antibodies show that neurofibrillary tangles and neurofilaments share antigenic determinants. *Nature*, **298**, 84–6.

Appel, S. H., (1981). A unifying hypothesis for the cause of amyotrophic lateral sclerosis, Parkinsonism and Alzheimer's disease. *Ann. Neurol.*, **10**, 499–505.

Ball, M. J. (1977). Neuronal loss, neuro-fibrillary tangles and granulovascular degeneration in the hippocampus with ageing and dementia. *Acta Neuropath. (Berl.)*, **37**, 111–18.

Ball, M. J. (1982). Limbic predilection in Alzheimer dementia: Is reactivated herpesvirus involved?. *Canad. J. Neurol. Sci.*, **9**, 303–6.

Barclay, L. L., Kheyfets, S., Zemcov, A., and McDowell, F. H. (1985). Genetic factors in Alzheimer's disease. *J. Neurol. (Suppl.)*, **232**, 61.

Bowen, D. M., and Davison, A. N. (1985). Importance of acetylcholine and tangle-bearing cortical neurones in Alzheimer's disease. *Proc. 5th Mtng Eur. Soc. Neurc*, **17**, 275–8.

Brody, H. (1955). Organization of cerebral cortex: III. A study of aging in the human cerebral cortex. *J. Comp. Neurol.*, **102**, 511–56.

Brun, A. (1983). An overview of light and electron microscopic changes. In Reisberg, B. (ed.), *Alzheimer's Disease*. The Free Press, New York, pp. 37–47.

Buell, S. J., and Coleman, P. D. (1979). Dendritic growth in the aged human brain and failure of growth in senile dementia. *Science*, **206**, 854–5.

Candy, J. M., Oakley, A. E., Klinowski, J., Carpenter, T. A., Perry, R. H., Atack, J. R., Perry, E. K., Blessed, G., Fairbairn, A., and Edwardson, J. A. (1986). Aluminosilicates contribute to senile plaque formation in Alzheimer's disease. *Lancet* (in press).

Cotman, C. W., and Scheff, S. W. (1979). Compensatory synapse growth in aged animals after neuronal death. *Mech. Aging and Devel.*, **9**, 103–11.

Damasio, H., Eslinger, P., Damasio, A. R., Rizzo, M., Huang, H. K., and Demeter, S. (1983). Quantitative computed tomographic analysis in the diagnosis of dementia. *Arch. Neurol.*, **40**, 715–19.

Dekaban, A. S. (1978). Changes in brain weights during the span of human life: Relation of brain weights to body heights and body weights. *Ann. Neurol.*, **4**, 345–56.

Fine, A., Dunnett, S. B., Bjorklund, A., and Iversen, S. D. (1985). Cholinergic ventral fore-brain grafts into the neocortex improve passive avoidance memory in a rat model of Alzheimer disease. *Proc. Nat. Acad. Sci. USA*, **82**, 5227–31.

Foster, N. L., Chase, T. N., Fedio, P., Patronas, N. J., Brooks, R. A., and Di Chiro, G. (1983). Alzheimer's disease: Focal cortical changes shown by positron emission tomo-graphy. *Neurology*, **33**, 961-5.

Francis, P. T., Palmer, A. M., Sims, N. R., Bowen, D. M., Davison, A. N., Esiri, M. M., Neary, D., Snowden, J. S., and Wilcock, G. K. (1985). Neurochemical studies of early-onset Alzheimer's disease. Possible influence on treatment. *New Eng. J.*, **313**, 7–11.

Geinisman, Y., Bondareff, W., and Telser, A. (1977). Transport of [3H] fucose labelled glycoproteins in the septo-hippocampal pathway of young adult and senescent rats. *Brain Res.*, **125**, 182–6.

Greenamyre, J. T., Young, A. B., Penney, J. B., D'Amato, C. J., Hicks, S. P., and Shoulson, I. (1985). Alterations in L-glutamate binding in Alzheimer's and Huntington's diseases. *Science*, **227**, 1496–9.

Hachinski, V. C. (1983). Differential diagnosis of Alzheimer's dementia: Multi-infarct dementia. In Reisberg, B. (ed.), *Alzheimer's Disease*. The Free Press, New York, 188–92.

Harman, D. (1981). The aging process. *Proc. Natl. Acad. Sci. USA*, **78**, 7124–8.

Henderson, G., Tomlinson, B. E., and Gibson, P. H. (1980). Cell counts in human cerebral cortex in normal adults throughout life using an image analysing computer. *J. Neurol. Sci.*, **46**, 113–36.

Hubbard, B. M., and Anderson, J. M. (1981). A quantitative study of cerebral atrophy in old age and senile dementia. *J. Neurol. Sci.*, **50**, 135–45.

Hubbard, B. M., and Anderson, J. M. (1986). Age-related variations in the neurone content of the cerebral cortex in senile dementia of Alzheimer type. *Neuropath. & Appl. Neuro-biol.* (in press).

Ishii, T. (1966). Distribution of Alzheimer's neurofibrillary changes in the brain stem and hypothalamus of senile dementia. *Acta Neuropathol. (Berl.)*, **6**, 181–7.

Konigsmark, B. W., and Murphy, E. A. (1970). Neuronal populations in the human brain. *Nature*, **228**, 1335–6.

Li, J. C., and Kaminskas, E. (1985). Deficient repair of DNA lesions in Alzheimer's disease fibroblasts. *Biochem & Biophys. Res. Comm.*, **129**, 733–8.

McKhann, G., Drachman, D., Folstein, M., Katzman, R., Price, D., and Stadlan, E. M. (1984). Clinical diagnosis of Alzheimer's disease: Report of the NINCDS–ADRDA work group under the auspices of dept. of health and human services task force on Alzheimer's disease. *Neurology*, **34**, 939–44.

Mann, D. M. A., Neary, D., Yates, P. O., Lincoln, J., Snowden, J. S., and Stanworth, P. (1981). Alterations in protein synthetic capability of nerve cells in Alzheimer's disease. *J. Neurol. Neurosurg. Psychiat.*, **44**, 97–103.

Mann, D. M. A., Yates, P. O., and Marcyniuk, B. (1984). Changes in nerve cells of the nucleus basalis of Meynert in Alzheimer's disease and their relationship to ageing and to the accumulation of lipofuscin pigment. *Mechanisms Ageing and Develop.*, **25**, 189–204.

Mann, D. M. A., Yates, P. O., and Marcyniuk, B. (1985). Some morphometric observations on the cerebral cortex and hippocampus in presenile Alzheimer's disease, senile dementia of Alzheimer type and Down's syndrome in middle age. *J. Neurol. Sci.*, **69**, 139–59.

Masters, C. L., Multhaup, G., Simms, G., Pottgiesser, J., Martins, R. N., and Beyreuther, K. (1985a). Neuronal origin of a cerebral amyloid: neurofibrillary tangles of Alzheimer's disease contain the same protein as the amyloid of plaque cores and blood vessels. *EMBO, J.*, **4** (in press).

Masters, C. L., Simms, G., Weinman, N. A., Malthaup, G., McDonald, B. L., and Beyreuther, K. (1985b). Amyloid plaque core protein in Alzheimer disease and Down syndrome. *Proc. Nat. Acad. Sci. USA*, **82**, 4245–9.

Monagle, R. D., and Brody, H. (1971). The effects of age upon the main nucleus of the inferior olive in the human. *J. Comp. Neurol.*, **155**, 61–6.

Mountjoy, C. Q., Roth, M., Evans, N. J. R., and Evans, H. M. (1983). Cortical neuronal counts in normal elderly controls and demented patients. *Neurobiol. of Aging*, **4**, 1–11.

Nieto-Sampedro, M., Manthrope, M., Barbin, G., Varon, S., and Cotman, C. W. (1983). Injury-induced neuronotrophic activity in adult rat brain: correlation with survival of delayed implants in the wound cavity. *J. Neurosci.*, **3**, 2219–29.

Oldstone, M. B. A., Holmstoen, J., and Welsh, R. M. Jr. (1977). Alterations of acetylcholine enzymes in neuroblastoma cells persistently infected with lymphocytic choriomeningitis virus. *J. Cellular Physiol.*, 91, 459-72.

Pearce, B. R., Palmer, A. M., Bowen, D. M., Wilcock, G. K., Esiri, M. M., and Davison, A. N. (1984). Neurotransmitter dysfunction and atrophy of the caudate nucleus in Alzheimer's disease. *Neurochem. Path.*, 2, 221-3.

Pearson, R. C. A., Esiri, M. M., Hiorns, R. W., Wilcock, G. K., and Powell, T. P. S. (1985). Anatomical correlates of the distribution of the pathological changes in the neocortex in Alzheimer disease. *Proc. Natl. Acad. Sci. USA*, 82, 1-4.

Pearson, R. C. A., Gatter, K. C., and Powell, T. P. S. (1983b). Retrograde cell degeneration in the basal nucleus in monkey and man. *Brain Res.*, 261, 321-6.

Pearson, R. C. A., Sofroniew, M. V., Cuello, A. C., Powell, T. P. S., Eckenstein, F., Esiri, M. M., and Wilcock, G. K. (1983a). Persistence of cholinergic neurons in the basal nucleus in a brain with senile dementia of the Alzheimer's type demonstrated by immunohistochemical staining for choline acetyltransferase. *Brain Res.*, 289, 375-9.

Perry, E. K., Curtis, M., Dick, D. J., Candy, J. M., *et al.* (1985). Cholinergic correlates of cognitive impairment in Parkinson's disease – comparisons with Alzheimer's disease. *J. Neurol. Neurosurg. Psychiat.*, 48, 413-22.

Perry, R. H. (1984). Neuropathology of Dementia. In Pearce, J. M. S. (ed.), *Dementia: A Clinical Approach*. Blackwells, London, pp. 89-116.

Perry, R. H., Candy, J. M., Perry, E. K., Irving, D., Blessed, G., Fairbairn, A. F., and Tomlinson, B. E. (1982). Extensive loss of choline acetyltransferase activity is not reflected by neuronal loss in the nucleus of Meynert in Alzheimer's disease. *Neurosci. Lett.*, 33, 311-15.

Robison, S. H., Munzer, J. S., Tandan, R., Bradley, R. S., and Bradley, W. G. (1985). DNA repair replication of alkylated DNA is reduced in Alzheimer's disease cells. *J. Neurology (Suppl.)*, 232, 63.

Rossor, M. N. (1981). Parkinson's disease and Alzheimer's disease as disorders of the iso-dendritic core. *Brit. Med. J.*, 283, 1588-90.

Rubenstein, R., and Price, R. W. (1984). Early inhibition of acetylcholinesterase and choline acetyltransferase activity in herpes simplex virus type 1 infection of PC12 cells. *J. Neurochem.*, 42, 142-50.

Sajdel-Sulkowska, E. M., and Marotta, C. A. (1984). Alzheimer's disease brain: alterations in RNA levels and in a ribonuclease-inhibitor complex. *Science*, 225, 947-9.

Sasaki, H., Muramoto, O., Kanazawa, I., Arai, H., Kosaka, K., and Iizuka, R. (1985). Selective reduction of glutamate in the postmortem brains of Alzheimer's disease. *J. Neurology (Suppl. to vol. 232)*, 232, 11.

Schiebel, A. B., and Tomiyasu, U. (1978). Dendritic sprouting in Alzheimer's pre-senile dementia. *Exp. Neurol.*, 60, 1-8.

Schwab, M. E., Otten, U., Agid, Y., and Thoenen, H. (1979). Nerve growth factor (NGF) in the rat CNS: absence of specific retrograde axonal transport and tyrosine hydroxylase induction in locus coeruleus and substantia nigra. *Brain Res.*, 168, 473-83.

Selkoe, D. J., Abraham, C., and Rasool, C. G. (1985a). Molecular properties of paired helical filaments and senile plaque amyloid fibers in Alzheimer's disease. *30th Oholobiological Conf.*, 25.

Selkoe, D. J., Abraham, C., and Rasool, C. G. (1985b). *Basic and Therapeutic Strategies in Alzheimer's and other Age-related Neuropsychiatric Disorders*. Edited and published by the Israel Institute for Biological Research.

Sims, N. R., Bowen, D. M., Allen, S. J., Smith, C. C. T., Neary, D., Thomas, D. J., and Davison, A. N. (1983). Presynaptic cholinergic dysfunction in patients with dementia. *J. Neurochem.*, 40, 503-9.

Smith, C. C. T., Bowen, D. M., Francis, P. T., Snowden, J. S., and Neary, D. (1985). Putative amino acid transmitters in lumbar cerebrospinal fluid of patients with histologically verified Alzheimer's dementia. *J. Neurol. Neurosurg. Psychiat.*, 48, 469-72.

Sofroniew, M. V., Pearson, R. C. A., Eckenstein, F., Cuello, A. C., and Powell, T. P. S. (1983). Retrograde changes in cholinergic neurons in the basal forebrain of the rat following cortical damage. *Brain Res.*, 289, 370-4.

Sourander, P., and Sjogren, H. (1970). The concept of Alzheimer's disease and its clinical implications. In Wolstenholme, G. E. W. and O'Connor, M. E. (eds.) *Alzheimer's Disease and Related Conditions*. Churchill, London, pp. 11–32.

Terry, R. D., Peck, A., DeTeresa, R., Schechter, R., and Horoupian, D. S. (1981). Some morphometric aspects of the brain in senile dementia of the Alzheimer's type. *Ann. Neurol.*, **10**, 184–92.

Tomlinson, B. E. (1980). The structural and quantitative aspects of the dementias. In Roberts, P. J. (ed.), *Biochemistry of Dementia*. Wiley, Chichester, pp. 15–52.

Tomlinson, A. H., and Esiri, M. M. (1983). Herpes simplex encephalitis: Immunohistological demonstration of spread of virus via olfactory pathways in mice. *J. Neurol. Sci.*, **60**, 473–84.

Tomlinson, B. E., Irving, D., and Blessed, G. (1981). Cell loss in the locus coeruleus in senile dementia of Alzheimer type. *J. neurol. Sci.*, **49**, 419–28.

White, P., Hiley, C. R., Goodhardt, M. J., Carrasco, L., Keet, J. P., Williams, J. E. J., and Bowen, D. M. (1977). Neocortical cholinergic neurones in elderly people. *Lancet*, **i**, 668–70.

Whitehouse, P. J., Price, D. L., Struble, R. G., Clark, A. W., Coyle, J. T., and Delong, M. R. (1982). Alzheimer's disease and senile dementia: loss of neurons in the basal forebrain. *Science*, **215**, 1237–9.

Winblad, B., Adolfsson, R., Gottfries, C. G., Oreland, L., and Roos, E. B. (1978). Brain monoamines, monoamine metabolites and enzymes in physiological ageing and senile dementia. In Frigerio, A. (ed.), *Recent Developments in Mass Spectrometry in Biochemistry and Medicine*. Plenum, New York, pp. 253–67.

Wisniewski, H. M., and Merz, G. S. (1984). Neuropathology of the aging brain and dementia of the Alzheimer type. In Gaitz, C., and Samorajski, T. (eds.), *Aging 2000: Our Health Care Destiny*.

2

The 'Autocannibalism' of Choline-containing Membrane Phopholipids in the Pathogenesis of Alzheimer's Disease

R. J. Wurtman, J. Bluszajn and J.-C. Maire

Brains of patients with Alzheimer's disease exhibit an abundance of possible clues as to the aetiology of the disease and the pathophysiologic processes causing its signs and symptoms (Wurtman, 1985). These include: characteristic aggregations of abnormal proteins in neurons (neurofibrillary tangles) and extra-cellular spaces (plaques; amyloid); concentrations of a potentially neurotoxic environmental contaminant, aluminium, within affected neurons; and an abnormal aggregate, amyloid, which may itself constitute an infectious particle ('prion'). Additional clues as to the aetiology and pathogenesis of Alzheimer's disease may also be provided by the patient's family history — which sometimes reveals a strong genetic component to the disease — or by data, obtained using scanning devices, which show major reductions in brain blood flow and in oxygen and energy consumption.

All of these abnormal findings have spawned research programmes designed to test their contributions to the clinical findings of Alzheimer's disease. However, none has affected the conduct of research nearly so much as observations suggesting that Alzheimer's disease preferentially affects particular populations of neurons, which are distinguishable by the neurotransmitter that they produce and release. An overwhelming consensus now exists among investigators that: (a) certain acetylcholine-releasing brain neurons, the septal neurons projecting to the hippocampus and basal forebrain neurons innervating the cerebral cortices, are invariably decimated in Alzheimer's disease (Perry *et al.*, 1978; Bowen *et al.*, 1982; Wilcock *et al.*, 1982); (b) other neurons (for example, serotonin-releasing neurons in the raphe nucleus; noradrenergic neurons of the locus coeruleus; cortical somatostatin-releasing neurons) are also often afflicted but to a lesser extent; and (c) most neuronal populations are unaffected in the disease. If one or more groups of neurons are invariably damaged in Alzheimer's disease, then examination of their biochemical peculiarities may yield insights as to the disease's aetiology or to the pathogenetic process that ultimately causes the neurons to die. Moreover, if the deficient neurotransmitter can be implicated in the abnormal behaviours typical of the disease — like acetylcholine in memory loss, norepinephrine in the impaired ability to sustain attention, or serotonin in disturbances of mood or in aggressiveness — then drugs which substitute for the deficient transmitter or which increase its availability in synapses might be useful in treating the disease.

This article focusses on the first of these hopes, that is on the possibility that a particular biochemical property unique to cholinergic neurons underlies their special vulnerability in Alzheimer's disease. This property has to do with the ways that cholinergic neurons metabolise choline. All cells in the body incorporate free choline into phospholipid molecules (which, by the way, constitute the majority of all lipids present in neuronal membranes (Ansell, 1973)), like phosphatidylcholine (PC), sphingomyelin, and the 1-acetylcholine glycerophospholipids. However, cholinergic cells use choline for an additional purpose, i.e. both as a constituent of membrane phospholipids and as the precursor for acetylcholine, the neurotransmitter that they release into their synapses. (Indeed, when a cholinergic neuron is physiologically active, the rate at which it synthesises and releases acetylcholine depends upon its choline levels (Blusztajn and Wurtman, 1983).) We propose that their need to obtain choline for acetylcholine synthesis may sometimes cause cholinergic neurons to destroy their membranes, particularly when the neurons are firing frequently or when free choline is in relatively short supply: they may cannibalise the choline stored in the phospholipid 'reservoir', thus altering membrane composition (and, presumably, function) and even blocking the production of new membranes (Blusztajn and Wurtman, 1983).

Our hypothesis begs the question of the aetiology of the Alzheimer's disease, focussing instead on why cholinergic neurons are more likely than others to be damaged by the aetiologic factor. It applies equally well whether the aetiologic factor is present only in diseased cells or is distributed throughout the brain. The factor that presumably causes a choline deficiency might be a decrease in choline production (by *de novo* synthesis), a decrease in its uptake from the synaptic cleft and extracellular space, or an excessive utilisation of choline to form a particular phospholipid. Choline uptake might be impaired if the delivery of oxygen or glucose to the nerve terminals is deficient, this perhaps being secondary to a diffusion block caused by the perivascular amyloidosis that is characteristic of Alzheimer's disease (Mandybur, 1975). Alternatively, the hypothetical choline deficiency might simply result from its over-use for acetylcholine synthesis, as might happen if the firing frequency of vulnerable neurons is persistently enhanced, or if the presynaptic storage of acetylcholine is impaired. Once cholinergic terminals begin to deteriorate and to release less of the transmitter, it seems likely that surviving, 'healthy' terminals might start to release *more* acetylcholine – either because the firing frequencies of their neurons will increase or because release is no longer subject to presynaptic inhibition. Increased acetylcholine synthesis might also be expected to increase the demand for its precursor, choline, within 'healthy' terminals, a process which might ultimately lead to 'autocannibalism' in these terminals as well.

The choline obtained by 'autocannibalism' could derive from the general metabolic 'pool' of choline phospholipids, or perhaps from a pool specifically mobilised for that purpose. Membrane phospholipids like PC are compartmented in three ways: by their subcellular localisation (for example synaptic vesicles *v*. plasma membranes); by their fatty acid composition; and by their mode of synthesis (methylation of phosphatidylethanolamine *v*. incorporation of pre-existing choline via the CDP-choline or base-exchange pathways). Excessive destruction of membrane PC might lead to changes in membrane composition (for example in the ratios of PC to other phospholipids, or to proteins) or to a loss in total membrane surface. Either alteration could affect the neuron's functional properties and even its viability. Such changes would be most likely to occur in nerve terminals, the neuronal structures that are specialised for neurotransmitter synthesis and release, damaging them first and only later affecting cell bodies.

The 'autocannibalism' hypothesis of the pathogenesis of Alzheimer's disease is not presently supported by an overwhelming body of clinical or experimental evidence, however it is consistent with a number of observations.

1. It is the terminals of cholinergic neurons in the cerebral cortex, and not the perikarya in the basal forebrain, which apparently degenerate first in Alzheimer's disease (Pearson *et al.*, 1983; Perry *et al.*, 1985). This is consistent with the fact that most of the neurons' acetylcholine is formed in the pre-synaptic terminals.

2. Only long-axon cholinergic neurons are affected by the disease process; the short-axon interneurons in the striatum are spared. Perhaps the short-axon neurons can more easily resynthesize their membranes because choline phospholipids are more readily available to them through axoplasmic transport (Abe *et al.*, 1973; Droz *et al.*, 1981). This transport would occur over a considerably shorter distance than that separating cholinergic perikarya in the nucleus basalis or septum from terminals in the frontoparietal cortex or hippocampus.

3. Choline is synthesized in brain neurons, *de novo*, by a multienzymatic pathway; the terminal steps in this pathway, catalysed by phosphatidyl-ethanolamine N-methyltransferase (PeMT), involve the stepwise methylation of phosphatidylethanolamine (PE) to PC using S-adenosylmethionine (SAM) as methyl donor. This newly formed PC is hydrolysed to free choline by a number of phospholipases and other hydrolases. We found that free choline constituted

23 % of the total PC synthesized by synaptosomal PeMT (from ^{3}H-methyl-SAM) during a 30-minute incubation period. Furthermore, the enrichment of the free choline pool with newly formed [3H] -choline was fifty-fold greater than that of the PC pool with newly formed [3H] -PC (Blusztajn and Wurtman, 1981). Thus the relatively small amount of PC synthesized *de novo* in nerve terminals may have a considerably faster turnover than the bulk of synaptosomal PC, possibly because this PC preferentially provides free choline for acetylcholine synthesis.

4. To determine whether an endogenous choline source (perhaps PC) in brain tissue can support acetylcholine synthesis in the absence of free choline, we measured acetylcholine release from rat striatal slices superfused with or without choline (Maire *et al.*, 1983). In the absence of free choline, acetylcholine was released spontaneously at a rate of 7.5 ± 1.3 pmol/mg protein/min (mean ± S.D.). Electrical field stimulation (15 Hz for 30 min) accelerated this release (25.6 ± 5.9 pmol/mg protein/min), and addition of choline (20 μM) to the superfusate significantly enhanced both the spontaneous (22.7 ± 5.7 pmol/mg protein/min) and the electrically evoked (37.4 ± 6.7 pmol/mg protein/min) release of the transmitter. Although the amount of acetylcholine in the tissue did not depend on extracellular choline concentration in this concentration range, the choline contents of the slices did increase as choline levels in the superfusate were raised. In the absence of exogenous choline, the combined efflux of free choline plus acetylcholine into the superfusate was 75 pmol/mg protein/min; the decrease in free choline plus acetylcholine within the tissue, however, was only 16 pmol/mg protein/min. Thus an endogenous pool of bound choline must have provided additional free choline for acetylcholine synthesis, and to maintain tissue choline and acetylcholine levels. The only known compounds whose pool sizes would be sufficient for this purpose are the choline-containing phospholipids. It appears that the choline liberated from striatal phospholipids must first enter the extra-cellular space and then be transported into cholinergic neurons by the high-affinity choline uptake system: addition of hemicholinium-3 (which blocks this uptake process) to the superfusate suppressed electrically evoked acetylcholine release and decreased striatal acetylcholine levels, even as compared with acetylcholine release from, and levels in, tissues that had been incubated without free choline.

Choline efflux from the isolated, perfused chicken heart was found to be enhanced by cholinesterase inhibitors or by muscarinic cholinergic agonists, and blocked by muscarinic antagonists (Corradetti *et al.*, 1983). This choline also apparently originates from the hydrolysis of tissue phospholipids. The rate at which this hydrolysis occurs appears to be modulated by cholinergic activity.

5. Stimulation of the preganglionic trunk of the cat's superior cervical ganglion for 20 min at 20, 4 or 1 Hz decreased the number of synaptic vesicles in cholin-ergic nerve terminals by 75, 54 or 56 %, respectively (Birks, 1974), without altering ganglionic acetylcholine contents (Birks and MacIntosh, 1961). This finding was interpreted as suggesting that the choline phospholipids in vesicular membranes were the source of the choline for acetylcholine synthesis. When, in

a similar experiment, the cat's superior cervical ganglion was stimulated for a shorter period, PC levels and the number of synaptic vesicles in presynaptic terminals did not fall. However, if the ganglion was also exposed to hemicholinium-3, the number of synaptic vesicles decreased after stimulation to 18 % of control, while ganglionic PC levels fell to 69 % of control (Parducz *et al.*, 1976). (Other phospholipids were not affected.) These observations indicate that when adequate extracellular choline is not available (after inhibition of its uptake by hemicholinium-3) vesicular PC is used to supply choline for acetylcholine synthesis.

No information is available concerning the possibility that neuronal choline-phospholipids provide choline for acetylcholine synthesis in human brain, nor that this process is pathologically accelerated in Alzheimer's disease. It is conceivable that brain regions rich in diseased cholinergic terminals might exhibit reductions in the ratio of PC to other phospholipids. However, a reduction would not occur if, for example, the terminal's failure to sustain adequate PC levels caused it simply to stop producing PC-containing membranes — a possibility that appears compatible with the preferential loss of cholinergic terminals over perikarya in Alzheimer's disease.

The hypothesised ability of the choline-phospholipids in cholinergic terminals to serve both as a structural component and as a reservoir for an important molecule of lower molecular weight (free choline) is not, of course, unique. Circulating albumin both contributes to the maintenance of colloid osmotic pressure and provides free amino acids when protein consumption is inadequate; bone is both a structural unit and a vast reservoir for calcium. Protein malnutrition can cause edema when too much albumin is broken down to provide free amino acids; calcium malnutrition can cause osteomalacia and bone breakage when bone is demineralised to provide the blood with free calcium. If our hypothesis concerning the reservoir functions of neuronal choline-phospholipids is correct, then consumption of supplemental choline — as such or as dietary PC (lecithin) — might serve an important nutritional function in patients with Alzheimer's disease, providing their diseased cholinergic neurons with some protection against 'autocannibalism' of their choline-containing membrane.

References

Abe, T., Haga, T., and Kurokawa, M. (1973). Rapid transport of phosphatidylcholine occurring simultaneously with protein transport in the frog sciatic nerve. *Biochem. J.*, 136, 731–40.

Ansell, G. B. (1973). Phospholipids and the nervous system. In Ansell, G. B., Hawthorne, J. N. and Dawson, R. M. C. (eds.), *Form and Function of Phospholipids*. Elsevier, Amsterdam, 377–422.

Birks, R. I. (1974). The relationship of transmitter release and storage to the fine structure in a sympathetic ganglion. *J. Neurocytol.*, 3, 133–60.

Birks, R. I., and MacIntosh, F. C. (1961). Acetylcholine metabolism of a sympathetic ganglion. *Can. J. Biochem. Physiol.*, 39, 787–827.

Blusztajn, J. K., and Wurtman, R. J. (1981). Choline biosynthesis by a preparation enriched in synaptosomes from rat brain. *Nature*, **290**, 417–18.

Blusztajn, J. K. and Wurtman, R. J. (1983). Choline and cholinergic neurons. *Science*, **221**, 614–20.

Bowen, D. M., Benton, J. S., Spillane, J. A., Smith, C. C. T., and Allen, S. J. (1982). Choline acetyltransferase activity and histopathology of frontal neocortex biopsies of demented patients. *J. neurol. Sci.*, **57**, 191–202.

Corradetti, R., Lindmar, R., and Loffelholz, K. (1983). Mobilization of cellular choline by stimulation of muscarinic receptors in isolated chicken heart and rat cortex *in vivo*. *J. Pharmacol. exp. Ther.*, **226**, 826–32.

Droz, B., Brunetti, M., DiGiambernadino, L., Koenig, H. L., and Porcellati, G. (1981). Axonal transport of phosphoglycerides to cholinergic synapses. In Pepeu, G. (ed.), *Cholinergic Mechanisms*. Plenum Press, New York, 377–86.

Maire, J.-C., Tacconi, M. T., and Wurtman, R. J. (1983). Source of choline for the release of choline and acetylcholine from brain slices. *Soc. Neurosci.*, **9**, 283.8 (abstract).

Mandybur, T. I. (1975). The incidence of cerebral amyloid angiopathy in Alzheimer's disease. *Neurology (Minneap.)*, **25**, 120–6.

Parducz, A., Kiss, Z., and Joo, F. (1976). Changes of the phosphatidylcholine content and the number of synaptic vesicles in relation to neurohumoral transmission in sympathetic ganglia. *Experientia*, **32**, 1520–1.

Pearson, R. C. A., Sofroniew, M. V., Cuello, A. C., Powell, T. P. S., Eckenstein, S., Esiri, M. M., and Wilcock, G. K. (1983). Persistence of cholinergic neurons in the basal nucleus in a brain with senile dementia of the Alzheimer's type demonstrated by immunohisto-chemical staining for choline acetyltransferase. *Brain Research*, **289**, 375–9.

Perry, R. H., Candy, J. M., Perry, E. K., Irving, D., Blessed, G., Fairbairn, A. F., and Tomlinson, B. E. (1985). Extensive loss of choline acetyltransferase activity is not reflected by neuronal loss in the nucleus of Meynert in Alzheimer's disease. *Neurosci. Lett.*, **33**, 311–15.

Perry, E. K., Tomlinson, B. E., Blessed, G., Bergman, K., Gibson, P. H., and Perry, R. H. (1978). Correlations of cholinergic abnormalities with senile plaques and mental test scores in senile dementia. *Brit. J. Med.*, **2**, 1458–9.

Wilcock, G. K., Esiri, M. M., Bowen, D. M., and Smith, C. C. T. (1982). Alzheimer's disease: correlation of cortical choline acetyltransferase activity with the severity of dementia and histological abnormalities. *J. neurol. Sci.*, **57**, 407–17.

Wurtman, R. J. (1985). Alzheimer's disease. *Scientific American*, **252**, 62–75.

3

Future Prospects Offered by Positron Emission Tomography for the Study of Alzheimer's Disease

J. C. Baron

1.1 Introduction

Positron emission tomography (PET) is a unique research tool in clinical neurosciences since it provides non-invasive, quantitative, *in vivo* autoradiography in humans (Phelps and Mazziotta, 1985). Hence, following administration to the subject of trace doses of a compound labelled with a positron-emitting radiopharmaceutical, images that quantitatively represent the distribution of the tracer in a cross-section of the brain can be obtained. The detection device necessary to collect the photons is specific in that it makes use of the physical characteristics of the paired photons that result from positron annihilation to generate high resolution, quantitative tomographic cuts. The availability of the positron emitters ^{15}O, ^{11}C, ^{13}N and ^{18}F allows hundreds of chemicals (including O_2, CO_2, CO, H_2O, sugars, amino-acids, neurotransmitters, drugs, peptides and hormones) to be labelled at high specific radioactivity (Comar *et al.*, 1982).

1.2 Applications and Limitations of PET

The classical autoradiographic approach can be applied to PET in order to study *in vivo* variables such as local cerebral glucose utilisation (using either ^{11}C-2-deoxy-D-glucose or ^{18}F-2-fluoro-deoxy-D-glucose), blood perfusion (using $H_2^{15}O$, ^{11}C-iodoantipyrine, etc.), intracellular pH (using ^{11}C-DMO), or blood volume (using ^{11}CO or $C^{15}O$). In addition, the short half-life of ^{15}O (2 min) led to the design of original, 'dynamic steady-state' models to measure local cerebral blood flow and oxygen consumption (Jones *et al.*, 1976).

Neuropharmacology is another field of application of PET, due to the unique possibility of measuring the local concentrations of labelled drugs in brain tissue. This approach has been applied to drugs such as phenytoin and valproate, in order to study their pharmacokinetics in both normal and abnormal tissue (*see* Baron *et al.*, 1983). Labelled drugs have also been used as specific radioligands in order to study *in vivo* different central neurotransmitter receptors such as the dopamine, serotonin, benzodiazepine and opiate receptors (Baron and Mazière, 1986). Using appropriate ligands administered in trace amounts, one can demonstrate *in vivo* that they bind specifically to their brain receptors, showing a specific regional distribution of the tracer. For example, the neuroleptic high-affinity antagonist ligand, spiperone, has been shown to accumulate more in the striatum than in the cerebellum (Figure 3.1). The dose-dependent inhibition or displacement of the ligand by an unlabelled competitor, the stereo-specificity of this displacement and the saturability of the *in vivo* ligand accumulation itself, all correlate with the known pharmacological properties of the dopamine receptor.

Another unique advantage of PET is to provide the time course of the tracer in any given region of the brain with a temporal resolution of less than one second. This is a considerable advantage over classical autoradiography, since it allows the actual local measurement of the rate constants of the radiopharmaceutical. Hence, a combination of PET and the Sokoloff method using labelled 2-deoxy-D-glucose to measure local cerebral glucose utilisation can be applied to pathological conditions such as cerebral ischaemia. The local tracer accumulation curve can be fitted to a three-compartment model in order to determine the actual rates of both transport across the blood–brain barrier and phosphorylation and, hence, the rate of local glucose utilisation (Huang *et al.*, 1980; Baron *et al.*, 1984). This interpretation assumes a constant relationship between the behaviour of glucose and that of the glucose analogue. Recent developments have shown that this relationship, the so-called 'lumped constant', can be measured regionally by PET using an additional study with ^{11}C-methyl-glucose (Gjedde *et al.*, 1985). A different approach to the measurement with PET of glucose utilisation uses the regional cerebral kinetics of intravenously administered ^{11}C-D-glucose (Raichle *et al.*, 1977), a method which avoids the problem of the 'lumped constant' but which is subject to errors due to the rapid metabolism of labelled glucose in brain, blood, and peripheral organs.

The kinetic approach has also been applied to the essential amino acids L-methionine and L-leucine, both labelled with ^{11}C (Bustany *et al.*, 1981; Phelps *et al.*, 1984). These authors demonstrated that in baboons the behaviour of ^{11}C-L-methionine in brain could be accurately described by a three-compartment model including plasma, a free-methionine pool in tissue (essentially the extracellular space), and a bound-methionine pool in tissue (essentially *de novo*

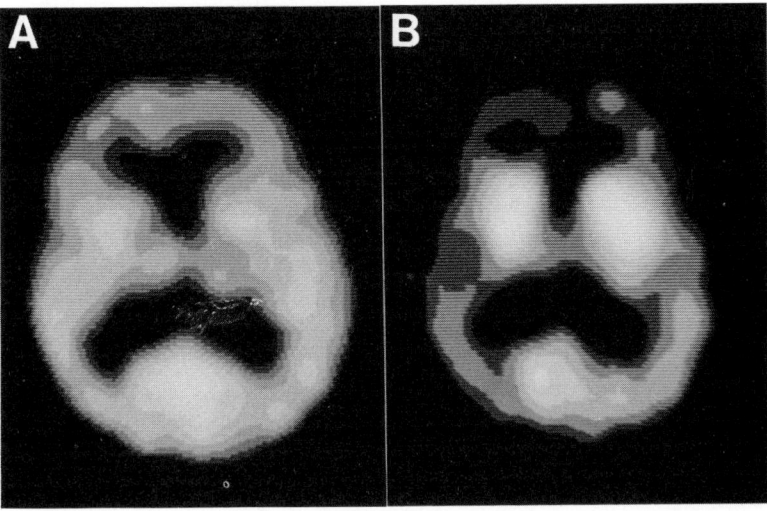

Figure 3.1 PET images of a normal human subject, performed at the level of the basal ganglia 15 min (image A) and 4.5 h (image B) after intravenous injection of a tracer dose (~ 1 μg) of the potent neuroleptic bromospiperone labelled with the positron emitter [76]Br. The early image shows a distribution of tracer reflecting passive penetration into brain tissue as a function of local perfusion. The later image shows redistribution of tracer which has accumulated in the striatum relative to the cortical mantle, in accordance with the high density of dopaminergic receptors in the former but not in the latter structure (from Mazière et al., 1985).

protein incorporation), while other possible fates of the tracer (e.g. demethylation, transmethylation) were negligible (Bustany and Comar, 1985). Since the breakdown of proteins in brain is a slow process relative to the duration of the study (~45 min), the return of protein-incorporated ^{11}C-L-methionine back to the free pool can be neglected, and the model simplifies to a three rate-constant situation similar to that of the 2-deoxyglucose Sokoloff paradigm. Accordingly, ^{11}C-L-methionine has been used to infer the rate of local protein synthesis in human brain in vivo (Bustany and Comar, 1985).

The brain kinetics of radioligands can be used to estimate quantitative parameters of specific binding to brain receptors in vivo, although there is as yet no general model that describes faithfully each particular radioligand–receptor interaction (Mintun et al., 1984; Syrota et al., 1984; Baron and Mazière, 1986). In addition, these models are limited in that they are not designed to provide both the affinity constant (K_d) and the receptor density (B_{max}). The interpretation of in vivo clinical PET studies of radioligands has so far relied on semi-quantitative indexes of specific binding. Thus, for example, the striatum/cerebellum radioactive concentration ratio has been used to assess dopaminergic receptor function in the striatum using labelled spiperone derivatives (Wong et al., 1984;

Baron *et al.*, 1985; Mazière *et al.*, 1985). The validity, under certain conditions, of this index has, however been amply demonstrated (Wong *et al.*, 1984).

Another promising application of PET has been developed over the last eight years at McMaster University (Canada), where the function of the presynaptic dopamine terminals has been studied using ^{18}F-labelled 6-fluoro-L-DOPA (Garnett *et al.*, 1983). Through elegant experimental validation studies, these authors were able to demonstrate that this compound behaves as an L-DOPA analogue, undergoing specific re-uptake at dopamine terminals in brain tissue (a process that results in its accumulation in the striatum and, to a lesser extent, in the frontal cortex). On the other hand, this compound is much less subject to further metabolism than L-DOPA, and is therefore suitable for the study of the regional brain kinetics of dopaminergic processes *in vivo*.

The limitations of PET should, however, be emphasised. Most positron emitters are cyclotron produced, and their fast physical decays (^{25}O: $t_{1/2}$ = 2 min; ^{11}C: $t_{1/2}$ = 2 min) require the availability of a medical cyclotron very close to the positron camera. In addition, labelling methods are sometimes difficult to develop, and many pharmaceutical compounds cannot, as yet, be labelled. Finally, the need for appropriate spatial and temporal data sampling has led to the development of sophisticated, high-cost positron cameras. To run such equipment, and to analyse the data correctly requires a large team of highly trained people. These considerations help explain why PET centres are so few, why they drain a large amount of public funds, and why they have been restricted so far to clinical research applications. It therefore follows that the research protocols need be very rigorous and methodologically sound in order to optimise the cost–benefit ratio of PET.

1.3 PET in Alzheimer's Disease and Normal Ageing

The potential applications of PET to the study of Alzheimer's disease (AD) are summarised in Table 3.1. Each one of these approaches is a whole long-term project in itself, and it is clear that several years at least will be necessary in order to achieve significant progress in this area.

Methodological problems, however, are also likely to slow down PET research in AD. Patient selection must be rigorous and follow the guidelines of the DSM III and of the NIH Research Committee (McKhann *et al.*, 1984) but this is an exacting task, and one which apparently selects a particular subgroup from the clinical spectrum of AD. In addition, the definition of a control group is itself a matter of debate, as it is not clear whether AD patients should be compared to very healthy aged persons or to a 'normal' population that may include various minor ailments (e.g. benign senescent forgetfulness) that are part of 'normal' ageing. A further problem is how to distinguish the primary effects of AD itself on the PET parameter being measured (usually glucose utilisation), from the

Table 3.1 Investigations of Alzheimer's disease with PET

Oxygen consumption Glucose utilisation →	Neuronal function and reactivity to cognitive stimulation
Perfusion ————————→	Vascular factors
Precursors Specific receptors →	Neurotransmission systems
Amino-acids ————————→	Protein synthesis
Human and animal models ————→	Pharmacology of 'pro-mnesic' drugs
Other approaches ————————→	Blood–brain barrier Intracellular pH Extracellular space Glial marker? Neurotoxic compounds?

secondary effects due to the different cognitive perception of the study environment as a result of AD.

Another problem more specific to PET is related to the cortical atrophy that is frequently associated with AD (Alavi and De Leon, 1985), since it is not possible to differentiate brain tissue from cerebro-spinal fluid (CSF) within the regions analysed. In order to minimise this problem, cortical atrophy may be quantified using X-ray computerised tomography in addition to PET scanning (Herscovitch et al., 1984), but the method of data correction between the two systems is yet to be developed. A final limitation of PET studies is data analysis since, as for autoradiography, there is no standardised method for defining regions of interest on the multiple digitalised brain images that are produced from a single PET study (Mazziotta, 1984).

Despite several reports on the effects of AD on the cerebral metabolism of oxygen and glucose, the effects of normal ageing on these parameters is still debated. Thus, several groups found that normal ageing is associated with a small but significant reduction in overall brain oxygen consumption (Frackowiak et al., 1980; Pantano et al., 1984) and glucose utilisation (Kuhl et al., 1982a), while other reports, sometimes from the same laboratories, claim no significant change in these parameters (Duara et al., 1983, 1984; Frackowiak and Gibbs, 1983; Hawkins et al., 1983a; De Leon et al., 1984). These discrepancies illustrate differences in selection criteria for normality, and are consistent with previous findings using the Kety–Schmidt technique (see Smith, 1984; Pantano et al., 1984), indicating that very healthy aged people may maintain normal cerebral metabolic rate, while more 'normal' ageing entails a small reduction in cerebral metabolism. Differences in experimental set-up (e.g. sensory input) during PET study may also account, in part, for these discrepancies, particularly since age-related effects on the visual and auditory processes have been shown to affect brain metabolic activity (Smith, 1984). The symmetrical metabolic reductions seen in normal ageing seem preferentially to affect the prefrontal, perisylvian and parieto-occipital cortex (Kuhl *et al.*, 1982a; Pantano *et al.*, 1984; Chawluck *et al.*, 1985). Data concerning white matter indicates a decrease in glucose utilisation but a preservation of oxygen consumption, suggesting possible alterations in the oxidative phosphorylation process of glial cells with ageing. Finally, the small changes seen in the perfusion–metabolism coupling may reflect age-related modifications of brain capillaries (Frackowiak and Gill, 1983). They may also imply a slightly reduced perfusion reserve capacity. It is worth noting that the regional metabolic data provided by PET are expressed per unit of brain volume, so that a maintained volumetric glucose utilisation rate in the presence of reduced total brain mass indicates, in fact, a decreased overall brain metabolism (Creasey and Rapoport, 1985).

There have been numerous PET studies of cerebral metabolism in probable AD patients (Frackowiak *et al.*, 1981; Benson *et al.*, 1983; De Leon *et al.*, 1983; Foster *et al.*, 1983, 1984; Friedland *et al.*, 1983b, 1985; Chase *et al.*, 1984; Haxby *et al.*, 1985; Alavi and De Leon, 1985; Chawluck *et al.*, 1985; Kuhl *et al.*, 1985; Metter *et al.*, 1985). They all concur in that there is a decreased overall cerebral metabolic rate of both oxygen and glucose, this decrement being roughly proportional to the severity of dementia. Another important feature has been the preferential location of this metabolic impairment in the parieto-temporo-occipital associative cortex (Figure 3.2) with relative preservation of the primary visual and sensory motor cortex, prefrontal cortex, anterior cingulum, basal ganglia, thalamus and cerebellum. Due to inadequate spatial resolution, there is little information on the medial-temporal cortex and hippocampus. A final important aspect of AD has been the significant prevalence of right–left metabolic asymmetry, particularly affecting the parieto-temporo-occipital cortex. Statistically significant clinical correlations have been demonstrated between these relatively focal metabolic impairments (Foster *et al.*, 1983, 1984; Chase *et al.*, 1985; Haxby *et al.*, 1985), indicating an association between right parieto-temporal metabolism and visuo-spatial tasks on the one hand, and between left temporo-parietal metabolism and verbal tasks on the other hand. Patients with predominant memory impairment show symmetrically depressed cortical metabolic rate. The parietal/cerebellum metabolic ratio has emerged as the index best correlated with severity of dementia (Kuhl *et al.*, 1985).

The mechanisms underlying these metabolic alterations in cerebral cortex of AD patients seem chiefly related to neuronal lesions (neuronal loss and neuro-fibrillary tangles) which are known to display a cortical regional distribution pattern somewhat similar to that described above for PET metabolic impairment (Brun and Englund, 1981). It is therefore likely that PET of brain metabolism provides a mapping of neuronal dysfunction and histopathology *in vivo*. It is,

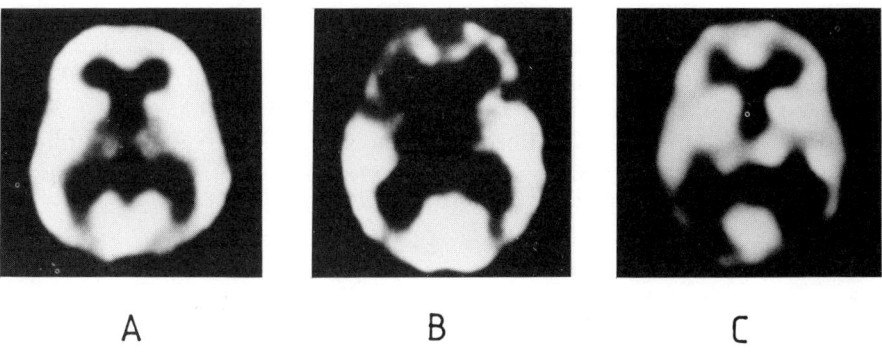

A   B   C

Figure 3.2   PET images displaying the local cerebral glucose utilisation at the basal ganglia level, obtained using the ^{18}F-fluoro-2-deoxy-D-glucose *in vivo* autoradiographic paradigm. These images were obtained from: (A) a normal control; (b) a patient with subcortical dementia (progressive supranuclear palsy); and (C) a patient with Parkinson's disease and Alzheimer's type dementia. Compared to the metabolic pattern seen in the control subject, there is a striking bilateral reduction in the metabolic rate affecting the prefrontal cortex in subcortical dementia, and the parieto-temporal cortex in Alzheimer's type dementia.

however, important to stress that PET studies have so far concentrated on advanced, typical AD cases conforming to strict research selection criteria. A prospective study of patients with early cognitive impairments, and follow-up with repeated PET studies ending with postmortem neuropathological assessment may help establish the early clinical correlates, prognostic value, and natural history of the focal metabolic changes in AD.

Another approach in metabolic measurements which is still in its infancy aims at studying brain function dynamically, using cognitive or sensory activation to assess how AD affects the cortical integrated functions, with reference to normal, age-matched, and education-matched controls. A recent study reported abnormal inter-correlations of glucose consumption among various brain regions in AD patients studied in a 'resting' condition (Metter *et al.*, 1984).

In order to investigate cortical metabolism in subcortical dementia, we studied six patients with progressive supranuclear palsy (PSP), a subcortical degenerative disorder that gives rise to a typical, frontal-lobe subcortical dementia (D'Antona *et al.*, 1985). Despite lack of significant neuronal degeneration in the cortex in PSP, we found a striking bilateral prefrontal cortex hypometabolism (Fig. 3.2) which we interpret as being due to loss of subcortico-cortical afferents. This study is important since it provides the first *in vivo* evidence in support of the concept of subcortical dementia (Albert *et al.*, 1974). Subcortical lesions are thought to play a major role in the development of dementia in AD, Parkinson's disease (PD), Huntington's disease (HD) and Wilson's disease (WD) (Cummings and Benson, 1984). In both AD and PD, lesions of the cholinergic and adrenergic systems are implicated, while in PD, lesions of the dopaminergic meso-corticolimbic system are also involved. In HD and WD, on the other hand, the sub-cortical regions implicated are the basal ganglia. In contrast to PSP, however, frontal cortex hypometabolism has not been a prominent feature in PET studies of either AD or demented patients with PD, HD or WD (Kuhl *et al.*, 1982b, 1984; Hawkins *et al.*, 1983b). Recently, Kuhl *et al.* (1985) reported a striking similarity in the pattern of regional alterations in cerebral glucose utilisation between AD and demented PD patients. These results would suggest a marked dissimilarity in the metabolic correlates of dementia between PSP and other degenerative processes. A marked bifrontal hypometabolism has occasionally been reported in probable AD patients (Frackowiak *et al.*, 1981; Benson *et al.*, 1983), particularly in advanced cases, although the clinical correlates of this pattern were not described. Recently, Metter *et al.* (1985) suggested a con-tinuum in the gradient of antero-posterior cortical hypometabolism in AD patients. Whether the frontal cortex hypometabolism in some AD patients reflects predominantly subcortical dementia (as in PSP) or preferential cortical degeneration (Gustafson *et al.*, 1985) remains to be established. In this context, it is worth noting that experimental lesions of the subcortico-cortical cholin-ergic systems in rats lead to marked ipsilateral cortical hypometabolism (London *et al.*, 1984). If it can be transposed to baboons, this approach may provide a useful primate model of AD-like cholinergic deafferentation for studying the *in vivo* metabolic effects of so-called 'pro-mnesic' drugs with PET.

There is only one, brief report of a ^{11}C-L-methionine PET study of AD patients (Bustany and Comar, 1985). These preliminary findings suggest that early AD is already reflected in a 20 % decrease in protein synthesis rate in the cerebral cortex, while more advanced cases show up to 75 % decrease, particu-larly in parieto-temporal and/or frontal cortex. The cortical protein synthesis rate therefore appears to be a very sensitive parameter in AD and may perhaps be altered long before glucose utilisation is impaired, especially if the hypo-thesis suggesting that AD is primarily a disease of nucleic acids is true (Mann, 1982; Sajdel-Sulkowska and Marotta, 1984).

There are as yet no PET studies of central receptors in AD. It is feasible to study the 5-HT and dopamine receptors in the cerebral cortex and the striatum, respectively, but no reliable PET method has yet been developed to investigate the muscarinic receptors in the cerebral cortex. Using both ^{11}C-methyl-spiperone and [76]Br-bromospiperone, a highly significant loss of striatal dopaminergic receptors has been demonstrated in normal ageing (Wong *et al.*, 1984; Mazière *et al.*, 1985). These studies not only confirm *in vivo* the results obtained post-mortem (Severson *et al.*, 1982), but also serve to illustrate the reliability and the sensitivity of these PET methods. Furthermore, we have shown a highly significant loss of [76]Br-bromospiperone binding sites in the striatum of seven patients with PSP (Baron *et al.*, 1985), in agreement with post-mortem data (Bokobza *et al.*, 1984). This provides an explanation for the lack of benefit from L-DOPA and DA agonists in this condition despite reduced nigro-striatal dopaminergic function. Such methods will be important for our better understanding of the effects of normal ageing on the dopaminergic systems, particularly if coupled to the ^{18}F-fluoro-DOPA method (Leenders et al., 1984).

In addition to the latter technique, other presynaptic markers of different neurotransmission systems are currently being developed for brain PET studies. Thus, choline has been labelled with ^{11}C, but the preliminary results indicate that poor blood-brain barrier penetration and large non-specific binding may limit its use as a marker of cortical cholinergic terminals (Friedland et al., 1983a).

References

Alavi, A., and De Léon, M. J. (1985). Studies of the brain in aging and dementia with positron emission tomography and X-ray computed tomography. In Reivich, M., and Alavi, A. (eds.), *Positron Emission Tomography*. A. R. Liss, New York, 273–90.

Albert, M. L., Feldman, R. G., and Willis, A. L. (1974). The subcortical dementia of progressive supranuclear palsy. *J. Neurology Neurosurgery and Psychiatry*, 37, 121–30.

Baron, J. C., and Mazière, B. (1986). Positron emission tomography studies of central receptors in humans. In Battistin, L. (ed.), *PET and NMR: Neurochemistry in vivo*. A. R. Liss, New York, (In press).

Baron, J. C., Mazière, B., Loc'h, C., Sgouropoulos, P., Bonnet, A. M., and Agid, Y. (1985). Progressive supranuclear palsy: loss of striatal dopamine receptors demonstrated in vivo by positron tomography. *Lancet*, i, 1163–4.

Baron, J. C., Roeda, D., Munari, C., Crouzel, C., Chodkiewizc, J. P., and Comar, D. (1983). Brain regional pharmacokinetics of ^{11}C-labelled diphenyl hydantoin: positron emission tomography in humans. *Neurology (Cleveland)*, 33, 580–5.

Baron, J. C., Rougemont, D., Soussaline, F., Bustany, P., Crouzel, C., Bousser, M. G., and Comar, D. (1984). Local interrelationships of cerebral oxygen consumption and glucose utilization in normal subjects and in ischemic stroke patients: a positron tomography study. *J. Cereb. Blood Flow Metab.*, 4, 140–9.

Benson, D. F., Kuhl, D. E., Hawkins, R. A., Phelps, M. E., Cummings, J. L., and Tsai, S. Y. (1983). The fluorodeoxyglucose ^{18}F scan in Alzheimer's disease and multi-infarct dementia. *Arch. Neurol., (Chicago)*, 40, 711–14.

Bokobza, B., Ruberg, M., Scatton, B., Javoy-Agid, F. and Agid, Y. (1984). ^{3}H-spiperone binding, dopamine and HVA concentrations in Parkinson's disease and supranuclear palsy. *Eur. J. Pharmacol.*, 99, 167–75.

Brun, A., and Englund, E. (1981). Regional pattern of degeneration in Alzheimer's disease: neuronal loss and histopathological grading. *Histopathology*, 5, 549–64.

Bustany, P., and Comar, D. (1985). Protein synthesis evaluation in brain and other organs in humans by PET. In Reivich, M. and Alavi, A. (eds.), *Positron Emission Tomography*. A. R. Liss, New York, 183–201.

Bustany, P., Sargent, T., Soudubray, J. A., Henry, J. F., and Comar, D. (1981). Regional human brain uptake and protein incorporation of ^{11}C-L-methionine studied in vivo with PET. *J. Cereb. Blood Flow Metabol.*, 1, Suppl. 1, 517–18.

Chase, T. N., Fedio, P., Foster, N. L., Brooks, R., Dichiro, G., and Mansi, L. (1984). Wechsler Adult intelligence scale performance. *Arch. Neurol. (Chicago)*, 41, 1244–7.

Chawluk, J., Alavi, A., Hartig, H., et al. (1985). Altered patterns of regional cerebral glucose metabolism in aging and dementia. *J. Cereb. Blood Flow Metabol.*, 5, 5121–2.

Comar, D., Berridge, M., Mazière, B., and Crouzel, C. (1982). Radiopharmaceuticals labelled with positron emitting radioisotopes. In Ell, P. J. (ed.), *Emission Computed Tomography*. Oxford University Press, Oxford, 42–90.

Creasey, H., and Rapoport, S. I. (1985). The Ageing human brain. *Ann. Neurol.*, 17, 2–10.

Cummings, J. L., and Benson, D. F. (1984). Subcortical dementia: review of an emerging concept. *Arch. Neurol. (Chicago)*, 41, 874–9.

D'Antona, R., Baron, J. C., Samson, Y., Serdaru, M., Viader, F., Agid, Y., and Cambier, J. (1985). Subcortical dementia: Frontal cortex hypometabolism detected by positron tomography in patients with progressive supranuclear palsy. *Brain*, **108**, 785–99.

Duara, R., Grady, C., Haxby, J., *et al.* (1984). Human brain glucose utilisation and cognitive function in relation to age. *Ann. Neurol.*, **16**, 702–13.

Duara, R., Margolin, R. A., Robertson-Chabo, E. A., *et al.* (1983). Cerebral glucose utilisation as measured with positron emission tomography in 21 resting healthy men between the ages of 21 and 83 years. *Brain*, **106**, 761–75.

Foster, N. L., Chase, T. N., Fedio, P., Patronas, N. J., Brooks, R. A., and Di Chiro, G. (1983). Alzheimer's disease: focal cortical changes shown by positron emission tomography. *Neurology, (Cleveland)*, **33**, 961–5.

Foster, N. L., Chase, T. N., Mansi, L., Brooks, R., Fedio, P., Patronas, N. J., and Di Chiro, G. (1984). Cortical abnormalities in Alzheimer's disease. *Ann. Neurol.*, **16**, 649–54.

Frackowiak, R. S. J., and Gibbs, J. M. (1983). The pathophysiology of Alzheimer's disease studied with positron emission tomography. In *Biological aspects of Alzheimer's disease*, Cold Spring Harbor, Banbury Report, **15**, 317–27.

Frackowiak, R. S. J., Lenzi, G. L., Jones, T., and Heather, J. D. (1980). Quantitative measurement of regional cerebral blood flow and oxygen metabolism in man, using ^{15}O and positron emission tomography: theory, procedure and normal values. *J. Comput. Assist. Tomogr.*, **4**, 727–36.

Frackowiak, R. S. J., Pozzilli, C., Legg, N. J., Du Boulay, G. H., Marshall, J., Lenzi, G. L., and Jones, T. (1981). Regional cerebral oxygen supply and utilisation in dementia: a clinical and physiological study with oxygen-15 and positron tomography. *Brain*, **104**, 753–78.

Friedland, R. P., Budinger, T. F., Koss, E., and Oder, B. A. (1985). Alzheimer's disease: anterior–posterior and lateral hemispheric alteration in cortical glucose utilisation. *Neurosci. Lett.*, **53**, 235–40.

Friedland, R. P., Mathis, C. A., Budinger, T. F., Mayer, B. R., and Rosen, M. (1983a). Labelled choline and phosphorylcholine: Body distribution and brain autoradiography. *J. nucl. Med.*, **24**, 812–15.

Friedland, R. P., Budinger, T. F., Ganz, E., Yano, Y., Mathis, C. A., Koss, B., Ober, B. A., Huesman, R. H., and Derenzo, S. E. (1983a). Regional cerebral metabolic alterations in dementia of Alzheimer type: positron emission tomography with ^{18}F-fluorodeoxyglucose. *J. Computer. Assis. Tomography*, **7**, 590–8.

Garnett, E. S., Firnau, G., and Nahmias, C. (1983). Dopamine visualized in the basal ganglia of living man. *Nature*, **305**, 137.

Gjedde, A., Wienhard, K., Heiss, W. D., Kloster, G., Diemer, N. H., Herholz, K., and Pawlik, G. (1985). Comparative regional analysis of 2-fluorodeoxyglucose and methylglucose uptake in brain of four stroke patients. With special reference to the regional estimation of the lumped constant. *J. Cereb. Blood Flow Metabol.*, **5**, 163–78.

Gustafson, L., Brun, A., Holmkvist, F., and Risberg, J. (1985). Regional cerebral blood flow in degenerative frontal lobe dementia of non-Alzheimer's type. *J. Cereb. Blood Flow Metabol.*, **5**, Suppl. 1, 5141–2.

Hawkins, R. A., Mazziotta, J. C., Phelps, M. E., *et al.* (1983a). Cerebral glucose metabolism as a function of age in man: influence of the rate constants in the fluorodeoxyglucose technique. *J. Cereb. Blood Flow Metabol.*, **3**, 250–3.

Hawkins, R. A., Phelps, M. E., Mazziotta, J. C., and Kuhl, D. E. (1983b). A study of Wilson's disease with F-18 FDG and positron tomography. *J. Cereb. Blood Flow Metabol.*, **3**, 498–9.

Haxby, J. V., Duara, R., Grady, C. L., Cutler, N. R., and Rapoport, S. I. (1985). Relations between neuropsychological and cerebral metabolic asymmetries in early Alzheimer's disease. *J. Cereb. Blood Flow Metabol.*, **5**, 193–200.

Herscovitch, P., Gado, M., Mintun, M. A., and Raichle, M. E. (1984). The necessity for correcting for cerebral atrophy in global positron emission tomography measurement. *Monogr. Neural. Sci.*, **11**, 93–7.

Huang, S. C., Phelps, M. E., Hoffman, E. J., Sideris, K., Selin, C. J., and Kuhl, D. E. (1980). Noninvasive determination of local cerebral metabolic rate of glucose in man. *American J. Physiol.*, **238**, 69–82.

Jones, T., Chesler, D. A., and Ter-Pogossian, M. M. (1976). The continuous inhalation of oxygen-15 for assessing regional oxygen extraction in the brain of man. *Brit. J. Radiol.*, **49**, 339–43.

Kuhl, D. E., Metter, E. J., and Riege, W. H. (1984). Patterns of local cerebral glucose utilization determined in Parkinson's disease by the ^{18}F-fluorodeoxyglucose method. *Annals Neurology*, **15**, 419–24.

Kuhl, D. E., Metter, E. J., Riege, W. H., and Phelps, M. E. (1982a). Effects of human aging on patterns of local cerebral glucose utilization determined by the ^{18}F-fluorodeoxyglucose method. *J. Cereb. Blood Flow Metabol.*, **2**, 163–71.

Kuhl, D. E., Phelps, M. E., Markham, C. H., Metter, E. J., Riege, W. H., and Winter, J. (1982b). Cerebral metabolism and atrophy in Huntington's disease determined by 18FDG and computed tomographic scan. *Ann. Neurol.*, **12**, 425–34.

Kuhl, D. E., Metter, E. J., Benson, F., Wesson-Ashford, J., Riege, W. H., Fujikawa, D. G., Markham, C. H., *et al.* (1985). Similarities of cerebral glucose metabolism in Alzheimer's disease and Parkinsonian dementia. *J. Cereb. Blood Flow Metabol.*, **5**, Suppl. 1, 169–70.

Leenders, K. L., Herold, S., Brooks, D. J., *et al.* (1984). Presynaptic and postsynaptic dopaminergic systems in human brain. *Lancet*, ii, 110–11.

De Leon, M. F., Ferris, S. H., George, A. E., Reisberg, B., Christman, D. R., Kricheff, S. S., and Wolf, A. P. (1983). Computed tomography and positron emission transaxial tomography evaluations of normal aging and Alzheimer's disease. *J. Cereb. Blood Flow Metabol.*, **3**, 391–4.

De Leon, M. J., George, A. E., Ferris, S. H., *et al.* (1984). Positron emission tomography and computed tomography assessments of the aging human brain. *J. Comput. Assist. Tomog.*, **8**, 88–94.

London, E. D., McKinney, M., Dam, M., Ellis, A., and Coyle, J. T. (1984). Decreased cortical glucose utilization after ibotenate lesions of the rat ventromedial globus pallidus. *J. Cereb. Blood Flow Metabol.*, **4**, 381–90.

McKhann, G., Drachman, D., Folstein, M., Katzman, R., Price, D., and Stadlan, E. M. (1984). Clinical diagnosis of Alzheimer's disease. *Neurology*, **34**, 939–44.

Mann, D. M. A. (1982). Nerve cell protein metabolism and degenerative disease. *Neuropath. Appl. Neurobiol.*, **8**, 161–76.

Mazière, B., Loc'h, C., Baron, J. C., Sgouropoulos, P., D'Antona, R., and Cambon, H. (1985). In vivo quantitative imaging of dopamine receptors in human brain using positron tomography and [76]Br-bromospiperone. *Eur. J. Pharmacol.*, **114**, 267–72.

Mazziotta, J. C. (1984). Physiologic neuroanatomy: New brain imaging methods present a challenge to an old disciple. *J. Cereb. Blood Flow Metabol.*, **4**, 481–3.

Metter, E. J., Riege, W. H., Kameyama, M., Kuhl, D. E. and Phelps, M. E. (1984). Cerebral metabolic relationship for selected brain regions in Alzheimer's, Huntington's and Parkinson's diseases. *J. Cereb. Blood Flow Metabol.*, **4**, 500–6.

Metter, E. J., Riege, W. H., Benson, D. F., Phelps, M. E., and Kuhl, D. E. (1985). Variability of regional cerebral glucose metabolism in Alzheimer's disease patients as compared to controls. *J. Cereb. Blood Flow Metabol.*, **5**, Suppl. 1, 127–8.

Mintun, M. A., Raichle, M. E., Kilbourn, M. R., Wooten, G. F. and Welch, M. J. (1984). A quantitative model for the in vivo assessment of drug binding sites with positron emission tomography. *Ann. Neurol.*, **15**, 217–27.

Pantano, P., Baron, J. C., Lebrun-Grandie, P., Duquesnoy, N., Bousser, M. G., and Comar, D. (1984). Regional cerebral blood flow and oxygen consumption in human aging. *Stroke*, **15**, 635–41.

Phelps, M. E., Barrio, J. R., Huang, S. C., Keen, R. E., Chugani, H., and Mazziotta, J. C. (1984). Criteria for the tracer kinetic measurement of cerebral protein synthesis in humans with positron emission tomography. *Ann. Neurol.*, **15**, 192–202.

Phelps, M. E., and Mazziotta, J. C. (1985). Positron emission tomography: human brain function and biochemistry. *Science*, **228**, 799–809.

Raichle, M. E., Welch, M. J., Grubb, R. L., Higgins, C. S., and Larson, K. B. (1977). Measurement of regional substrate utilization rate by emission tomography. *Science*, **199**, 986–7.

Sajdel-Sulkowska, E., and Marotta, C. (1984). Alzheimer's disease brain: alterations in RNA levels and in a ribonuclease-inhibitor complex. *Science*, **225**, 947–9.

Severson, J. A., Marcusson, J., Winbled, B., and Finch, C. E. (1982). Age-correlated loss of dopaminergic binding sites in human basal ganglia. *J. Neurochem.*, **39**, 1623–31.

Smith, C. B. (1984). Aging and changes in cerebral energy metabolism. *Trends Neurosci.*, 203–8.

Syrota, A., Paillotin, G., Davy, J. M., and Aumont, M. C. (1984). Kinetics of in vivo binding of antagonists to muscarinic cholinergic receptor in the human heart studied by positron emission tomography. *Life Sciences*, **35**, 837–45.

Wong, D. F., Wagner, H. N., Dannals, R. F., *et al.* (1984). Effects of age on dopamine and serotonin receptors measured by positron tomography in the living human brain. *Science*, **226**, 1393–6.

4

The Neuronal Cytoskeleton and Neurofibrillary Tangles

B. H. Anderton, J.-P. Brion, J. Flament-Durand, M. C. Haugh,
J. Kahn, C. C. J. Miller, A. Probst and J. Ulrich

4.1 Introduction

Dementia of the Alzheimer type, or Alzheimer's disease, has a characteristic brain histopathology comprising neurofibrillary tangles, senile neuritic plaques, granulovacuolar bodies and Hirano bodies. A correlation between the number of tangles, the extent of the cholinergic deficit and the degree of dementia has been found (Wilcock *et al.*, 1982). Tangles are composed of bundles of 10–13 nm filaments which appear to be twisted about each other in pairs with a crossover roughly every 80 nm; these filaments are known as paired helical filaments (PHFs) (Kidd, 1963; Wisniewski *et al.*, 1976). The tangles are present in, and appear to fill, affected neuronal perikarya of the hippocampus and other cortical and subcortical areas but the PHFs are also found as small aggregates in the swollen neurites present in the periphery of the senile plaques (Kidd, 1963, 1964; Terry *et al.*, 1964; Gonatas *et al.*, 1967).

Alzheimer type tangles consisting of PHFs are also a feature of several other diseases, including Down's syndrome, postencephalitic Parkinson's disease, dementia pugilistica, subacute sclerosing panencephalitis, Parkinson-dementia complex and Hallevorden–Spatz syndrome (Wisniewski *et al.*, 1979). Some tangles contain straight filaments approximately 15 nm in diameter (Hirano *et al.*, 1968; Yagishita *et al.*, 1981; Okamoto *et al.*, 1982). Straight 15 nm filaments are the predominant filamentous component of the neuronal inclusions characteristic of Pick's disease (Rewcastle *et al.*, 1968; Towfighi, 1972; Wisniewski *et al.*, 1972; Brion *et al.*, 1973). What relationship, if any, exists between PHFs and straight filaments is unknown but it has been a widespread assumption that PHFs are some abnormal form of the neuronal cytoskeleton.

The cytoskeleton is composed of three fibrous organelles. These are microtubules 24 nm in diameter, 6–7 nm microfilaments and 10 nm intermediate filaments (Lazarides 1980, 1982; Anderton 1981, 1982). The intermediate filaments are subdivided into five tissue-related types and are represented by neurofilaments in neurones. Kidd (1963) suggested that PHFs may be derived from neurofilaments because of their similar diameters, the chemical composition of PHFs, however, remains unresolved.

4.2 Physical and Chemical Properties of PHFs

PHFs and their constituent subunits have not yet been prepared in homogeneous form. An important discovery made by Selkoe and colleagues was to show that many PHFs are resistant to the common protein denaturing and solubilising agents such as sodium dodecyl sulphate (SDS), urea or guanidinium hydrochloride (Selkoe *et al.*, 1982a). This property was exploited for preparing fractions enriched in PHFs, the PHFs still retaining their characteristic ultrastructural appearance. Iqbal *et al.* (1984) have claimed that these insoluble PHFs can be partially solubilised by sonication and prolonged extraction with SDS, although the proportion which dissolves depends on the brain specimen and can vary from 2 to 90 % of the total isolated PHFs. Those proteins which were extracted by this harsh treatment still possessed a strong tendency to reaggregate but several components were resolved on SDS gels, the major bands having molecular weights of 57,000 and 62,000, with several minor bands smaller than 57,000 molecular weight. None of these polypeptides corresponded in size to any known cytoskeletal proteins.

Yen and Kress (1983) have reported that isolated PHFs can be disrupted by treatment with proteases and a proportion of the SDS-insoluble material extracted in formic acid. This is similar to the finding of Masters *et al.* (1985), in that amyloid protein from senile plaque cores which is resistant to SDS and urea can also be solubilised by formic acid. However, it is not clear if the entire PHFs are dissolved since an amorphous residue was left and it is not known if there is variability from brain to brain (Yen and Kress, 1983). The possibility that non-disulphide covalent cross-linking of PHF constituents has a role in tangle formation and maturation as was suggested by Selkoe *et al.* (1982a,b) remains, although a more thorough assessment of the solubility properties of PHFs in solvents such as formic acid is required.

One possible cross-link which might be introduced into PHFs is an isodipeptide bond between lysine and glutamine side chains catalysed by calcium-dependent transglutaminase (Selkoe *et al.*, 1982b). We have found that all three neurofilament triplet proteins (apparent molecular weights 200,000, 160,000 and 70,000) are substrates *in vitro* for purified transglutaminase but that the insoluble PHFs are not a substrate (Anderton *et al.*, 1985; Miller and Anderton, 1985). This could be because all potential sites for transglutaminase in PHFs are already participating in cross-links. Preliminary immunocytochemical studies have indicated that transglutaminase may be a component of tangle-bearing neurones (unpublished observation).

4.3 Ultrastructure of Isolated PHFs, Neurofilaments and Microtubules

Microtubules and neurofilaments are the predominant polymeric components of the neuronal cytoskeleton. Although actin is present in neurones, microfilaments are rare and the actin is probably present as monomers and short filaments close to the plasma membrane (Anderton, 1982). Immunocytochemical studies have implicated neurofilaments and microtubules, but not (so far) microfilaments, in tangle composition (*see* Section 4.4). Ultrastructural studies have, as a result, concentrated on comparing PHFs with neurofilaments and microtubules.

Wisniewski and Wen (1985) and Wischik *et al.* (1985) have pointed out that PHFs do not resemble ultrastructurally neurofilaments or microtubules and have a different substructure (Fig. 4.1). Wischik *et al.* (1985) have shown that the structural subunit of PHFs does not seem to be fibrous, which would make them quite different from neurofilaments. Neurofilaments, along with all intermediate filaments, contain alpha-helical protein sequences which form the filament backbone (Geisler *et al.*, 1983). Isolated neurofilaments are often seen to fray at the ends like a piece of frayed rope, whereas the PHFs are blunt-ended. However, the alpha-helical domain of all the intermediate filament proteins so far examined, including neurofilaments, has a total mass of only about 40,000d, with the rest of the flanking polypeptide domains being non-helical and possibly external to the filament core.

4.4 Antibody Staining of Neurofibrillary Tangles and PHFs

Immunocytochemical studies on tangles *in situ* have indicated that they may contain microtubule (but not, so far, tubulin) antigens (Grundke-Iqbal *et al.*, 1979; Yen *et al.*, 1981; Kosik *et al.*, 1984; Perry *et al.*, 1985) and neurofilament antigens (Gambetti *et al.*, 1980; 1983; Ihara *et al.*, 1981; Anderton *et al.*, 1982, 1985; Autilio-Gambetti *et al.*, 1983; Elovaara *et al.*, 1983; Forno *et al.*, 1983; Rasool and Selkoe, 1984; Rasool *et al.*, 1984; Perry *et al.*, 1985). However, not all neurofilament and microtubule antibodies stain tangles, and this demonstrates that the neurofilaments and microtubule-associated proteins which contribute to the tangle inside affected neurones are structurally aberrant (Gambetti *et al.*, 1980; Kahn *et al.*, 1980; Yen *et al.*, 1981; Probst *et al.*, 1983; Kosik *et al.*, 1984; Perry *et al.*, 1985). Furthermore, several of the tangle-reactive neuro-

38

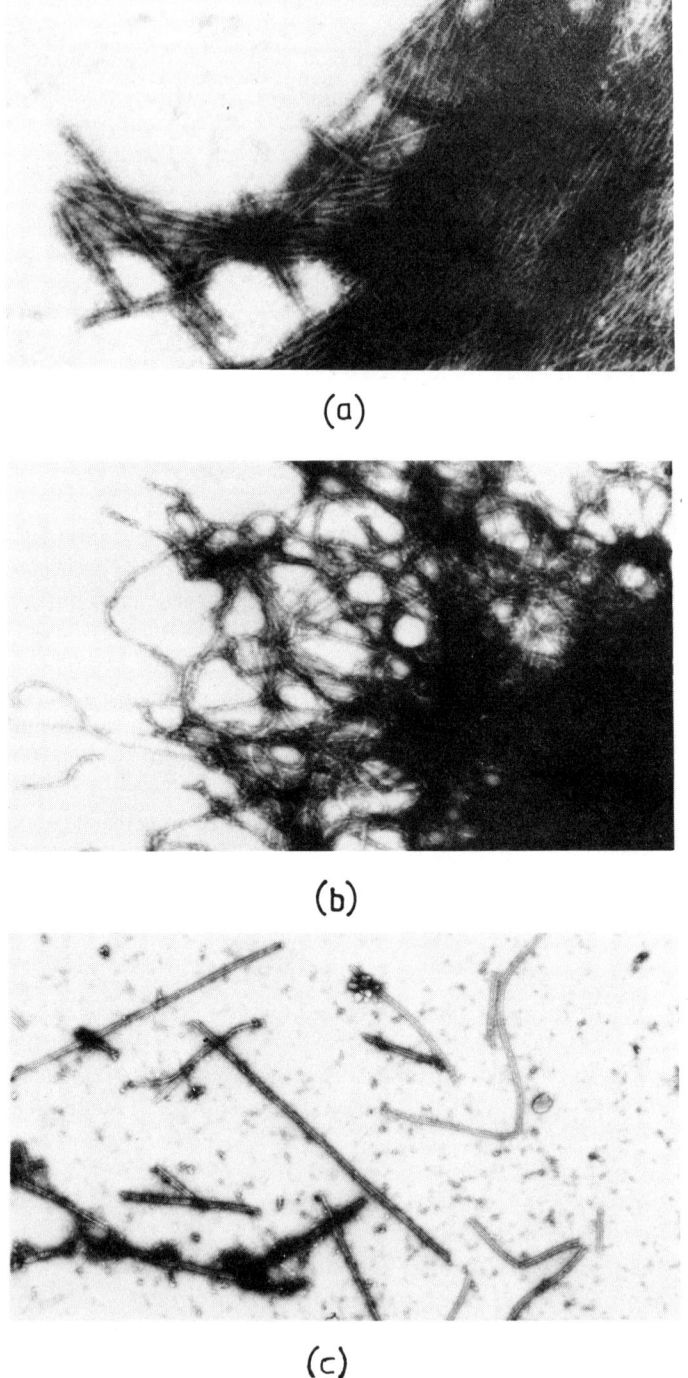

(a)

(b)

(c)

Fig. 4.1 Electron micrographs of negatively stained, isolated (a) PHFs, (b) bovine neurofilaments, and (c) bovine microtubules.

filament antibodies are directed against the largest or heavy neurofilament polypeptide (NF-H), and this protein has been shown to be absent from the perikaryon of pyramidal cells of the hippocampus and may be present only in axonal neurofilaments (Shaw et al., 1981). Certainly, pyramidal cell perikarya which do not contain a tangle only stain very weakly with neurofilament antibodies, and so there is an abnormal accumulation of these neurofilament epitopes within the cell bodies of affected neurones.

Another type of tangle-reactive antibody has been produced by immunising with the SDS-insoluble fraction which is enriched in PHFs. Both monoclonal and polyclonal antibodies, called anti-PHFs, have been prepared (Ihara et al., 1983; Grundke-Iqbal et al., 1984; Wang et al., 1984; Brion et al., 1985). These antibodies do not stain normal neurones and they have not been found to react with any cytoskeletal proteins nor consistently with any other brain components. One anti-PHF serum has been reported to label the polypeptides extracted from PHFs by prolonged SDS-treatment (Grundke-Iqbal et al., 1984). When Alzheimer brain is gently disrupted and treated with SDS, a fraction enriched in apparently morphologically intact tangles as well as probable tangle fragments can be isolated. These SDS-insoluble tangles are stained strongly by the anti-PHF antibodies but some of the tangle-reactive neurofilament and microtubule-associated antibodies fail to stain these structures (Kosik et al., 1984; Rasool et al., 1984; Rasool and Selkoe, 1984). However, other such antibodies do still stain the isolated tangles (Table 4.1 and Fig. 4.2) (Anderton et al., 1985; Perry et al., 1985). This finding has led to the assumption that the cytoskeleton does not contribute to the PHFs but that it has become trapped within or stuck to the aggregated PHFs. Even if this were the case, the staining of tangles in situ by only some, but consistently the same, neurofilament and microtubule antibodies independent of the Alzheimer case, is still significant and implies a disturbance of the cytoskeleton. We have therefore attempted to identify ultrastructurally the distribution of the epitopes within tangles and PHFs which are recognised by our tangle-reactive neurofilament monoclonal antibodies. However, pertinent to this question are immunoytochemical results on Pick bodies. Pick bodies which contain predominantly straight filaments have also been studied with neurofilament and anti-PHF antibodies. We found that the same neurofilament antibodies which stain Alzheimer tangles in situ also stain Pick bodies (Fig. 4.3), and neurofilament antibodies which fail to stain tangles do not stain Pick bodies (Table 4.1) (Probst et al., 1983). Rasool and Selkoe (1985) have confirmed these findings and have also shown that anti-PHF antibodies stain Pick bodies. These results imply that the selective retention of neurofilament epitopes and the presence of PHF epitopes are not simply determined by the morphology of PHFs but are related to some other properties common to the PHFs of Alzheimer tangles and the straight filaments of Pick bodies.

Monoclonal antibodies RT97, BF10 and 8D8 have been used to label tangles in situ by the indirect immunogold method, and observations made by electron microscopy (Table 4.1 and Fig. 4.4). The results show that it is the PHFs per se

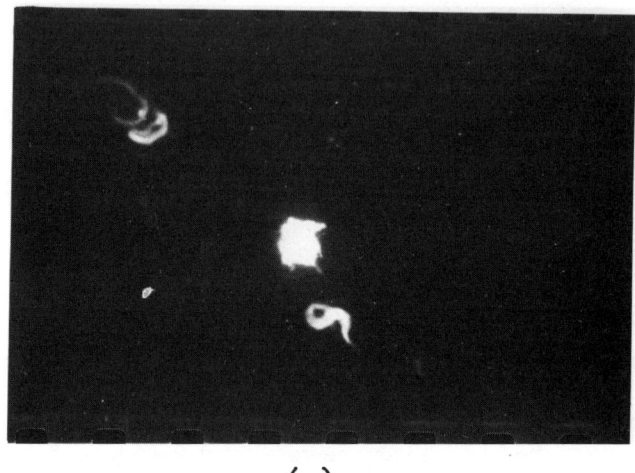

(a)

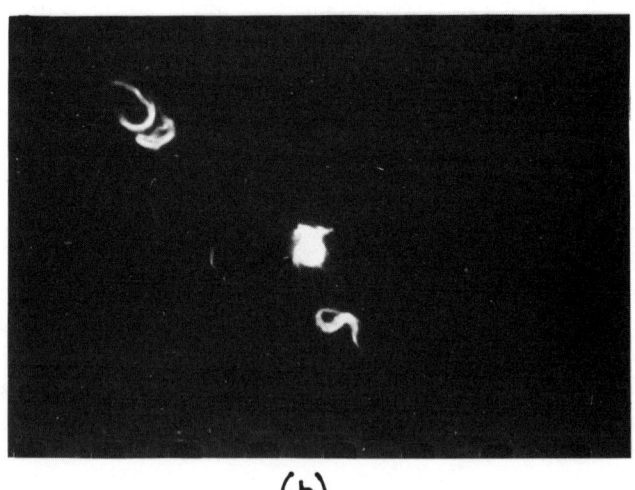

(b)

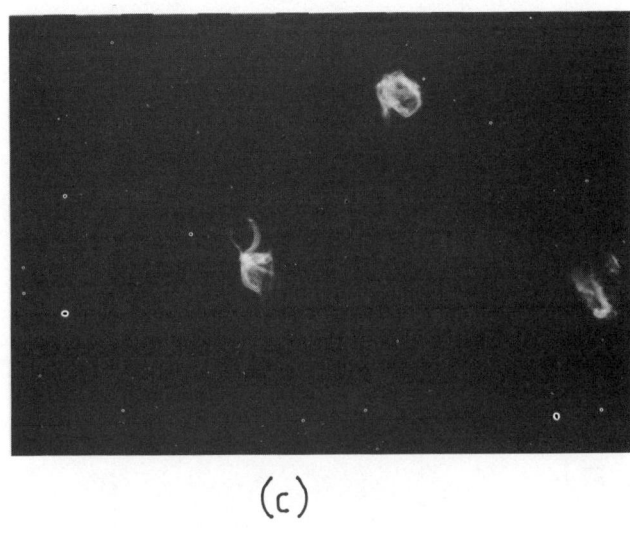

(c)

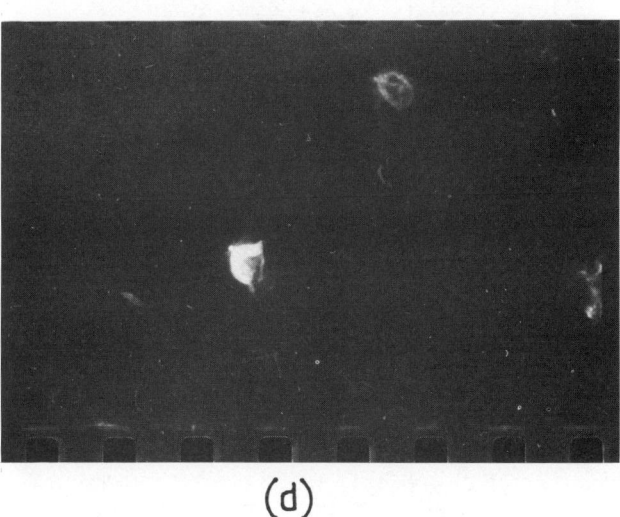

(d)

Fig. 4.2 Double immunofluorescence microscopy of SDS-insoluble isolated neurofibrillary tangles stained with (a, c) anti-PHF, (b) 8D8, (d) RT97. In (a) and (c) the second antibody was FITC-conjugated goat anti-rabbit Ig, and in (b) and (d) the second antibody was Texas Red goat anti-mouse Ig.

Table 4.1 Antibody staining of Alzheimer tangles, Pick bodies and isolated PHFs by neurofilament antibodies

Antibody	Principal neurofilament antigen	Light microscope				Electron microscope	
		Staining of neurofilaments	Staining of Pick bodies in situ	Staining of Alzheimer tangles in situ	Staining of SDS-isolated tangles	Labelling of PHFs in situ	Labelling of isolated PHFs
Monoclonals							
8D8	NF-H	+	+	+	>90 %	+	>90 %
RT97	NF-H	+	+	+	20–50 %	+	20–50 %
1215	NF-H	+	ND	+	20–50 %	ND	20–50 %
BF10	NF-M	+	+	+	1 %	+	ND
147	NF-H	+	–	–	0 %	–	0 %
Polyclonals							
anti-NF-H	NF-H	+	–	–	ND	ND	ND
anti-NF-M	NF-M	+	–	–	ND	ND	ND

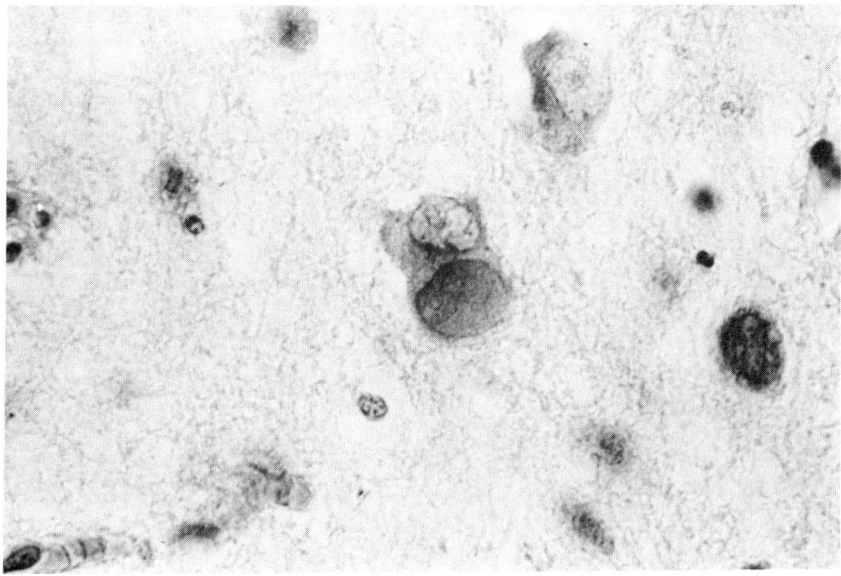

Fig. 4.3 A Pick body stained by RT97. Peroxidase was the detection method using the ABC staining protocol.

and not simply admixed neurofilaments which were labelled by these antibodies. This result confirms an earlier study with RT97 using immunoperoxidase to localise the binding site for RT97 (Kahn *et al.*, 1984). SDS-insoluble, isolated PHFs have also been investigated by immunogold and negative staining in the electron microscope. Monoclonal antibody 8D8 labelled more than 90 % of the PHFs and in double-labelling experiments with an anti-PHF serum, there was competition between the antibodies. This competition demonstrates that both antibodies recognise (Fig. 4.5) the same structures. The intensities of immuno-fluorescence on the isolated tangles and the densities of gold particles on isolated PHFs in the electron microscope for 8D8 and the anti-PHF antibodies were comparable, thus suggesting that the 8D8 epitope is not a minor contaminant. Monoclonal antibodies RT97 and 1215 labelled only a proportion of the PHFs and this often had a patchy distribution (Fig. 4.5). Furthermore, the proportion labelled varied from brain to brain. Antibody BF10 labelled hardly any isolated PHFs. These results are similar to those of Perry *et al.* (1985), who also showed by electron microscopy that certain neurofilament antibodies labelled PHFs and not contaminating straight filaments.

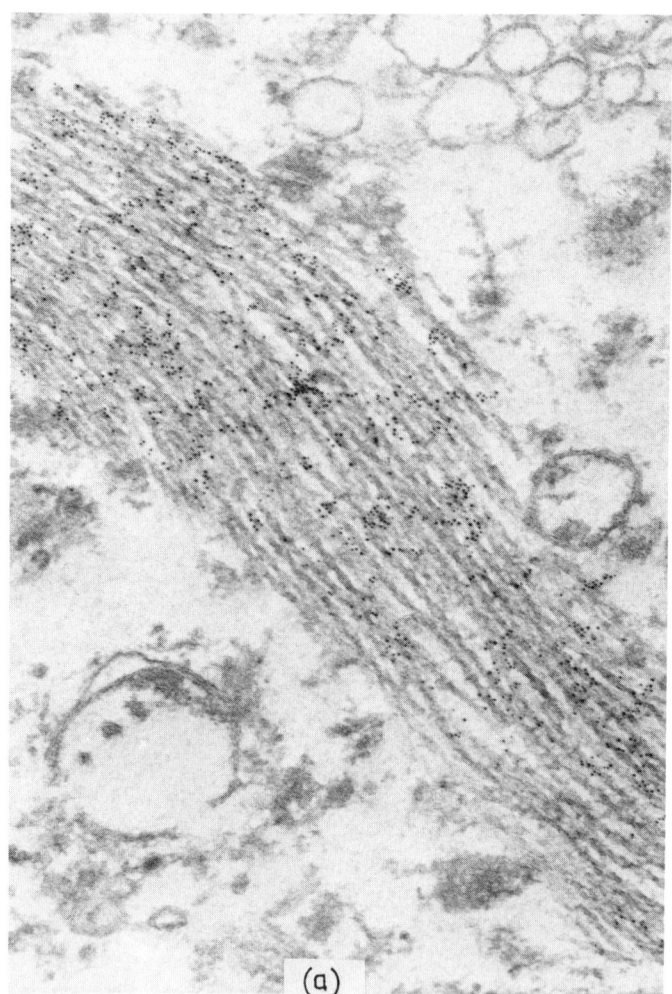

(a)

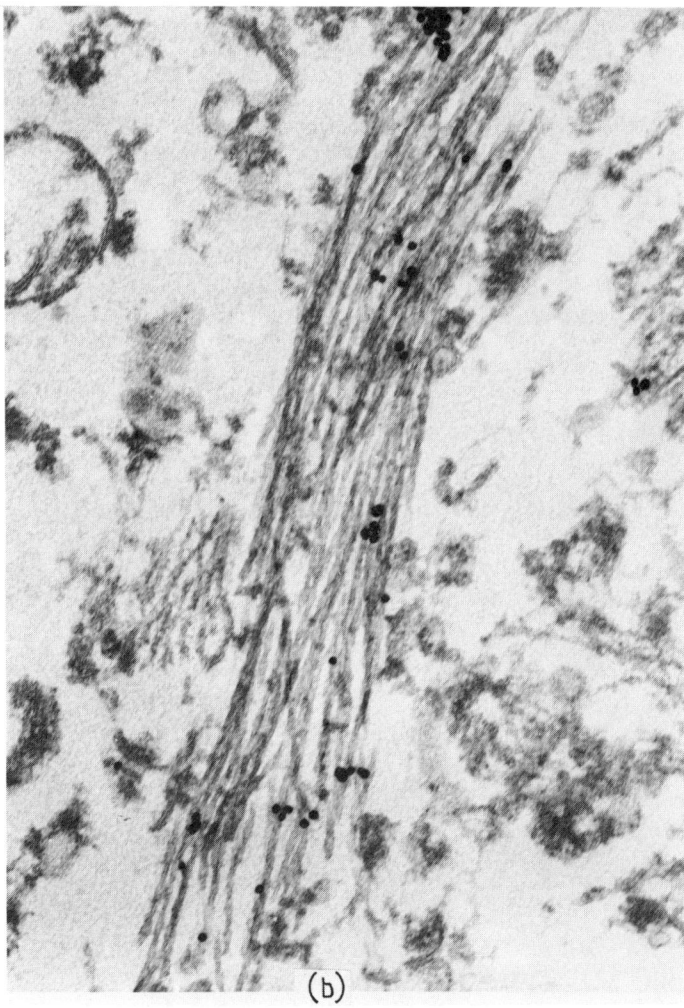

Fig. 4.4 Immunogold labelling of neurofibrillary tangles *in situ* with: (a) anti-PHF; (b) RT97; (c) 8D8; and (d) BF10. 5 nm gold particles conjugated to goat anti-rabbit Ig were used in (a), and 15 nm particles conjugated to goat anti-mouse Ig were used for (b–d). All antibodies labelled PHFs and did not label admixed straight filaments. Labelling by the monoclonal antibodies was less dense than with anti-PHF because of a loss of epitopes due to the specimen processing before application of primary antibodies.

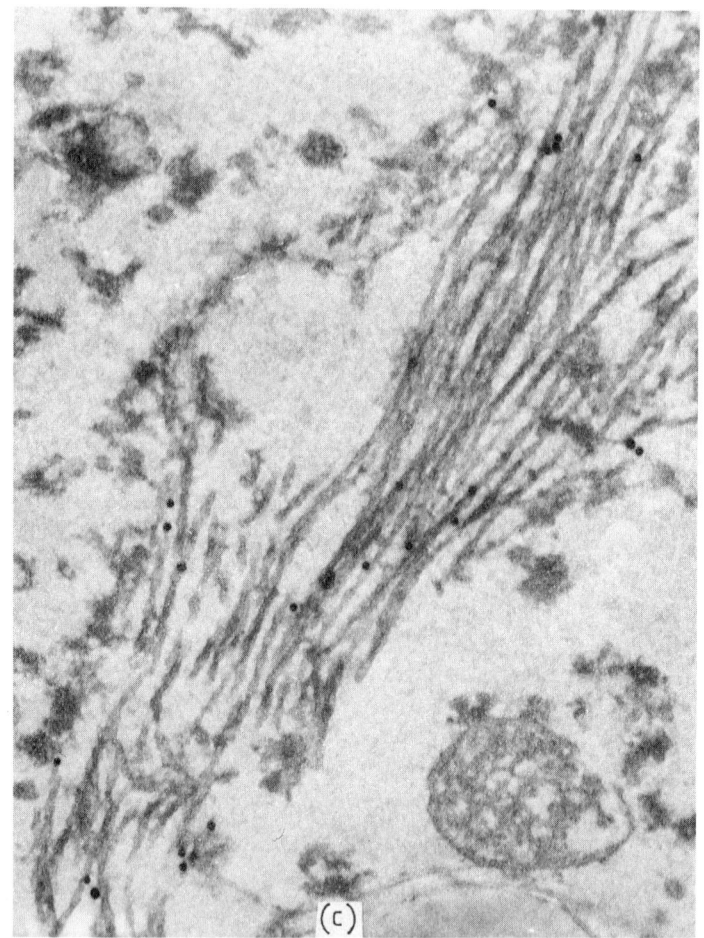

(c)

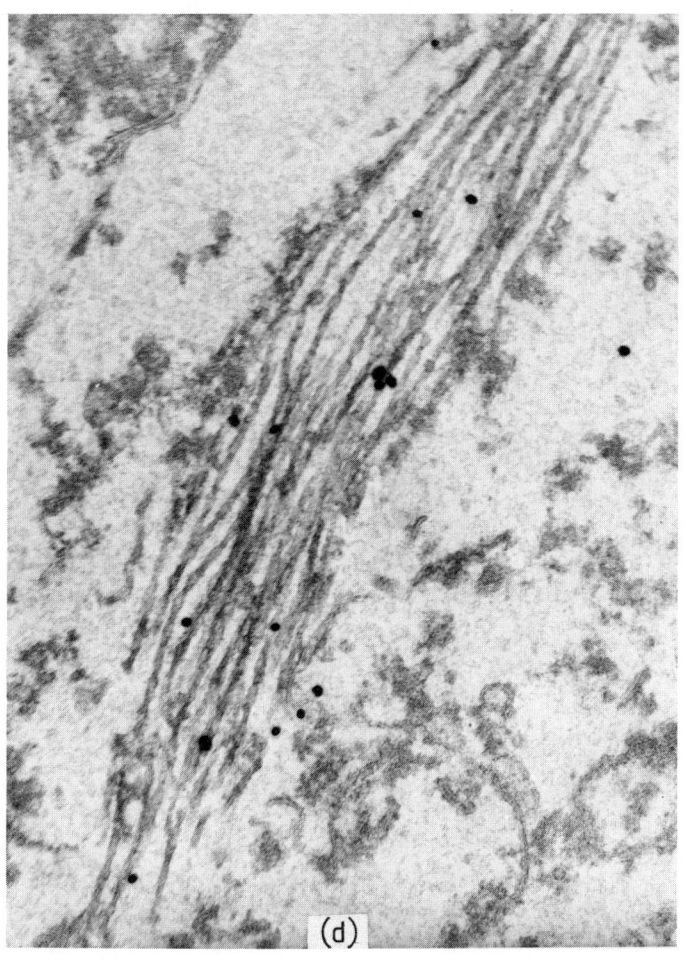

Fig. 4.4 (cont'd.).

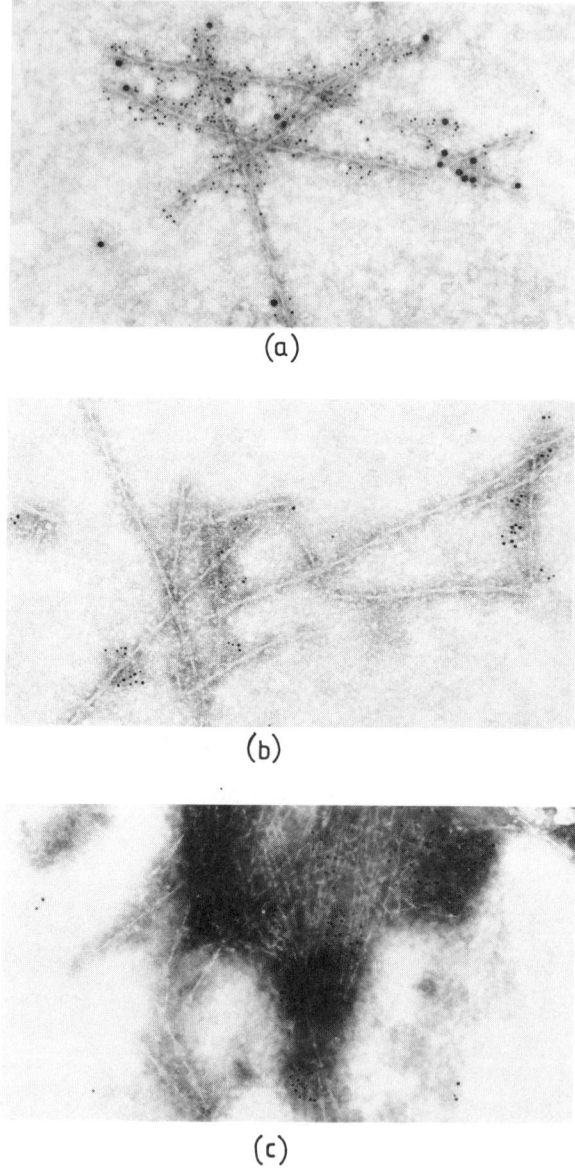

Fig. 4.5 Immunogold labelling of isolated PHFs with: (a) anti-PHF and 8D8 (double staining); (b) RT97; and (c) 1215. Anti-PHF was localised with 15 nm gold particles conjugated to goat anti-rabbit Ig, and 8D8, RT97 and 1215 with 5 nm gold particles conjugated to antibody. Note the patchy labelling with RT97 and 1215 compared with the more uniform labelling with 8D8.

4.5 Conclusions

Paired helical filaments are clearly not simply a collapsed form of the neuronal cytoskeleton. Their ultrastructure, physico-chemical properties and antigenic properties argue against this possibility. However, there is a general accord that tangles *in situ* are labelled by selected neurofilament and microtubule-associated antibodies. There are also now independent findings that some of these epitopes are retained in the insoluble residue. We propose that the cytoskeleton is disrupted, possibly by a raised level of intracellular calcium ions which could cause microtubules to be depolymerised and proteolytic degradation of neurofilaments. Some neurofilament fragments could then be stably incorporated into the PHFs (e.g. 8D8 epitope) and others could loosely be associated with PHFs (e.g. BF10 epitope), such that on isolation some are lost and others retained. This does not exclude additional PHF constituents such as a derepressed gene product or an extraneous infectious agent, either of which might be the anti-PHF antigens. However, the epitopes recognised by anti-PHF antibodies might equally be novel, arising as a result of gross modification of cytoskeletal components. After all, the SDS-insoluble residue has apparently been stripped of some neurofilament epitopes (e.g. BF10, *see* Table 4.1), and so might represent the most extensively modified component of the tangle. Chemical changes to neurofilaments, such as proteolysis, could also result in a loss of the helical domains, and the PHFs would therefore contain the non-helical tail pieces in a new conformation. It is now important to devise methods for solubilising or fragmenting PHFs so that peptides can be sequenced, since this will be the way to identify the extent of homologies between PHFs and other proteins.

Acknowledgement

This work was supported by the Medical Research Council and The Wellcome Trust.

References

Anderton, B. H. (1981). Intermediate filaments: a family of homologous structures. *J. Muscle Res. Cell Motil.*, 2, 141–66.

Anderton, B. H. (1982). The neuronal cytoskeleton: proteins and pathology. In Smith, W. T., and Cavanagh, J. B. (eds.), *Recent Advances in Neuropathology, Vol. 2*. Livingstone, Edinburgh, pp. 29–51.

Anderton, B. H., Haugh, M. C., Kahn, J., Miller, C., Probst, A., and Ulrich, J. (1985). The nature of neurofibrillary tangles. In Traber, J., and Gispen, H. (eds.), *Senile Dementia of Alzheimer Type, Advances in Applied Neurological Sciences, Vol. 2*. Springer-Verlag, Berlin Heidelberg, pp. 205–16.

Anderton, B. H., Breinburg, D., Downes, M. J., Green, P. J., Tomlinson, B. E., Ulrich, J., Wood, J. N., Kahn, J. (1982). Monoclonal antibodies show that neurofibrillary tangles and neurofilaments share antigenic determinants. *Nature*, 298, 84–6.

Autilio-Gambetti, L., Gambetti, P., Crane, R. C. (1983). Paired helical filaments: related-ness to neurofilaments shown by silver staining and reactivity with monoclonal anti-bodies. *Banbury Reports 15: Biochemical Aspects of Alzheimer's Disease.* Cold Spring Harbor Laboratory, Cold Spring Harbour, pp. 117–24.

Brion, S., Mikol, J., and Osimaras, A. (1983). Recent findings in Pick's disease. In Zimmermann, H. M. (ed.) *Progress in Neuropathology, Vol. 2.* Grune and Stratton, New York, pp. 421–52.

Brion, J. P., Couck, A. M., Passareiro, E., and Flament-Durand, J. (1985). Neurofibrillary tangles of Alzheimer's disease: an immunohistochemical study. *J. Submicrosc. Cytol.,* 17, 89–96.

Elovaara, I., Paetau, A., Lehto, V.-P., Dahl, D., Virtanen, I., and Palo, J. (1983). Immuno-cytochemical studies of Alzheimer neuronal perikarya with intermediate filament anti-sera. *J. Neurol. Sci.,* 62, 315–26.

Forno, L. S., Strefling, A. M., Sternberger, L. A., Sternberger, N. H., and Eng, L. F. (1983). Immunocytochemical staining of neurofibrillary tangles and of the periphery of Lewy bodies with a monoclonal antibody to neurofilaments. *J. Neuropathol. Exp. Neurol.,* 42, 342.

Gambetti, P., Autilio-Gambetti, L., Perry, G., Shecket, G., and Crane, R. C. (1983). Anti-bodies to neurofibrillary tangles of Alzheimer's disease raised from human and animal neurofilament fractions. *Lab. Invest.,* 49, 430–5.

Gambetti, P., Velasco, M. E., Dahl, D., Bignami, A., Roessmann, U., and Sindely, S. P. (1980). Alzheimer neurofilament tangles: an immunohistochemical study. In Amaducci, L., Davison, A. N., and Antuono, P. (eds.), *Aging of the Brain and Dementia (Aging, Vol. 13).* Raven, New York, 55–68.

Geisler, N., Kaufman, E., Fischer, S., Plessman, U., and Weber, K. (1983). Neurofilament archi-tecture combines structural principles of intermediate filaments with carboxy-terminal extensions increasing in size between triplet proteins. *EMBO J.,* 2, 1295–302.

Gonatas, N. K., Anderson, W., and Evangelista, I. (1967). The contribution of altered synapses in the senile plaque: an electron microscope study in Alzheimer's dementia. *J. Neuropathol. Exp. Neurol.,* 26, 25–39.

Grundke-Iqbal, K., Iqbal, K., Tung, Y.-C., and Wisniewski, H. M. (1984). Alzheimer paired helical filaments: immunochemical identification of polypeptides. *Acta Neuropathol.,* 62, 259–67.

Grundke-Iqbal, K., Johnson, A. B., Wisniewski, H. M., Terry, R. D., and Iqbal, K. (1979). Evidence that Alzheimer neurofibrillary tangles originate from neurotubules. *Lancet,* I, 578–80.

Hirano, A., Dembitzeer, H. M., Kurland, L. T., and Zimmermann, H. M. (1968). The fine structure intraganglionic alterations. Neurofibrillary tangles, granulovacuolar bodies and 'rod-like' structures as seen in Guam amyotrophic lateral sclerosis and Parkinsonism-dementia complex. *J. Neuropathol. Exp. Neurol.,* 27, 167–82.

Ihara, Y., Abraham, C., and Selkoe, D. J. (1983). Antibodies to paired helical filaments in Alzheimer's disease do not recognise normal brain proteins. *Nature,* 304, 727–30.

Ihara, Y., Nukina, N., Sugita, H., and Toyokura, Y. (1981). Staining of Alzheimer's neuro-fibrillary tangles with antiserum against 200K components of neurofilament. *Proc. Jap. Acad.,* 57B, 152–6.

Iqbal, K., Zaidi, T., Thompson, C. H., Merz, P. A., and Wisniewski, H. M. (1984). Alzheimer paired helical filaments: bulk isolation, solubility, and protein composition. *Acta Neuro-pathol.,* 62, 167–77.

Kahn, J., Green, P. G., Thorp, R., and Anderton, B. H. (1980). Immunohistochemistry of neurofilaments in Alzheimer's disease. *J. Clin. Exp. Gerontol.,* 2, 199–210.

Kahn, J., King, T., Anderton, B. H., Oyanagi, S., Haga, S., and Ishii, T. (1984). Immuno-electron microscopy of rat neurofilaments and Alzheimer type neurofibrillary tangles. *Neuropathol. Appl. Neurobiol.,* 10, 306.

Kidd, M. (1963). Paired helical filaments in electron microscopy of Alzheimer's disease. *Nature,* 197, 192–3.

Kidd, M. (1964). Alzheimer's disease – an electron microscopical study. *Brain,* 87, 307–20.

Kosik, K. S., Duffy, L. K., Dowling, M. M., Abraham, C., McCluskey, A., and Selkoe, D. J. (1984). Microtubule-associated protein 2: monoclonal antibodies demonstrate the selective incorporation of certain epitopes into Alzheimer neurofibrillary tangles. *Proc. Natl Acad. Sci. USA*, **81**, 7941–5.

Lazarides, E. (1980). Intermediate filaments as mechanical integrators of cellular space. *Nature*, **283**, 249–56.

Lazarides, E. (1982). Intermediate filaments: a chemically heterogeneous, developmentally regulated class of proteins. *Annu. Rev. Biochem.*, **51**, 219–50.

Masters, C. L., Sims, G., Weinman, N. A., Bayreuther, K., Multhaup, G., and McDonald, B. L. (1985). Amyloid plaque core protein in Alzheimer's disease and Down's syndrome. *Proc. Natl Acad. Sci. USA*, **82**, 4245–9.

Miller, C. C. J., and Anderton, B. H. (1985). Neurofilaments and Alzheimer neurofibrillary tangles as substrates for transglutaminase. *Biochem. Soc. Trans.* (in press).

Okamoto, K., Hirano, A., Yamaguchi, H., and Hirai, S. (1982). The fine structure of eosinophilic stages of Alzheimer's neurofibrillary tangles. *Clin. Neurol. (Tokyo)*, **22**, 840–6.

Perry, G., Rizzuto, N., Autilio-Gambetti, L., and Gambetti, P. (1985). Paired helical filaments from Alzheimer disease patients contain cytoskeletal components. *Proc. Natl Acad. Sci. USA*, **82**, 3916–20.

Probst, A., Anderton, B. H., Ulrich, J., Kohler, R., Kahn, J., and Heitz, P. U. (1983). Pick's disease: an immunocytochemical study of neuronal changes. Monoclonal antibodies show that Pick bodies share antigenic determinants with neurofibrillary tangles and neurofilaments. *Acta Neuropathol.*, **60**, 175–82.

Rasool, C. G., and Selkoe, D. J. (1984). Alzheimer's disease: exposure of neurofilament immunoreactivity in SDS-insoluble paired helical filaments. *Brain Res.*, **322**, 194–8.

Rasool, C. G., and Selkoe, D. J. (1985). Sharing of specific antigens by degenerating neurons in Pick's disease and Alzheimer's disease. *New Eng. J. Med.*, **312**, 700–5.

Rasool, C. G., Abraham, C., Anderton, B. H., Haugh, M., Kahn, J., and Selkoe, D. J. (1984). Alzheimer's disease: immunoreactivity of neurofibrillary tangles with anti-neurofilament and anti-paired helical filament antibodies. *Brain Res.*, **310**, 249–60.

Rewcastle, N. B., Ball, C. B., and Ball, M. J. (1968). Electron microscopic structure of the 'inclusion bodies' in Pick's disease. *Neurology*, **18**, 1205–13.

Selkoe, D. J., Abraham, C., and Ihara, Y. (1982b). Brain transglutaminase: *in vitro* cross-linking of human neurofilament proteins into insoluble polymers. *Proc. Natl Acad. Sci. USA*, **79**, 6070–4.

Selkoe, D. J., Ihara, Y., and Salazar, F. J. (1982a). Alzheimer's disease: insolubility of partially purified paired helical filaments in sodium dodecyl sulphate and urea. *Science*, **215**, 1243–5.

Shaw, G., Osborn, M., and Weber, K. (1981). An immunofluorescence microscopical study of the neurofilament triplet proteins, vimentin and glial fibrillary acidic protein within the adult rat brain. *Eur. J. Cell Biol.*, **26**, 68–82.

Terry, R. D., Gonatas, N. F., and Weiss, M. (1964). Ultrastructural studies in Alzheimer's presenile dementia. *Am. J. Pathol.*, **44**, 269–97.

Towfighi, J. (1972). Early Pick's disease. *Acta Neuropathol.*, **21**, 224–31.

Wang, G. P., Grundke-Iqbal, I., Kascsak, R. J., Iqbal, K., and Wisniewski, H. M. (1984). Alzheimer neurofibrillary tangles: monoclonal antibodies to inherent antigen(s). *Acta Neuropathol.*, **62**, 268–75.

Wilcock, G. K., Esiri, M. M., Bowen, D. M., and Smith, C. C. T. (1982). Alzheimer disease. Correlation of cortical choline acetyltransferase activity with severity of dementia and histological abnormalities. *J. Neurol. Sci.*, **57**, 407–17.

Wischik, C. M., Crowther, R. A., Stewart, M., and Roth, M. (1985). Subunit structure of paired helical filaments in Alzheimer's disease. *J. Cell Biol.*, **100**, 1905–12.

Wisniewski, H. M., and Wen, G. Y. (1985). Substructure of paired helical filaments from Alzheimer's disease neurofibrillary tangles. *Acta Neuropath. (Berl.)*, **66**, 173–6.

Wisniewski, H. M., Coblentz, J., and Terry, R. D. (1972). Pick's disease. A clinical and ultrastructural study. *Arch. Neurol.*, **26**, 97–108.

Wisniewski, H. M., Narang, H. K., and Terry, R. D. (1976). Neurofibrillary tangles of paired helical filaments. *J. Neurol. Sci.*, **27**, 173–81.

Wisniewski, K., Jervis, G. A., Moretz, R. C., and Wisniewski, H. M. (1979). Alzheimer neurofibrillary tangles in diseases other than senile dementia and presenile dementia. *Ann. Neurol.*, **5**, 288–94.

Yagishita, S., Itoh, Y., Nan, W., and Amano, N. (1981). Reappraisal of the fine structure of Alzheimer's neurofibrillary tangles. *Acta Neuropathol.*, **54**, 239-46.

Yen, S.-H., Gaskin, F., and Terry, R. D. (1981). Immunocytochemical studies of neuro-fibrillary tangles. *Am. J. Pathol.*, **104**, 77-89.

Yen, S.-H., and Kress, Y. (1983). The effect of chemical reagents or proteases on the ultra-structure of paired helical filaments. In (Katzman, R. (ed.), *Banbury Reports 15*, Cold Spring Harbor Laboratory, pp. 155-65.

5

Neurochemical and Behavioural Effects Following Lesions of the Nucleus Basalis in the Rat

G. Pepeu, F. Casamenti, F. Pedata, F. Orzi, G. Diana and E. Palumbo

5.1 Introduction

Immunohistochemical and histochemical evidence demonstrates that the nucleus basalis of Meynert (Nb) is the major source of cholinergic innervation to the frontal and parietal cortex in all mammalian species so far investigated (Pepeu *et al.*, 1985a). The Nb is part of a complex system of magnocellular neuclei of the basal forebrain characterised by intense staining for cholineacetyltransferase (ChAT) and acetylcholinesterase (AChE) (Bigl *et al.*, 1982). The various cholinergic neurons of the basal forebrain form a continuum along the ventral portion of the telencephalon and are not always aggregated into discrete nuclei: in some instances they are admixed with ChAT negative cells. The rostral components of this system consist of the medial septal nucleus, nuclei of the diagonal band of Broca and magnocellular preoptic nucleus. These nuclei have been designated Ch1 and Ch2 by Mesulam *et al.* (1983) in an attempt to provide a simpler classification. Ch3 includes the cholinergic neurons of the horizontal limb of the diagonal band of Broca. Ch4 is the larger and more loosely aggregated of these nuclei, including the nucleus basalis of Meynert, which partly overlaps the so called area innominata (Lamour *et al.*, 1982a), the nucleus of the ansa peduncolaris, and the nucleus of the ansa lenticularis. The most constant feature of the Ch4 neurons is their closeness to the medioventral portion of the globus pallidus. The vast majority of the cholinergic neurons of this region appear to innervate relatively discrete areas of the cortex, and an essential rostracaudal topography has been observed for these projections (Bigl *et al.*, 1982). Basal forebrain neurons projecting to the frontal cortex were found primarily in Nb (Woolf *et al.*, 1983).

Functional evidence also demonstrates that the Nb projects to the neocortical mantle. Electrical stimulation of the Nb increases acetylcholine (ACh) release from the cerebral cortex (Pepeu, 1983). The local injection of a GABA agonist in the Nb decreases ACh turnover in the frontal and parietal cortices (Wood and Richard, 1982) and depresses high affinity choline uptake (HACU) in the frontal cortex (Wenk, 1984).

A loss of cholinergic neurons of the basal forebrain nuclei including the Nb, is the most consistent neurochemical change detected in Alzheimer's disease (Price *et al.*, 1985). The degeneration and death of these neurons is the cause of the decrease in cortical ChAT (Terry and Davies, 1980) and presynaptic cholinergic disfunction (Sims *et al.*, 1983). A relationship has been demonstrated between the decrease in ChAT activity and the severity of cognitive function impairment (Sims *et al.*, 1980).

The alteration of the cortical and hippocampal cholinergic system appears therefore to be an important pathogenetic cause of cognitive deficits associated with senile dementia of Alzheimer's type, since the role of brain cholinergic mechanisms in memory and cognition is widely supported (Bartus *et al.*, 1982).

The attempts to correct the cholinergic deficits by pharmacological treatment with directly or indirectly acting cholinomimetics have been rather disappointing (Bartus *et al.*, 1982). The search for new agents effective in senile dementia needs appropriate animal models for screening new molecules. These reasons have prompted many investigators in recent years to reproduce in the rat lesions of the Nb of the type found in senile dementia of Alzheimer's type.

5.2 Lesions of the Nucleus Basalis

Initially, unilateral electrolytic lesions were placed in the Nb of the rat in the ventromedial region of the globus pallidus, with the purpose of detecting and investigating the origin of the cholinergic fibres ascending to the cortex (Kelly and Moore, 1978; Johnston *et al.*, 1979; Lehmann *et al.*, 1980; Hartgraves *et al.*, 1982). Later, the behavioural and electrocortical changes brought about by the destruction of the cholinergic fibres were investigated with unilateral (Lo Conte *et al.*, 1982a,b; Casamenti *et al.*, 1985) or bilateral (Miyamoto *et al.*, 1985) electrolytic lesions of the basal forebrain. Since electrolytic lesions also destroy 'en passant' fibres as shown by small but statistically significant decreases in cortical serotonin and homovanillic acid levels (Pepeu *et al.*, 1985), neurotoxic lesions are more frequently used. Survival rates after bilateral neurotoxic lesions are also generally higher than following electrolytic lesions. Kainic acid was used by Johnston *et al.* (1979), Lehman *et al.* (1980) and Friedman *et al.* (1983). Ibotenic acid was used by Flicker *et al.* (1983), Wenk *et al.* (1984b), Hepler *et al.* (1985) and Murray and Fibiger (1985). We owe to Wenk *et al.* (1984b) the most detailed description of the bilateral lesion procedure using ibotenic acid, of the size and placement of the lesions resulting in a large destruction of cholinergic neurons and of the post-operative care which makes it possible to obtain a good survival rate. Unilateral electrolytic or neurotoxic lesion of the Nb in the rat are followed by a prompt recovery and no mortality. After bilateral lesions the rats need a few days of forced feeding since they neither eat or drink spontaneously (Salamone *et al.*, 1984).

5.3 Neurochemical Changes Induced by the Lesions

5.3.1 Changes of Presynaptic Cholinergic Markers

The decrease in cortical and hippocampal ChAT activity has been used generally as a measure of the destruction of the cholinergic neurons following the lesion of the Nb. Dependent on the size and placement of the lesions and on the cortical area investigated, the decrease may range from 58 % in the frontal cortex (Hartgraves *et al.*, 1982) to 17 % in the occipital cortex (Friedman *et al.*, 1983). No larger decreases have been so far reported. It should be mentioned that cholinergic interneurons have been demonstrated in rat cerebral cortex and that they account for approximately 30 % of the total cortical ChAT (Lewey *et al.*, 1984; McGeer *et al.*, 1984).

If the lesion is confined to the Nb ChAT activity in the hippocampus is not reduced. However, if the lesion is extended rostrally to include the diagonal band, a decrease in ChAT activity of the ventral hippocampus can be found (Wenk *et al.*, 1984b).

A slow but complete recovery in cortical ChAT activity within three months after a unilateral neurotoxic lesion has been demonstrated by Wenk and Olton (1984), and within 6 months after a unilateral electrolytic lesion by Pepeu *et al.* (1985). The recovery can be accelerated, particularly in the posterior cortical areas, by the administration of GM1 ganglioside for 22 days after the lesion (Casamenti *et al.*, 1985).

Lesions of the Nb also bring about a 40 % decrease in cortical high affinity choline uptake (HACU) (Johnston *et al.*, 1979; Pedata *et al.*, 1982; Wenk and Olton, 1984) 4-10 days following the lesion. However, Pedata *et al.* (1982) demonstrated that, after a unilateral electrolytic lesion, HACU undergoes a rapid recovery and returns almost to normal values within 20 days in both frontal and occipital areas. A similar recovery was observed by Wenk and Olton (1984) 4 weeks after an ibotenic acid lesion. The recovery occurred within 4 days if the rats are treated daily with GM1 ganglioside (Pedata *et al.*, 1984). The rate of HACU can be considered not only as a marker of the presence of cholinergic nerve endings but also as an indication of their activity. Wenk *et al.* (1984b) demonstrated that behaviour alters HACU in cortical and hippocampal nerve endings. The rapid recovery of HACU observed in the lesioned animals could therefore indicate an increase in activity of the cholinergic neurons spared by the lesion.

An indication of the degeneration of the cortical cholinergic fibres following lesions of the forebrain nuclei is also given by the decrease in acetylcholinesterase (AChE) activity in the cerebral cortex. Wenk *et al.* (1980), using histochemical and biochemical techniques, demonstrated an 80 % decrease in AChE activity seven days after unilateral electrolytic lesions in the frontal cortex of the rat; their lesions were particularly extensive. A decrease of approximately 40 % in AChE activity was found by Altman *et al.* (1985) 2 weeks after a unilateral ibotenic acid lesion of the Nb and of 21-26 % by Lehman *et al.* (1980) after either kainic acid or electrolytic lesions.

The most direct consequence of the destruction of cholinergic fibres ascending to the cerebral cortex is a decreased availability of neurotransmitter at the nerve endings. Twenty days after the lesion, the spontaneous ACh release from the cerebral cortex in freely moving rats shows a decrease ranging from 18 to 40 % according to the size and placement of the lesion (Lo Conte *et al.*, 1982a, 1982b). Furthermore, the increase in ACh release induced by scopolamine, amphetamine and cholecistokinin is strongly reduced (Pepeu *et al.*, 1986).

ACh levels also show a 30-40 % reduction one week after lesion (Johnston *et al.*, 1979; Pepeu *et al.*, 1985), followed by a partial recovery within the next two weeks. However, 20 days after the lesion ACh turnover still shows a 50 % decrease in both frontal and parietal areas (Pepeu *et al.*, 1985).

5.3.2 Changes of Postsynaptic Cholinergic Markers

Muscarinic receptors are located on both presynaptic cholinergic nerve endings and postynaptic membranes. The latter localisation is presumably the most extensive. Two weeks following bilateral neurotoxic lesions of the Nb, Altman *et al.* (1985) found no change in the total number of muscarinic binding sites. A similar finding was reported by McKinney and Coyle (1982) after determining the total number of binding sites 5 weeks post-lesion. On the other hand, this could merely be an apparent lack of change resulting from a increase in high affinity binding sites which follows an initial small but significant reduction in low affinity binding sites (McKinney and Coyle, 1982). The lesion of the Nb therefore induces complex adaptative changes in cortical ACh receptors. This is also demonstrated by a transient but large increase in the number of neurons excited by ACh observed by Lamour *et al.* (1982b) two weeks after lesion.

5.3.3 Changes in Other Neurotransmitter Systems

A small but statistically significant decrease in serotonin and homovanillic acid levels was found in the cerebral cortex of rats with a unilateral electrolytic lesion of the Nb (Pepeu *et al.*, 1985), indicating a damage to '*en passant*' serotoninergic and dopaminergic fibres. No significant changes in noradrenaline levels were detected, however (Casamenti *et al.*, 1985). On the other hand (according to Johnston *et al.* (1979)), unilateral neurotoxic lesions of the Nb did not modify the cortical levels of noradrenaline, serotonin and GABA, the uptake of noradrenaline and GABA, and the activity of glutamate decarboxylase, tyrosine hydroxylase and histidine decarboxylase. This indicates that monoaminergic and GABAergic fibres were not damaged by the lesion.

5.3.4 Metabolic Changes

Table 5.1 shows the changes in glucose utilisation induced in the cerebral hemisphere by a unilateral kainic acid lesion of the Nb. Glucose utilisation was measured according to the ^{14}C deoxyglucose method of Sokoloff *et al.* (1977). Four days after the lesion a statistically significant decrease in the rate of glucose metabolism was detected in the frontal, somatosensory and parietal cortical areas. In the auditory and visual cortices, hippocampus and caudate nucleus there was also a small and not statistically significant decrease. This widespread decrease in glucose utilisation may indicate that the effects of the lesion on the frontal and parietal cortex are associated with a still incomplete surgical recovery. Fourteen days after the lesion a statistically significant decrease in glucose utilisation was detected only in the frontal cortex.

Our results are strictly comparable with those obtained by London *et al.* (1984). The latter authors observed a complete disappearance of the asymmetry in glucose metabolic rate within 28–32 days after the lesion.

Table 5.1 Effect of unilateral kainic acid lesions of the nucleus basalis on regional cerebral metabolic rates for glucose expressed as μmol/100 g/min $\pm$ S.E.M.

Hemisphere Regions	Days after lesion					
	4			14		
	Contro-lateral	Kainate injected		Contro-lateral	Kainate injected	
Cortex:						
Frontal	86 ± 6	54 ± 10*	−38 %	88 ± 7	72 ± 8*	−18 %
Somato-sensory	91 ± 4	56 ± 14*	−38 %	84 ± 4	72 ± 10	−14 %
Parietal	92 ± 7	58 ± 10*	−37 %	84 ± 8	85 ± 3	+ 2 %
Auditory	117 ± 9	102 ± 17	−12 %	90 ± 19	93 ± 22	+ 3 %
Visual	104 ± 9	97 ± 7	− 7 %	76 ± 8	86 ± 5	+13 %
Hippocampus	71 ± 8	66 ± 18	− 8 %	53 ± 1	49 ± 4	− 8 %
Caudate n.	86 ± 8	69 ± 9	−20 %	85 ± 5	83 ± 6	− 2 %

Each value is the mean of 3–4 rats.
*Statistically significant difference: $P < 0.05$. ChAT activity measured in the frontal cortex by the method of Fonnum (1975) 4 days post-lesion showed a 37 ± 5 % decrease ipsilaterally to the lesion.

5.4 Electroencephalographic Changes

Differences exist between the electrocortical changes brought about by unilateral electrolytic lesions of neurotoxin lesions of the Nb. In the first case, two weeks after the lesion a decrease in total electrical activity recorded from the ipsilateral cerebral cortex was observed (Lo Conte et al., 1982a). The spectrum analysis shows that even though the reduction involved all frequencies, the high frequency bands are more affected.

Conversely (according to Steward et al. (1984)), in rats with kainic acid lesions the initial bilateral depression of the cortical electrical activity tended to disappear within two weeks and the electrocorticogram was characterised by large, irregular, slow activity reminiscent of the electrocortical pattern following atropine administration. This large, irregular, slow activity was abolished by pilocarpine. It appears, therefore, that while the depression of electrical activity results from unspecific damage to 'en passant' fibres or non-cholinergic nuclei, the reduction of fast activity results from the loss of the cholinergic input to the cerebral cortex.

There are no reports of electrocortical changes induced by bilateral lesions of the Nb.

5.5 Behavioural Effects of the Lesions of Nucleus Basalis

Once the rats have recovered from surgery and initial unspecific damage, the decrease of the cholinergic input to the cerebral cortex brought about by the electrolytic or neurotoxic lesion of the Nb is associated with no changes in spontaneous behaviour (Flicker et al., 1983; Altman et al., 1985).

Conversely, even unilateral lesions of the Nb, which only reduce ChAT activity by 30-40 % in the ipsilateral cortex, are followed by a marked impairment in the acquisition and retention of conditioned behaviours. The types of impairment so far reported are listed in Table 5.2. From their analysis it appears that there is no difference between the behavioural effects of electrolytic and neurotoxic lesions of the Nb. Furthermore, the disruption of passive avoidance acquisition brought about by bilateral lesions is more profound than that caused by a unilateral lesion (Pepeu et al., 1985). Similarly, only bilateral lesions placed in the Nb after training impair retention of an active avoidance response (Miyamoto et al., 1985). Finally, training the lesioned rats to more complex tasks reveals an impairment of spatial memory and an impairment of either trial-dependent working memory (Hepler et al., 1985) or long-term reference memory (Murray and Fibiger, 1985), according to the task performed.

A partial recovery of the behavioural impairment caused by lesions of the Nb was obtained by repeated administrations of physostigmine (Murray and Fibiger, 1985) or GM1 ganglioside (Casamenti et al., 1985). In the latter case, the behavioural improvement was associated with a partial recovery in cortical ChAT activity.

Table 5.2 Conditioned behaviours disrupted by lesions of the nucleus basalis

Type of lesion	Type of behaviour	Reference
Unilateral electrolytic	Active avoidance: acquisition, no effect on retention	Lo Conte *et al.* (1982a)
Bilateral, electrolytic	Active avoidance: acquisition and retention	Miyamoto *et al.* (1985)
Bilateral, ibotenic	Active avoidance: acquisition, no effect on extinction	Flicker *et al.* (1983)
Unilateral, electrolytic	Passive avoidance: acquisition	Lo Conte *et al.* (1982a)
Bilateral, electrolytic	Passive avoidance: acquisition and retention	Miyamoto *et al.* (1985)
Bilateral, ibotenic kainic	Passive avoidance: acquisition, and retention	Flicker *et al.* (1983) Friedman *et al.* (1983) Altman *et al.* (1985), Pepeu *et al.* (1985b) Miyamoto *et al.* (1985)
Bilateral, electrolytic	Discrimination of rewarded alternation (T maze)	Hepler *et al.* (1985)
Bilateral, ibotenic	Discrimination of rewarded alternation (T maze)	Salamone *et al.* (1984) Hepler *et al.* (1985)
Bilateral, ibotenic	Acquisition of spatial memory task (radial maze)	Murray and Fibiger (1985)

5.6 Conclusions

It is somewhat naive to consider the rat with a lesion of the Nb as a model of Alzheimer's disease. Even if the degeneration of the basal forebrain cholinergic system is the most consistent neurochemical observation, changes in mono-amine systems, decrease in somatostatin levels and morphological alterations, including neurofibrillary tangles and plaques, together with the severe impairment of memory and cognition (Price *et al.*, 1985), make Alzheimer's disease an extremely complex picture of which the Nb lesioned rats are a pale and partial image.

We believe, however, that the lesions of the Nb are important for three main reasons. First, they are a useful tool for investigating the anatomy of the cholinergic pathways ascending to the cortex. Second, the electrocortical and behavioural changes induced by the lesions make it possible to unravel the functional role of the cortical cholinergic system. Third, the demonstration that a partial recovery of the electrocortical and behavioural changes can be obtained by drug treatments makes the lesioned rats suitable for the screening of drugs potentially active in pathological conditions characterised by an impairment of the basal forebrain cholinergic system, of which Alzheimer's disease is the most important example.

References

Altman, H., Crosland, R. D., Jenden, D. J., and Berman, R. F. (1985). Further characterizations of the nature of the behavioural and neurochemical effects of lesions to the nucleus basalis of Meynert in the rat. *Neurobiol. Aging*, 6, 125–30.

Bartus, R. T., Dean, R. L., Beer, B., and Lippa, A. S. (1982). The cholinergic hypothesis of geriatric memory dysfunction. *Science*, 217, 408–17.

Bigl, V., Woolf, N. J., and Butcher, L. L. (1982). Cholinergic projections from the basal forebrain to frontal, parietal, temporal, occipital, and cingulate cortices: a combined fluorescent tracer and acetylcholinesterase analysis. *Brain Res. Bull.*, 8, 727–49.

Casamenti, F., Bracco, L., Bartolini, L., and Pepeu, G. (1985). Effects of ganglioside treatment in rats with a lesion of the cholinergic forebrain nuclei. *Brain Res.*, 338, 45–52.

Flicker, C., Dean, D. R., Watkins, D. L., Fisher, S. K., and Bartus, R. T. (1983). Behavioural and neurochemical effects following neurotoxic lesions of a major cholinergic input to the cerebral cortex in the rat. *Pharmacol. Biochem. Behav.*, 19, 309–12.

Fonnum, F. (1975). A rapid radiochemical method for the determination of choline acetyltransferase. *J. Neurochem.*, 24, 407–9.

Friedman, E., Lerer, B., and Kuster, J. (1983). Loss of cholinergic neurons in the rat neocortex produces deficits in passive avoidance learning. *Pharmacol. Biochem. Behav.*, 19, 309–12.

Hartgraves, S. L., Mensah, P. L., and Kelly, P. H. (1982). Regional decrease of cortical choline acetyltransferase after lesions of the septal area and in the area of nucleus basalis magnocellularis. *Neuroscience*, 7, 2369–76.

Hepler, D. J., Olton, D. S., Wenk, G. L., and Coyle, J. T. (1985). Lesions in the nucleus basalis magnocellularis and medial septal area of rats produce qualitatively similar memory impairments. *J. Neurosci.*, 5, 866–73.

Johnston, M. V., McKinney, M., and Coyle, J. T. (1979). Evidence for a cholinergic projection to neocortex from neurons in basal forebrain. *Proc. Natl Acad. Sci. USA*, 76, 5392–6.

Kelly, P. H., and Moore, K. E. (1978). Decrease of neocortical choline acetyltransferase after lesion of the globus pallidus in the rat. *Exp. Neurol.*, 61, 479–84.

Lamour, Y., Dutar, P., and Jobert, A. (1982a). Topographic organization of basal forebrain neurons projecting to the rat cerebral cortex. *Neurosci. Lett.*, 34, 117–22.

Lamour, Y., Dutar, P., and Jobert, A. (1982b). Spread of acetylcholine sensitivity in the neocortex following lesion of the nucleus basalis. *Brain Res.*, 252, 377–81.

Lehman, J., Nagy, J. I., Atmodja, S., and Fibiger, H. C. (1980). The nucleus basalis magnocellularis: the origin of a cholinergic projection to the neocortex of rat. *Neuroscience*, 5, 1161–74.

Lewey, A. I., Wainer, B. H., Rye, D. B., Mufson, E. J., and Mesulam, M. M. (1984). Choline acetyltransferase-immunoreactive neurons intrinsic to rodent cortex and distinction from acetylcholinesterase-positive neurons. *Neurosci.*, 13, 341–53.

Lo Conte, G., Bartolini, L., Casamenti, F., Marconcini Pepeu, I., and Pepeu, G. (1982a). Lesions of cholinergic forebrain nuclei: changes in avoidance behaviour and scopolamine actions. *Pharmac. Biochem. Behav.*, 17, 933–7.

Lo Conte, G., Casamenti, F., Bigl, V., Milaneschi, E., and Pepeu, G. (1982b). Effect of magnocellular forebrain lesions on acetylcholine output from the cerebral cortex, electrocorticogram and behaviour. *Arch. Ital. Biol.*, **120**, 176–88.

London, E. D., McKinney, M., Dam, M., Ellis, A., and Coyle, J. T. (1984). Decreased cortical glucose utilization after ibotenate lesion of the rat ventromedial globus pallidus. *J. Cer. Blood Flow Metab.*, **4**, 381–90.

McGeer, P. L., McGeer, E. G., and Peng, J. H. (1984). Choline acetyltransferase: purification and immunohistochemical localization. *Life Sci.*, **34**, 2319–38.

McKinney, M., and Coyle, J. T. (1982). Regulation of neocortical muscarinic receptors: effect of drug treatment and lesions. *J. Neurosci.*, **2**, 97–105.

Mesulam, M. M., Mufson, E. J., Wainer, B. H., and Lewey, A. I. (1983). Central cholinergic pathways in the rat: an overview based on an alternative nomenclature (Ch. 1–6). *Neuroscience*, **10**, 1185–201.

Miyamoto, M., Shintani, M., Nagaoka, A., and Nagawa, Y. (1985). Lesioning of the rat basal forebrain leads to memory impairments in passive and active avoidance tasks. *Brain Res.*, **328**, 97–104.

Murray, C. L. and Fibiger, H. C. (1985). Learning and memory deficits after lesions of the nucleus basalis magnocellularis: reversal by physostygmine. *Neuroscience*, **14**, 1025–32.

Pedata, F., Giovannelli, L., and Pepeu, G. (1984). GM1 ganglioside facilitates the recovery of high affinity choline uptake in the cerebral cortex of rats with a lesion of the nucleus basalis magnocellularis. *J. Neurosci. Res.*, **12**, 421–7.

Pedata, F., Lo Conte, G., Sorbi, G., Marconcini Pepeu, I., and Pepeu, G. (1982). Changes in high affinity choline uptake in rat cortex following lesions of the magnocellular forebrain nuclei. *Brain Res.*, **233**, 359–67.

Pepeu, G. (1983). Brain acetylcholine: an inventory of our knowledge on the 50th anniversary of its discovery. *T.I.P.S.*, **4**, 416–18.

Pepeu, G., Casamenti, F., Bracco, L., Ladinsky, H., and Consolo, S. (1985). Lesions of the nucleus basalis in the rat: functional changes. In Traber, J. and Gispen, W. H. (eds.), *Senile Dementia of the Alzheimer Type*. Springer Verlag, Berlin, pp. 305–15.

Pepeu, G., Casamenti, F., Pedata, F., Cosi, C., and Marconcini Pepeu, I. (1986). Are the neurochemical and behavioural changes induced by lesions of the nucleus basalis in the rat a model of Alzheimer's disease? *Progress Neuro-Psychopharmacol.* (in press).

Price, D. L., Whitehouse, P. J., and Struble, R. G. (1985). Alzheimer's disease. *Ann. Rev. Med.*, **36**, 349–56.

Salamone, J. D., Berat, P. M., Alpert, J. E., and Iversen, S. D. (1984). Impairment in T maze reinforced alternation performance following nucleus basalis magnocellularis lesions in rat. *Behav. Brain Res.*, **13**, 63–73.

Sims, N. R., Bowen, D. M., Smith, C. C. T., Flack, R. H. A., Davison, A. N., Snowden, J. S., and Neary, D. (1980). Glucose metabolism and acetylcholine synthesis in relation to neuronal activity in Alzheimer's disease. *Lancet*, i, 333–5.

Sims, N. R., Bowen, D. M., Allen, S. J., Smith, C. C. T., Neary, D., Thomas, D. J., and Davison, A. N. (1983). Presynaptic cholinergic disfunction in patients with dementia. *J. Neurochem.*, **40**, 503–9.

Sokoloff, L., Reivich, M., Kennedy, C., Des Rosiers, M., Patlak, C., Pettigrew, K., Sakurada, O. and Shinohara, M. (1977). ^{14}C-Deoxyglucose method for the measurement of local cerebral glucose utilization: theory, procedure and normal values in the conscious and anaesthetized albino rat. *J. Neurochem.*, **28**, 897–916.

Steward, D. J., Macfabe, D. F., and Wanderwolf, C. H. (1984). Cholinergic activation of the electrocorticogram: role of substantia innominata and effect of atropine and quinuclidinyl benzilate. *Brain Res.*, **322**, 219–32.

Terry, R. D., and Davies, P. (1980). Dementia of the Alzheimer type. *Ann. Rev. Neurosci.*, **3**, 77–95.

Wenk, G. L. (1984). Pharmacological manipulation of the substantia innominata–cortical cholinergic pathways. *Neurosci. Lett.*, **51**, 99–103.

Wenk, G., and Olton, D. S. (1984). Recovery of neocortical choline acetyltransferase activity following ibotenic acid injection into the nucleus basalis of Meynert in rats. *Brain Res.*, **293**, 184–6.

Wenk, H., Bigl, V., and Meyer, U. (1980). Cholinergic projections from magnocellular nuclei of the basal forebrain to cortical areas in rats. *Brain Res. Rev.*, **2**, 295–316.

Wenk, G., Hepler, D., and Olton, D. (1984a). Behavior alters the uptake of 3H choline into acetylcholinergic neurons of the nucleus basalis magnocellularis and medial septal area. *Behav. Brain Res.*, **13**, 129-38.

Wenk, G. L., Cribbs, B., and McCall, L. (1984b). Nucleus basalis magnocellularis: optimal coordinates for selective reduction of choline acetyltransferase in frontal neocortex by ibotenic acid injections. *Exp. Brain Res.*, **56**, 335-40.

Wood, P. L., and Richard, P. L. (1982). Gabaergic regulation of the substantia innominata-cortical cholinergic pathway. *Neuropharmacol.*, **21**, 969-72.

Woolf, N. J., Eckenstein, F., and Butcher, L. (1983). Cholinergic projections from the basal forebrain to the frontal cortex: a combined fluorescent tracer and immunohistochemical analysis in the rat. *Neurosci. Lett.*, **40**, 93-8.

6

In Search of Possible Markers and Models in Alzheimer's Disease

M. Briley, M. Brown, P. Chopin, X. Heral and C. Moret

6.1 Introduction

The search for therapeutic agents effective in Alzheimer's disease is hampered by two major problems. First, there is no specific animal model which reproduces the biochemical, morphological and behavioural characteristics of the disease. Thus drug screening tends to be based on the search for a biochemical activity considered to be necessary in the therapy of Alzheimer's disease. This is the case in the search for cholinomimetic agents as a replacement therapy for the defective cholinergic innervation in the cortex and hippocampus. The extrapolation from screening to clinical testing in these cases is, however, extremely uncertain. The second difficulty is that of diagnosis. Since Alzheimer's disease is a progressive, degenerative disease, any therapy would be expected to be most effective in the early stages when the deficiency is less marked and the cause possibly still reversible. Unfortunately, at this very early stage the symptoms of Alzheimer's disease are easily confused with those of various other psychiatric and neurological diseases such as depression and Parkinsonism, and even iatrogenic conditions such as subacute benzodiazepine toxicity.

6.2 Animal Models

6.2.1 Introduction

Choline acetyltransferase (ChAT) levels are significantly reduced in the brain of Alzheimer patients and there is very probably a major loss of cholinergic neurons in the nucleus basalis of Meynhert (Nb) (Coyle *et al.*, 1983). Indeed, the reduction of ChAT activity has been shown to be proportional to the severity of the dementia (Sims *et al.*, 1980). In order to mimic this situation in animals, lesions of the Nb have been carried out either by electrolytic lesion or by specific neurotoxic agents such as kainic acid or ibotenic acid (Flicker *et al.*, 1983) or the choline analogue AF-64A (Mantione *et al.*, 1981). Animals lesioned in this way do indeed show learning deficits analogous to those found in Alzheimer's disease (for a review, see Ch. 5), although the anatomo-histological characteristics of the disease such as the senile plaques and tangles are absent. The learning deficits appear to be sensitive to cholinergic agents, and recently Haroutunian *et al.* (1985) have shown that physostigmine could partially reverse the lesion-induced learning deficit. Whereas this model is undoubtedly useful for screening compounds which are aimed at replacing the cholinergic deficit, it gives no indications as to the basic causes of the pathology.

For a certain number of human diseases, analogous conditions have been found in animals either spontaneously or by selective breeding. The 'spontaneously hypertensive rat' and the 'obese rat' are classical examples. The spontaneous nature of these conditions suggests that their study could give some indications as to their origins or causes which may have some factors in common with the related human conditions.

Recently, Gage *et al.* (1984) showed that individual rats within an aged population develop cognitive impairment to a varying degree. Thus, in an attempt to find a 'natural' animal model for senile dementia, we have studied a population of 'aged' rats in order to investigate the possible existence of a subpopulation of animals with a spontaneous memory deficit.

6.2.2 Methods

Male Long-Evans rats (Janvier, France) were received in the laboratory at an age of 24 months. Due to their size and aggressive nature they were housed either singly or in pairs with free access to food and water. A 12 h light/12 h dark cycle (light 18.00–06.00) was used. Any rats showing physical disabilities such as blindness, arthritis or coordination problems were excluded from the study, as were any animals with obvious tumours. 'Aged' animals, used at ages of 33 to 35 months, were tested in a standard 'shuttle box' active avoidance paradigm between 09.00 and 12.00 for four consecutive days.

'Young' animals (3 to 6 months) were obtained from the same suppliers and were kept for at least 1 week under the same conditions as the 'aged' rats, housed five per cage, before being tested in the same experimental paradigm.

^{3}H-Quinuclidinyl benzylate (^{3}H-QNB) binding was measured using a method adapted from that of Yamamura and Snyder (1974). ^{3}H-Pirenzepine (^{3}H-Pz) binding was determined essentially as described by Watson *et al.* (1982).

Choline uptake was determined in a crude synaptosomal fraction (P_2 fraction) obtained from rat cortex. The synaptosomal suspension (400 μl) was preincubated for 5 min at 37 °C, and then ^{3}H-choline (60–90 Ci/mmol, New England Nuclear Chemicals) was added in a total volume of 500 μl.

The uptake process was stopped 2 min later by filtration through Whatman GF/C filters, which were rinsed and dried, and the radioactivity was counted in an Instagel scintillator (Packard). Specific uptake of ^{3}H-choline is defined as the difference between uptake in the absence and that in the presence of 10 μM hemicholinium.

6.2.3 Results

The avoidance scores of young rats increased over the four days, and although there was a certain dispersion in the individual values on the fourth day the population appeared homogeneous (Fig. 6.1). In contrast, the aged rat population was very heterogeneous. Six out of 14 rats had fourth day avoidance scores similar to those of the young rats, whereas the rest had scores essentially the same as on the first day (Fig. 6.1). Thus, 8 out of 14 of the old rats had an apparent total learning deficit in this paradigm.

Following testing in the shuttle box the aged rats were sacrificed and the cortex dissected. Total muscarinic binding (^{3}H-QNB), M_1 muscarinic binding (^{3}H-Pz), M_2 muscarinic binding (by difference) and choline uptake were measured in individual animals.

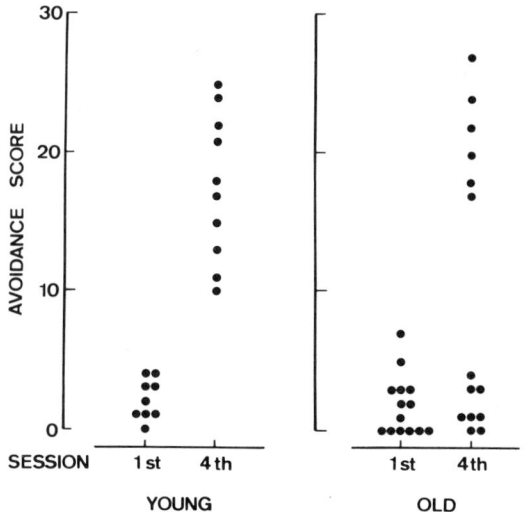

Fig. 6.1 Shuttle-box avoidance performance in 'young' and 'old' rats. 'Young' (3–6 months) and 'old' (33–35 months) rats were tested in a standard 'shuttle-box' paradigm for four consecutive days. The avoidance scores for the first and fourth days are given for each individual animal.

On the basis of the learning performances the rats were divided into two groups, 'normal learners' with a fourth day avoidance score of 15 or more and 'poor learners' with a score of less than 15. Statistical analysis of these two groups (Table 6.1) showed no difference in any of the biochemical parameters measured.

6.2.4 Conclusion

It has been shown that in a population of aged rats housed together under identical conditions approximately half had a serious learning deficit in a simple paradigm. The biochemical tests that were carried out suggest that this deficit was not linked to a cholinergic deficit. If these preliminary results are found in other groups of similarly aged animals, this spontaneous learning deficit may prove to be an interesting animal model of dementia. Although the very preliminary biochemical analyses presented here suggest that, in contrast to Alzheimer's disease, there is no apparent cholinergic deficit in these animals,

Table 6.1   Biochemical measurements in 'normal learner' and 'poor learner' aged rats

	Normal learners	Poor learners
Avoidance score	18.7 ± 4.1 ($n = 6$)	1.6 ± 0.6* ($n = 8$)
Total muscarinic binding ^{3}H-QNB (B_{max}) (fmole/mg protein) ^{3}H-QNB (K_d) (nM)	106.7 ± 7.2 ($n = 4$) 0.103 ± 0.014 ($n = 4$)	135.0 ± 17.0 ($n = 7$) 0.088 ± 0.016 ($n = 7$)
M_1 *muscarinic binding* ^{3}H-Pz (B_{max}) (fmole/mg protein) ^{3}H-Pz (K_d) (nM)	56.6 ± 13.7 ($n = 3$)	78.0 ± 8.6 ($n = 7$)
M_2 *muscarinic binding* ^{3}H-QNB–^{3}H-Pz (B_{max}) (fmole/mg protein)	51.6 ± 4.2 ($n = 3$)	56.9 ± 11.7 ($n = 7$)
Choline uptake V_{max} (fmole/mg tissue/2 min) K_m (μM)	67.7 ± 14.5 ($n = 5$) 0.101 ± 0.023 ($n = 5$)	76.5 ± 24.1 ($n = 5$) 0.157 ± 0.049 ($n = 5$)

'Normal' learners were defined as those animals with a fourth day avoidance score of 15 or more. 'Poor' learners had a fourth day avoidance score of less than 15. Statistical analyses were carried out using the Student-t test. *$p < 0.001$.

further studies are required to determine to what extent histological and bio-chemical characteristics found in these animals reflect those of human dementia.

6.3 Peripheral Markers

6.3.1 Introduction

The diagnosis of Alzheimer's disease is essentially a diagnosis by exclusion. Only post-mortem histopathology or the study of brain biopsy samples can give a categorical diagnosis of Alzheimer's disease (McKhann *et al.*, 1984). In Alzheimer's disease, any potential therapy can be expected to be more effective the earlier it is used in the degenerative process. This is true whether the therapy is sympto-matic or is aimed at the basic physiopathology. Thus a major problem facing anyone trying to test new potential drugs in Alzheimer's disease is the identi-fication of early stage Alzheimer patients. Indeed it is conceivable that the lack of therapeutic success of such 'logical' treatments as with choline is partially due to the exclusive use of 'advanced' Alzheimer patients.

Platelets have been shown to possess a remarkable number of receptors, enzymes and uptake mechanisms (Sneddon, 1973). Among these several have been found to be qualitatively similar to those in the brain. Monoamine oxidase activity (Sullivan *et al.*, 1979), the uptake of serotonin (Stahl and Meltzer, 1978) and the binding site for ^{3}H-imipramine (Langer and Briley, 1981) have been suggested to be quantitatively related to their cerebral counterparts. Thus it is possible that different biochemical markers in platelets may be of use in the early diagnosis of certain pathological conditions of the central nervous system.

Very little research has been carried out into the existence of cholinergic elements in platelets, although Green *et al.* (1972) described the high-affinity accumulation of choline in human platelets. In an attempt to find a peripheral marker that may be correlated with changes in the central cholinergic system, we have investigated the existence of cholinergic muscarinic receptors and ChAT-like activity in animal and human platelets.

6.3.2 Methods

Blood, obtained from rats (260 g), or rabbits (2 kg), was collected from the abdominal aorta under ether anaesthesia. Human blood was taken by venous puncture from healthy volunteers. Platelets were prepared essentially as pre-viously described by Briley *et al.* (1979).

^{3}H-QNB binding was carried out as described by Yamamura and Snyder (1974) for rat brain, with the exception that the incubation mixture was diluted into 5 ml ice-cold buffer immediately before filtration.

ChAT-like activity was measured as described by Fonnum (1975). The pellet obtained from the centrifugation of the platelet-rich plasma was resuspended in 10 mM EDTA (pH 7.4) to give a membrane concentration of about 30 mg protein/ml.

6.3.3 Results

[3]H-QNB was found to bind in a saturable manner to rat and human platelets, giving linear Scatchard plots (Figs. 6.2 and 6.3). The K_d values (Table 6.2) in rat and human platelets were similar but about 10 times greater than that measured in rat cortex. Specific ^{3}H-QNB binding in platelets from both species was inhibited by a series of cholinergic agonists and antagonists, with IC_{50} values similar to those determined in rat cortex (Table 6.3).

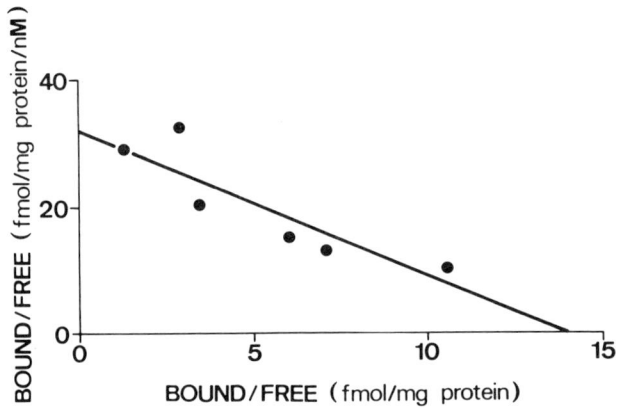

Fig. 6.2 Typical Scatchard plot of ^{3}H-QNB binding in rat platelets. ^{3}H-QNB binding was measured as described in the text. Each point is determined in duplicate. The line of best fit was determined by linear regression analysis using the method of least squares. The values of B_{max} and K_d for this particular experiment were 14 fmol/mg protein and 0.44 nM, respectively.

ChAT-like activity was found in platelets from rat, rabbit and man (Fig. 6.4). The enzyme activity and the total acetylcholine synthesized was lowest in platelets from the rat and greatest in human platelets (Fig. 6.4). Dilution of the platelet suspension gave reduced ChAT activity, with the reduction corresponding approximately to the dilution factor (Fig. 6.5). Heating the platelet suspension for 5 min at 50 °C reduced these activities by between 60 and 90 % (Fig. 6.5).

6.3.4 Conclusion

The preliminary results presented here suggest that at least two characteristics of the cholinergic synapse exist in animal and human platelets. In addition, choline has been shown to be actively taken up by human platelets in a concentration-

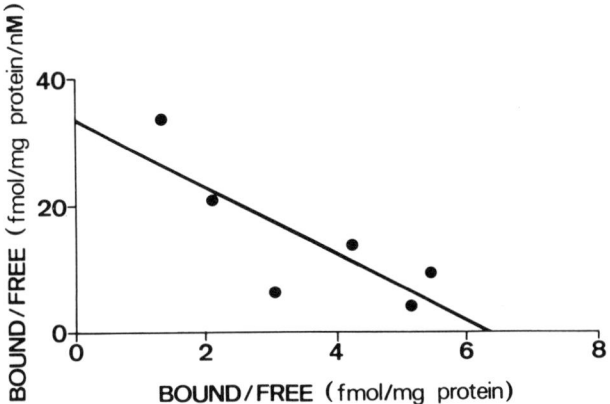

Fig. 6.3 Typical Scatchard plot of ^{3}H-QNB binding in human platelets. ^{3}H-QNB binding was measured as described in the text. Each point is determined in duplicate. The line of best fit was determined by linear regression analysis using the method of least squares. The values of B_{max} and K_d for this particular experiment were 6.4 fmol/mg protein and 0.18 nM, respectively.

Table 6.2   High-affinity ^{3}H-QNB binding to rat and human platelets

	Rat cortex	Rat platelets	Human platelets
K_d	0.048 ± 0.007 $n = 4$	0.46 ± 0.06 $n = 9$	0.39 ± 0.10 $n = 7$
B_{max}	93 ± 5 $n = 4$	24 ± 4 $n = 9$	6.3 ± 1.2 $n = 7$

The K_d values are expressed in nM and the B_{max} values as fmol/mg tissue in brain membranes and fmol/mg protein in platelet membranes. The data represent the means ± SEM of n Scatchard plots each of 6 points determined in duplicate.

Table 6.3   Inhibition of ^{3}H-QNB binding

	Rat cortex	Rat platelets	Human platelets
Scopolamine	1.4 ± 0.2	0.4 ± 0.2	1.7 ± 1.0
Pirenzepine	187 ± 8	450 ± 98	–
Atropine	3.0 ± 0.7	2.0 ± 0.5	1.1 ± 0.5
Oxotremorine	1200 ± 140	1175 ± 278	1600
Pilocarpine	9800 ± 3000	1725 ± 303	–

IC_{50} is the concentration required to inhibit 50 % of the specific ^{3}H-QNB binding at 0.06 nM for the cortex and 0.5 nM for the platelets. Values are the means of 2 to 5 values (± SEM, where $n = 3$ or more) determined from individual inhibition curves of 6 concentrations determined in duplicate.

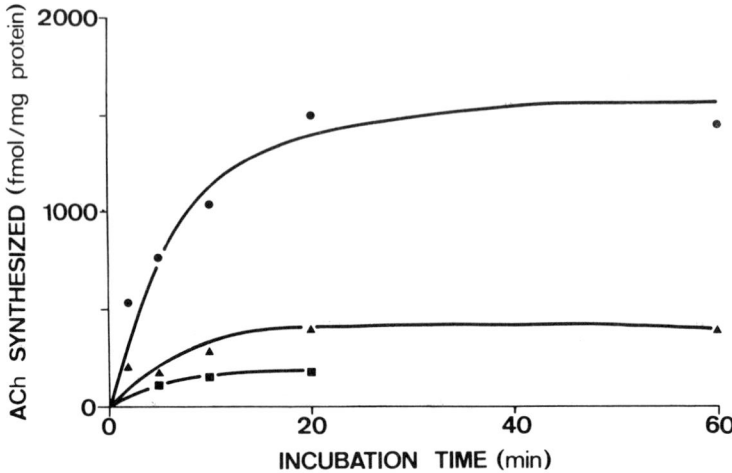

Fig. 6.4 Choline acetyltransferase-like activity in platelets. ChAT-like activity was measured by the method of Fonnum (1975). Platelets from rat (■), rabbit (▲) and man (●) were tested.

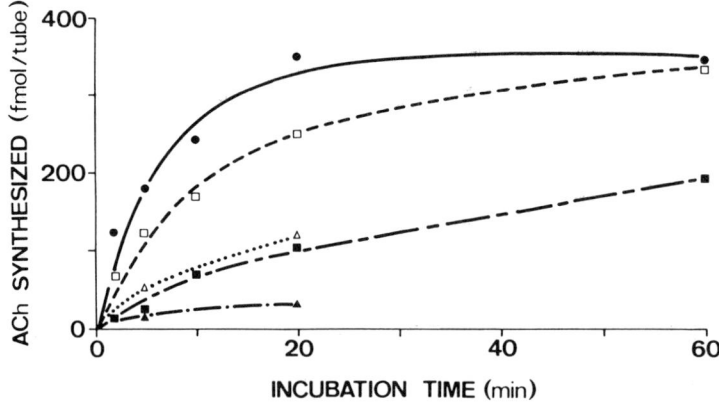

Fig. 6.5 Choline acetyltransferase-like activity in human platelets. ChAT-like activity was measured by the method of Fonnum (1975). Platelet membranes were used at a final concentration of 30 mg protein/ml (●), 12 mg protein/ml (□) or 2 mg protein/ml (■). Platelet membranes denatured by heating for 5 min at 50 °C were tested at 30 mg protein/ml (△) and 12 mg protein/ml (▲).

dependent manner, with kinetics and inhibitor selectivity resembling those of choline uptake into central cholinergic neurons (Green *et al.*, 1972).

High-affinity ^{3}H-QNB binding sites appear to exist on rat and human platelets with pharmacological specificity similar to, if not identical with, that of central cholinergic muscarinic receptors. The density of these receptors is, however, extremely low and with the present tools and techniques their routine analysis in blood samples from Alzheimer patients does not seem feasible. A ChAT-like activity appears to exist in platelets from the three species tested. It remains to be verified that the ^{3}H-acetyl group is in fact transferred to the added choline and not to other possible endogenous acetyl group acceptors. Whatever the precise nature of this activity it seems to be quantitatively sufficient for precise analysis in small blood samples.

These preliminary results suggest that blood platelets possess a number of biochemical activities in common with central cholinergic neurons. In view of the ease with which platelets can be repeatedly analysed in patients and the importance of the cholinergic system in Alzheimer's disease, the further investigation of this approach would appear worthwhile. To what extent the platelet may represent a useful probe in Alzheimer's disease remains, however, to be determined.

References

Briley, M., Raisman, R., and Langer, S. Z. (1979). Human platelets possess high-affinity binding sites for ^{3}H-imipramine. *Europ. J. Pharmacol.*, 58, 347-8.

Coyle, J. T., Price, D. L., and Dehong, M. R. (1983). Alzheimer's disease: A disorder of cortical cholinergic innervation. *Science*, 219, 1184-90.

Flicker, C., Dean, R. L., Watkins, D. L., Fisher, S. K., and Bartus, R. T. (1983). Behavioral and neurochemical effects following neurotoxic lesions of a major cholinergic input to the cerebral cortex in the rat. *Pharmacol. Biochem. Behav.*, 18, 973-81.

Fonnum, F. (1975). A rapid radiochemical method for the determination of choline acetyltransferase. *J. Neurochem.*, 24, 407-9.

Gage, F. H., Kelly, P. A. T., and Björklund, A. (1984). Regional changes in brain glucose metabolism reflect cognitive impairments in aged rats. *J. Neuroscience*, 4, 2856-65.

Green, A. R., Boullin, D. J., Massarelli, R., and Hanin, I. (1972). Can the platelet be used as a model for the cholinergic nerve ending? *Life Sciences*, 11, 1049-58.

Haroutunian, V., Kanof, P., and Davis, K. L. (1985). Pharmacological alleviation of cholinergic lesion induced memory deficits in rats. *Life Sciences*, 37, 945-52.

Langer, S. Z., and Briley, M. (1981). High-affinity ^{3}H-imipramine binding: A new biological tool for studies in depression. *Trends in Neurosci.*, 4, 28-31.

McKhann, G., Drachman, D., Folstein, M., Katzman, R., Price, D., and Stadlan, E. M. (1984). Clinical diagnosis of Alzheimer's disease. *Neurology*, 34, 939-43.

Mantione, C. R., Fisher, A., and Hanin, I. (1981). AF64A Neurotoxicity: A potential animal model of central cholinergic hypofunction. *Science*, 213, 579-80.

Sandberg, K., Schnaar, R. L., McKinney, M., Hanin, I., Fisher, A., and Coyle, J. T. (1985). AF64A: An active site directed irreversible inhibitor of choline acetyltransferase. *J. Neurochem.*, 44, 439-45.

Sims, N. R., Bowen, D. M., Smith, C. I., Flack, R. H., Davison, A. N., Snowden, J. S., and Neary, D. (1980). Glucose metabolism and acetylcholine synthesis in relation to neuronal activity in Alzheimer's disease. *Lancet*, i, 333-5.

Sneddon, J. M. (1973). Blood platelets as a model for monoamine containing neurons. *Prog. Neurobiol.*, 1, 151-98.

Stahl, S. M., and Meltzer, H. Y. (1978). A kinetic and pharmacological analysis of 5-hydroxytryptamine transport by human platelets and platelet storage granules: Comparison with central serotonergic neurons. *J. Pharmac. Exp. Therap.*, 205, 118-32.

Sullivan, J. L., Cavenar, J. O., Maltbie, A. A., Lister, P., and Zung, W. W. K. (1979). Familial biochemical and clinical correlates of alcoholics with low platelet monoamine oxidase activity. *Biol. Psychiatry*, 14, 385-94.

Watson, M., Roeske, W. R., and Yamamura, H. I. (1982). ^{3}H-Pirenzepine selectively identifies a high affinity population of muscarinic cholinergic receptors in the rat cerebral cortex. *Life Sci.*, **31**, 2019–23.
Yamamura, H. I., and Snyder, S. H. (1974). Muscarinic cholinergic binding in rat brain. *Proc. Nat. Acad. Sci.*, **71**, 1725–9.

7

Neurotransmitter Systems in Alzheimer's Disease

S. de St Hilaire-Kafi, C. Bouras and J. Constantinidis

7.1 Introduction

First described in 1907, Alzheimer's disease (AD) is a neuropathological disorder that causes progressive dementia with deterioration of memory and all cognitive functions in advanced cases. The brain pathology of AD consists of the presence of senile plaques and neurofibrillary tangles (Wisniewsky and Terry, 1976; Constantinidis *et al.*, 1978; Constantinidis and Tissot, 1979). Many studies on post-mortem brains of AD patients have consistently shown evidence of neurotransmitter impairment.

7.2 Acetylcholine (ACH)

In the basal forebrain, the nucleus basalis of Meynert (a principal source of cholinergic innervation of the neocortex) has shown a decrease in the number of neurons and their nucleolar volume in AD (Whitehouse *et al.*, 1981, 1982; Perry *et al.*, 1982; Rossor *et al.*, 1982a; Tagliavini and Pilleri, 1983). Decreased levels of choline acetyltransferase (ChAT) — the enzyme that synthesizes acetylcholine (ACh) — and acetylcholinesterase (AChE) — the degradative enzyme of ACh — have been reported in the cortex and hippocampus (Davies, 1979; Carlsson *et al.*, 1980; Rossor *et al.*, 1980b; Yates *et al.*, 1980; Perry *et al.*, 1982). In AD, both enzymes ChAT and AChE are markedly reduced in the frontal, parietal, temporal and occipital cortex, in the hippocampus, in the mammillary body and in the nucleus caudatus (Davies, 1979). The important degenerative effect of the cholinergic nerve terminals, originated in the diagonal band of Broca and the nucleus basalis of Meynert, in the formation of some neuritic plaques has also been suggested (Perry *et al.*, 1982; Struble *et al.*, 1982). In recent years the severity of psychological dysfunction in AD has been suggested to be a reflection of the changes in cholinergic markers (Sims *et al.*, 1983). Thus cholinergic drug therapies for geriatric amnesia and senile dementia were used in clinical research (Bartus *et al.*, 1982). On the mechanisms of memory processing, Flood *et al.* (1985) reported an improvement of test retention in mice after administration of arecholine and oxotremorine (both Ach agonists). Physostigmine, a cholinesterase inhibitor, has been used for improvement of memory and cognition in AD. In these results it was noted that the efficacy of physostigmine diminishes as AD progresses and the cholinergic degeneration continues. Therefore drug therapy, which has to alter presynaptic function, depends on the existence of intact cholinergic neurons (Davis *et al.*, 1983; Thal *et al.*, 1983).

7.3 Monoamines

The impaired functioning of the noradrenaline (NA) neuronal groups, particularly the NA cells of the locus coeruleus (LC), in AD has been extensively reviewed (Tomlinson *et al.*, 1981; Bondareff *et al.*, 1982; Mann *et al.*, 1982; Berger, 1984). These studies described a loss of NA neurons in the LC, a reduction of NA in the brain, and a significantly greater decrease of NA in the hypothalamus (up to 50 %).

There is also evidence that NA, dopamine-β-hydroxylase (DBH – a specific enzyme of NA synthesis), and 3-methoxy-4-hydroxyphenylethyleneglycol (MHPG – an NA metabolite), decrease significantly in the frontal, temporal, occipital, and hippocampic cortex (Berger *et al.*, 1980; Yates *et al.*, 1983a). From some laboratory studies on the function of the NA system, certain conclusions have, with some controversy, emerged. Iversen *et al.* (1983) reported a positive correlation between the loss of LC neurons and the decrease of the NA level in the temporal cortex. Meanwhile, Cross *et al.* (1983) have found no correlation between the neuronal loss and the decrease of cortical DBH activity or MHPG metabolite.

Dopamine (DA) activity in AD has not been extensively investigated. Adolfsson *et al.* (1979) and Mann *et al.* (1982) observed a slight decrease of DA in several cortical areas and in the striatum. Berger *et al.* (1980) reported an important reduction of DA in the frontal cortex in AD. Thus, DA activity is decreased in the nigro-striatal pathway and in the cerebral cortex (Adolfsson *et al.*, 1979; Carlsson and Winblad, 1976).

Serotonin (5-HT)-containing cells of the raphe nuclei in the brain stem and midbrain areas of AD patients were examined and the decrease of the uptake as well as the altered functional capacity of these neurons were reported (Gottfries *et al.*, 1969; Argentiero and Tavolato, 1980; Benton *et al.*, 1982). Mann and

Yates (1983) have observed that nucleolar volume and cytoplasmic RNA content in the cells of the nucleus supratrochlearis were significantly reduced as compared to controls. They also described changes in cell structure (tangle formation) together with a reduced functional capacity as the basis for the altered 5-HT metabolism. Differential losses of 5-HT_1 and 5-HT_2 receptors were reported in the neocortex, the hippocampus, and amygdala, whereas no changes occurred in the basal forebrain and basal ganglia (Cross et al., 1984a). The same group reported that in AD patients the losses of 5-HT_1 receptors are age-related, whereas losses of the 5-HT_2 receptors were greater but were not age-related. The concept of differences with respect to both development and ageing of the 5-HT system is in agreement with the recent work of Marcusson et al. (1984).

7.4 GABA

The distribution of GABA neurons in various parts of the central nervous system (CNS) has been described by Roberts et al. (1975) by means of glutamate decarboxylase (GAD) antibodies and immunochemistry. It has also been reported that in AD GAD decreases in the nucleus caudatus, remains unchanged in the putamen, and decreases in the thalamic and cortical areas (Bird and Iversen, 1974; Cote and Kremzner, 1974; McGeer and McGeer, 1976; Rossor et al., 1982a). This GAD decrease is correlated with the presence of neurofibrillary tangles in numerous neuronal bodies in the cortex and the hippocampus. In AD patients, a 70% decrease of GABA and a decrease in GABA receptors are found in the nucleus caudatus and the temporal and frontal cortex (Reisine et al., 1978; Rossor et al., 1982a). Nevertheless, Cross et al. (1984b) reported no changes in the GABA receptor binding in AD. Constantinidis (1982, 1983, 1984) related a clear and lasting improvement in AD patients in all their symptoms after administration of progabide (SL-76002), which can cross the blood–brain barrier (Bartholini et al., 1979). On the other hand, the coexistence of GABA with somatostatin (SS) in a subpopulation of GABAergic cell bodies in the cortex and the subcortical white matter (Schmechel et al., 1984) may explain the moderate decrease of GABA rate generally admitted (Berger, 1984), and the important paralleled SS cortical deficit.

7.5 Glutamate (GLU)

The hippocampic pyramidal neurons contain a large amount of GLU. In AD, the neurofibrillary tangles initially appear in the pyramidal neurons. Based on this knowledge, it has been hypothesised that GLU, as a neurotransmitter, might be involved in AD (Constantinidis, 1979; Constantinidis and Tissot, 1981). Tarbit et al. (1980), however, have found that in AD the hippocampic GLU level does not differ from that in the controls.

It must be mentioned that it is difficult to distinguish metabolic GLU from neurotransmitter GLU. Pearce *et al.* (1984) described the increased specific binding of L-(^{3}H) GLU to membranes of the caudate nucleus of AD brains as evidence of a change in GLU neurotransmission in this disease. They concluded that the positive relationship between the number of tangles in the neocortex and the values of GLU binding possibly reflects a change in GLU receptors in the caudate nucleus. Earlier, Smith *et al.* (1983) reported that potassium-evoked release of GLU from synaptosomes of AD neocortex is not significantly different from that of controls.

7.6 Aspartate

Smith *et al.* (1983) reported normal aspartate release from seven autopsied AD temporal cortices, but it is difficult to obtain an appropriate dosage of this neurotransmitter.

7.7 Neuropeptides

The wide distribution of peptides in the central nervous system (CNS) raises questions about their functional role in neurological diseases. In AD peptidic changes have been reported in post-mortem studies of human brain (Rossor and Emson, 1982).

In this review on neuropeptides, we will first discuss data from our laboratories on the morphological changes of somatostatin (SS) and substance P (SP) in AD.

7.7.1 Somatostatin

SS, a 28- and 14-amino-acid peptide that inhibits growth hormone release, is largely distributed in the mammalian CNS. SS is also found within cell bodies in both the cerebral cortex and hippocampus (Morrison *et al.*, 1983; Bouras *et al.*, 1985). In our study, post-mortem brain regions from three patients who died with a diagnosis of AD were compared with those of four control cases using the indirect immunohistofluorescence method of Coons (1958) and the peroxidase–antiperoxidase (PAP) method (Bouras *et al.*, 1984). Comparative investigation of the SS fluorescence or PAP immunoreactive intensity showed the following results.

In the hippocampus, a decrease of SS-positive neurons as well as in the intensity of specific SS-like immunoreactivity (SSLI) or in PAP staining were seen.

In the neocortex, the loss of SS-positive neuronal bodies, fibres and terminals affected all cortical layers and particularly the superficial cortical layers for the fibres and terminals. A decrease in the number of SS cell bodies and fibres was also found in the sub-cortical white matter.

An accumulation of SS-positive material was observed within, or close to, the corona of senile plaques (Fig. 7.1), and some of the cell bodies containing neuro-fibrillary tangles also showed a slight SS-positive fluorescence; this observation may suggest a participation of SS cell bodies in the pathogenesis of AD. On the other hand, a slight reduction in the density of SS-positive fibres and terminals was seen in the amygdaloid nuclear complex. In contrast, in the substantia innominata, an increase in the immunoreactive intensity of SS-positive fibres was observed (Fig. 7.2).

An important reduction in the number of SS-positive cell bodies and fibres was observed in the nucleus septi lateralis; in the nucleus septi medialis a decrease of the number of SS-positive fibres was also seen.

The mammilary bodies of the hypothalamus showed only a slight reduction in SS-positive fibres. There were no changes in the nucleus caudatus, the puta-men and the thalamus. Our morphological results are in agreement with those of radioimmunoassays of Rossor *et al.* (1980a), Davies *et al.* (1982), Ferrier *et al.* (1983), Sagar *et al.* (1984) and Armstrong *et al.* (1985).

These SS changes in AD suggest that ACh and SS possibly interact in some brain areas, especially in the substantia innominata (the major source of the

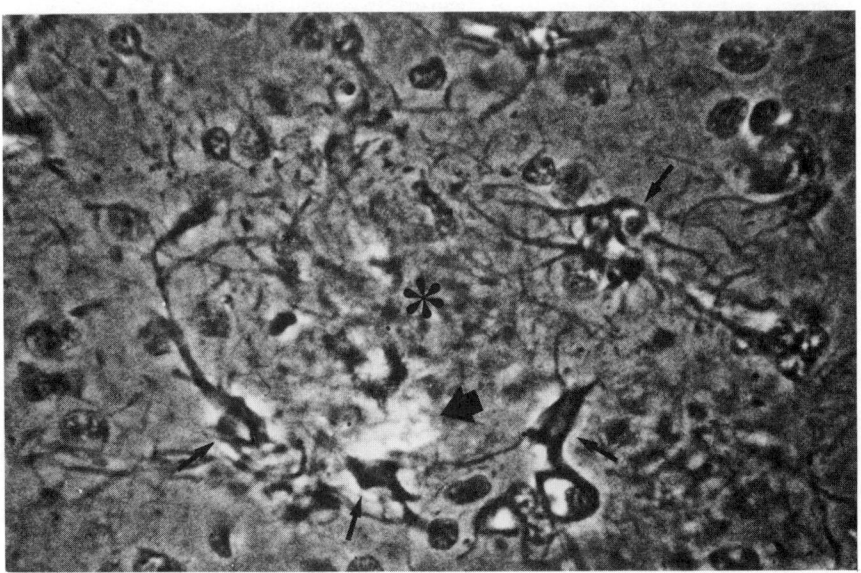

Fig. 7.1 Senile plaque in the zona moleculare of the fascia dentata in the hippocampus of an Alzheimer's disease case: Thick arrow = SS-positive amorphous material; asterisk = amyloid material of the senile plaque; and thin arrow = astrocytes encircling the senile plaque. Combined immunohistofluorescence and phase contrast methods. X 880.

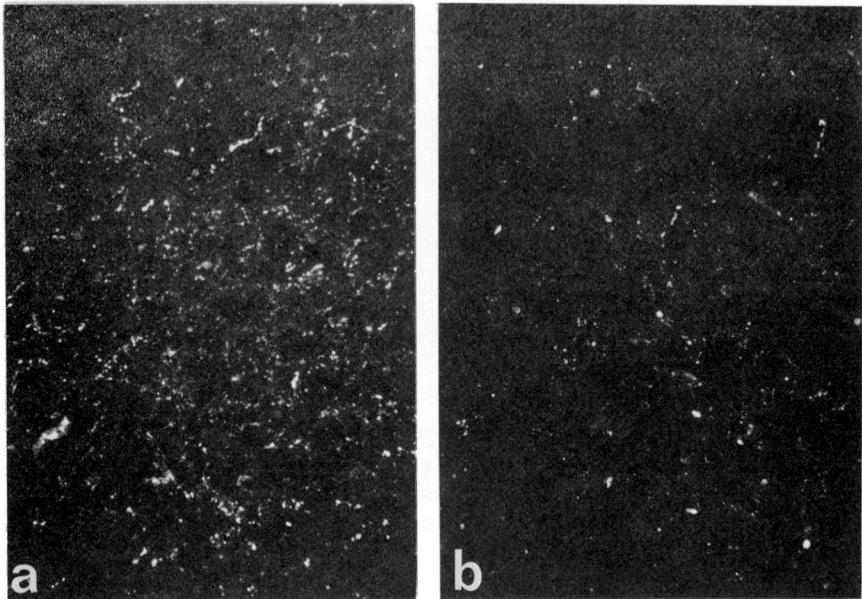

Fig. 7.2 Increased immunoreactive intensity of the SS-positive fibres in the substantia innominata in Alzheimer's disease (a), as compared to control (b).

cholinergic innervation of the cerebral cortex) and in the cortex. Malthesorenssen *et al.* (1978) described an influence on the ACh turnover and a decrease in ACh content in the cortex after intraventricular administration of SS. Thus, we suggest that the increased SS in the substantia innominata area in AD may influence ACh turnover and play a basic role in the important cortical ACh decrease. In a recent study Morrison *et al.* (1985) have postulated the relationship between SS and plaques. The high incidence of both plaques and SS in the cortex has been reported (Armstrong *et al.*, 1985; Morrison *et al.*, 1985; Bouras *et al.*, 1986). Nevertheless, the paralleled cortical deficit of SS and ACh is probably not due to the same causes, but would be in direct relation with the number of the senile plaques in the cortex. In our present study, the most important SS changes have been found in the more severe degenerative cases. On the other hand, there is a positive correlation between AChE activity and the number of the senile plaques in the cortex (Struble *et al.*, 1982). Moreover, the cortical SS deficit is observed not only in AD but in cases of Parkinson's disease with dementia (in contrast to non-dementia cases of the same neurological disorder). Thus it is probable that the diverse dementia syndromes of multiple degenerative causes may be accompanied by an SS cortical deficit (Agid *et al.*, 1983; Epelbaum *et al.*, 1983; Javoy-Agid *et al.*, 1984).

7.7.2 *Substance P*

It has been reported (Davies and Terry, 1981; Davies *et al.*, 1982) that somato-statin-like immunoreactivity (SSLI) material was decreased in the cerebral cortex of AD patients. Using a radioimmunoassay for SP, Crystal and Davies (1982) found a significant decrease of SPLI in the following eight regions: mid-frontal, inferior parietal, occipital, mid-temporal, superior temporal, inferior temporal, anterior cingulate and hippocampus. In their study, the SPLI mean in AD is approximately 43 to 68 % of that found in controls. Davies *et al.* (1982) observed significant reductions in the concentration of SPLI in the hippocampus, superior temporal, gyrus and mid-frontal cortex in AD. On the other hand, SP was signi-ficantly increased (+ 88 %) in the putamen and there were no changes in any other areas; SP was reduced by 25 % in the septum but this difference was not significant (Ferrier *et al.*, 1983). In contrast, no alteration of SP in AD has been reported (Coyle *et al.*, 1983; Yates *et al.*, 1983b; Sagar *et al.*, 1984). More recently, intense immunoreactivity for SP in the globus pallidus and substantia nigra in AD has been described (Grafe *et al.*, 1985).

By immunohistofluorescence technique, we observed a decrease of SP in the hippocampus (Fig. 7.3) as well as an increase of SP in the globus pallidus (Fig. 7.4) and in the substantia nigra (Fig. 7.5) in one case of AD, as compared

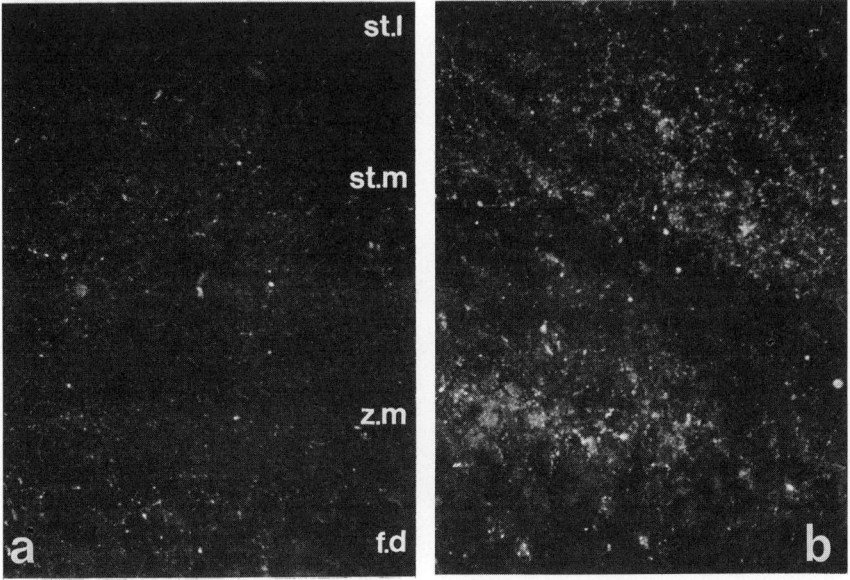

Fig. 7.3 Decreased SP-positive immunoreactive intensity in the hippocampus of an Alzheimer's disease case (a), as compared to control (b), by immunohistofluorescence method: f.d. = fascia dentata; z.m. zona moleculare of the fascia dentata; st. m. = stratum moleculare; st. l.: stratum lacunosum. × 105.

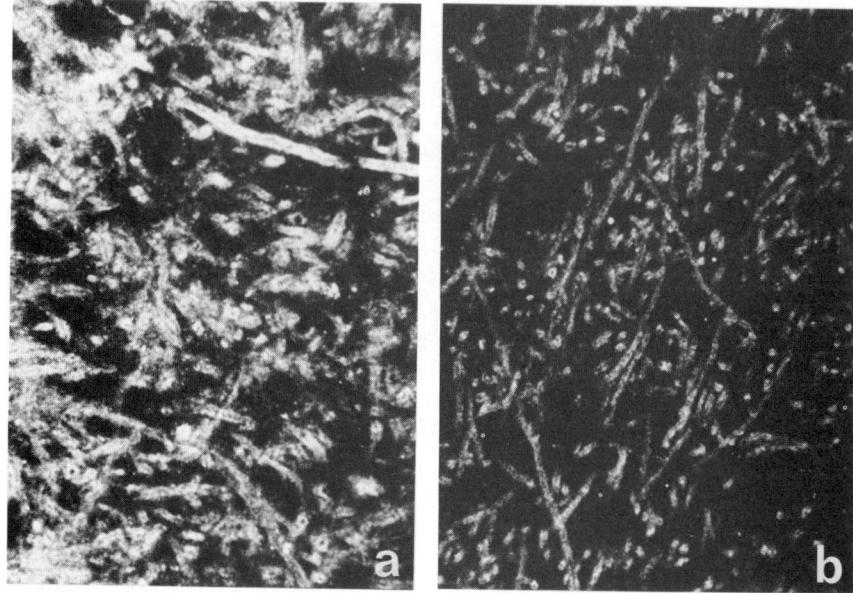

Fig. 7.4 Increased SP-positive immunoreactive intensity in the globus pallidus of an Alzheimer's disease case (a), as compared to control (b), by immunohistofluorescence method. × 270.

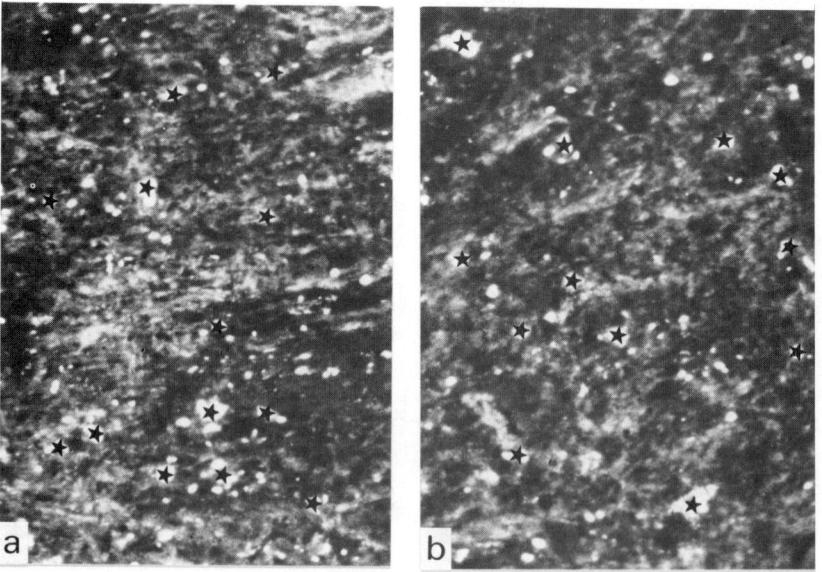

Fig. 7.5 Slight increase in SP-positive immunoreactive intensity in the substantia nigra of an Alzheimer's disease case (a), as compared to control (b), by immunohistofluorescence method. The star = non-specific fluorescence.

to four controls, which is in agreement with the findings by radioimmunoassay of Grafe *et al.* (1985).

7.7.3 Cholecystokinin (CCK-8)

CCK-8 has been found in high concentration in the mammalian brain (Larsson and Rehfeld, 1979; Sakamoto *et al.*, 1984), and also widely distributed in the human brain (Bouras and Constantinidis, 1984b). The presence of CCK-8 as a neurotransmitter in the CNS has naturally led to the investigation of the role of this peptide in AD. In the cerebral cortex of AD patients no change in the concentration of CCK-8 has been found (Rossor *et al.*, 1982b; Ferrier *et al.*, 1983; Sagar *et al.*, 1984). Differences in CCK-8 concentration were, however, reported in AD cases grouped according to post-mortem delay intervals of less than or more than 22 hours (Perry *et al.*, 1981). On the other hand, CCK-8 was administered either 0.02 mg/kg or 0.04 mg/kg intravenously in patients with diagnosed AD, and no change in their cognitive impairment was observed (Serby *et al.*, 1984). The authors reported that these treatments were ineffective in AD.

7.7.4 Neurotensin (NT)

Along with CCK-8, NT belongs to the group of peptides which do not change in the cerebral cortex in AD (Feuerstein, 1984). An extensive study of NT has shown a significant decrease of this peptide (by 56 %) in the septum in AD; no changes were seen in any other areas (Ferrier *et al.*, 1983). These authors found no relationship between NT in the septum and ACh in any brain area. Nevertheless, because of functional interactions between several peptides in the septum and ACh turnover in the hippocampus, they have proposed that reduced ACh synthesis may lead to secondary changes in NT levels in this region.

7.7.5 Thyrotropin-Releasing Hormone (TRH)

The distribution of TRH, a peptide restricted to the hypothalamus, has been investigated in post-mortem brain and spinal cord of AD cases. The 24 regions examined (Yates *et al.*, 1983b) showed that TRH is widely spread in the human brain and spinal cord in concentrations similar to those in rat brain. TRH was measured by the same authors in post-mortem brains of six AD cases and no significant differences were observed in TRH levels, as compared to controls.

7.7.6 Vasoactive Intestinal Peptide (VIP)

VIP, a 28-amino-acid neuropeptide, is widely distributed in the human brain (Bouras and Constantinidis, 1984a), including in the cortex, in the limbic cortical area, in the amygdala, in the hippocampus and in the hypothalamus. Its high concentration has also been reported in human cerebrospinal fluid (CSF) (Fahrenkrug and Schaffalittky de Muckadell, 1978; Emson, 1979).

Perry *et al.* (1981) have compared VIP immunoreactivity in the cerebral cortex of autopsied controls to that of autopsied AD patients. They reported no significant differences in VIP concentration in AD patients as compared to the control group. The regional distribution of VIP in control and AD brains showed that this peptide is non-significantly reduced in the septum in AD (Ferrier *et al.*, 1983). VIP-like immunoreactivity has also been measured by radioimmunoassay in 21 cerebral regions of seven AD patients. The results showed significant reductions of VIP in two cortical areas, the insula and angulate cortex (Arai *et al.*, 1984). This observation is in contrast with the results of the studies reviewed above in which VIP-containing neurons seemed to be intact in AD. On the other hand, the radioimmunoassay concentration of VIP in CSF in AD patients did not differ from that of controls (Wikkelso *et al.*, 1985). Finally, the coexistence of VIP and ACh in the cerebral cortex as well as in some peripheral nerves has been reported by Lundberg *et al.* (1979) and Eckenstein and Baughman (1984).

7.7.7 Neuropeptide Y (NPY)

NPY, a 36-amino-acid neuropeptide, has been shown to be widely distributed in the human brain (Adrian *et al.*, 1983). Allen *et al.* (1984) have examined NPY in four cortical areas and in the substantia innominata, hippocampus, septum, hypothalamus and three striatal areas in AD patients. They reported no changes in NPY in all these regions, including the four cortical areas, with the exception of the substantia innominata, where the NPY level was found to be significantly higher than in controls. A positive correlation between NPY and SS in the substantia innominata has been suggested by Allen *et al.* (1984). Subsequent studies by Chromwall *et al.* (1984) showed that SS and NPY may coexist in the human cerebral cortex.

7.8 Summary and Conclusion

A review of the literature concerning acetylcholine, monoamines, GABA, amino-acids and neuropeptides in Alzheimer's disease has been presented. In addition, in this work, changes in post-mortem brain material of three cases of Alzheimer's disease have been compared to four controls, using immunohisto-chemical methods for somatostatin and substance P.

The following modifications in the Alzheimer's disease cases were observed.

7.8.1 Somatostatin

(a) There was important reduction in the number of the somatostatin-positive cell bodies and fibres in the hippocampus, parahippocampic cortex and neo-cortex, especially in the parietal and frontal areas. A decrease in the number of the somatostatin cell bodies and fibres was also found in the sub-cortical white matter.

(b) Somatostatin-positive amorphous material was seen within or close to the corona of a number of senile plaques.

(c) An important decrease in the number of somatostatin cell bodies and fibres in the lateral septi nuclei and of the fibres in the medial septi nuclei was noted.

(d) There was an increase in the immunoreactive intensity of the somatostatin-positive fibres in the substantia innominata.

7.8.2 Substance P

(a) There was a significant increase in substance P immunoreactive intensity in the globus pallidus and in the substantia nigra.

(b) An important reduction in the number of the substance P fibres and terminals in the hippocampus, mainly in the molecular layer of the fascia dentata and the stratum moleculare, was seen.

From the present review, it can be concluded that a variety of neurotransmitters are altered in the Alzheimer's disease brain. A great number of them are certainly altered by the loss of neurons and the dysfunction in the interaction of the multiple neurotransmitter systems, which is partly responsible for the cognitive and behavioural disturbances in this neurological disorder. On the other hand, the diverse functional interactions in the brain within the various neurotransmitter systems, as was suggested between acetylcholine and somatostatin, seem to be very important. Moreover, some of these neurotransmitters may play a role in the pathogenesis of the Alzheimer's disease.

References

Adolfsson, R., Gottfries, C. G., Roos, B. E., and Winblad, B. (1979). Changes in brain catecholamines in patients with dementia of Alzheimer type. *Brit. J. Psychiat.*, 135, 216–23.

Adrian, T. E., Allen, J. M., Bloom, S. R., Ghatei, M. A., Rosser, M. N., Roberts, G. W., Crow, T. J., Tatemoto, K., and Polak, J. M. (1983). Neuropeptide Y distribution in the human brain. *Nature (Lond.)*, 306, 584–6.

Agid, Y., Ruberg, M., Dubois, B., and Javoy-Agid, F. (1983). Biochemical substrates of mental disturbances in Parkinson's disease. *Adv. Neurol.*, 40, 211–18.

Allen, J. M., Ferrier, I. N., Roberts, G. W., Cross, A. J., Adrian, T. E., Crow, T. J., and Bloom, S. R. (1984). Elevation of neuropeptide Y (NPY) in substantia innominata in Alzheimer's type dementia. *J. neurol. Sci.*, 64, 324–31.

Arai, H., Moroji, T., and Kosaka, K. (1984). Somatostatin and vasoactive intestinal polypeptide in postmortem brains from patients with Alzheimer-type dementia. *Neurosci. Lett.*, 52, 73–8.

Argentiero, V., and Tavolato, B. (1980). Dopamine (DA) and serotonin levels in the cerebrospinal fluid (CSF) in Alzheimer's presenile dementia, under basic conditions and after stimulation with cerebral cortex phospholipids. *J. Neurol.*, 224, 53–8.

Armstrong, D., LeRoy, S., Shields, D., and Terry, R. D. (1985). Somatostatin-like immuno-reactivity within neuritic plaques. *Brain Res.*, **338**, 71-9.

Bartholini, G., Lloyd, K. G., Worms, J., Constantinidis, J., and Tissot, R. (1979). GABA and GABAergic medication: relation to striatal dopamine function and Parkinsonism. In Poirier, L. J. *et al.*, (eds), *Advances in Neurology, Vol. 24*. Raven Press, New. York, p. 253.

Bartus, R. T., Dean, R. L., Beer, B., and Lippa, A. S. (1982). The cholinergic hypothesis of geriatric memory dysfunction. *Science*, **217**, 408-17.

Benton, J. S., Bowen, D. M., Allen, S. J., Haan, E. A., Davison, A. N., Neary, D., Murphy, R. P., and Snowden, J. S. (1982). Alzheimer's disease as a disorder of isodendritic core. *Lancet*, i, 456.

Berger, B. (1984). Anomalies des neurotransmitteurs dans la maladie d'Alzheimer. *Rev. Neurol (Paris)*, **140**, (10), 539-52.

Berger, B., Tassin, J. P., Rancurel, G., and Blanc, G. (1980). Catecholaminergic innervation of the human cerebral cortex in presenile and senile dementia. Histochemical and bio-chemical studies. In Usdin, E., Sourkes, T. L., and Youdim, M. G. H. (eds.), *Enzymes and Neurotransmitters in Mental Disease*. John Wiley & Sons, Chichester, pp. 317-28.

Bird, E. D., and Iversen, L. L. (1974). Huntington's chorea: post-mortem measurement of glutamic acid decarboxylase, choline acetyltransferase and dopamine in basal ganglia. *Brain*, **94**, 457-72.

Bondareff, W., Mountjoy, C. Q., and Roth, M. (1982). Loss of neurons of origin of the adrenergic projections to cerebral cortex (nucleus locus coeruleus) in senile dementia. *Neurobiology*, **32**, 164-8.

Bouras, C., and Constantinidis, J. (1984a). VIP distribution in the human brain (an immuno-histochemical study by fluorescence microscopy). *Collegium Internationale Neuro-Psychopharmacologicum, 14th Congress*, Florence, Italy, June 19-23. Book of Abstracts, Fidia Research Biomedical Information, P-348, 663.

Bouras, C., and Constantinidis, J. (1984b). Cholecystokinin distribution in the human brain (an immunohistochemical study by fluorescence microscopy). *Collegium Internationale Neuro-Psychopharmacologicum, 14th Congress*, Florence, Italy, June 19-23. Book of Abstracts, Fidia Research Biomedical Information, P-169, 485.

Bouras, C., Guntern, R., and Constantinidis, J. (1985). Somatostatin distribution in the human brain (An immunohistochemical study). In Moody, T. W., (ed.), *Neural and Endocrine Peptides and Receptors, 5th International Spring Symposium, Abstract Vol.*, Washington, Abstract No 108.

Bouras, C., Guntern, R., and Constantinidis, J. (1986). Somatostatin in dementias of Alzheimer type. In Burrows, G. D., and Norman, T. R. (eds.), *Clinical and Pharmaco-logical Studies in Psychiatric Disorders*, John Libbey, London, 293-305.

Bouras, C., Taban, C. H., and Constantinidis, J. (1984). Mapping of enkephalins in human brain. An immunohistofluorescence study on brains from patients with senile and presenile dementia. *Neuroscience*, **12** (1), 179-90.

Carlsson, A., and Winblad, B. (1976). Influence of age and time interval between death and autopsy on dopamine and 3-methoxytyramine levels in human basal ganglia. *J. neural Transm.*, **38**, 271-6.

Carlsson, A., Adolfsson, R., Aquilonius, S. M., Gottfries, C. G., Oreland, L., Svennerholm, L., and Winblad, B. (1980). Biogenic amines in human brain in normal aging, senile dementia and chronic alcoholism. In Goldstein, M., *et al.* (eds.), *Ergot Compounds and Brain Function Neuroendocrine and Neuropsychiatric Aspects*. Raven Press, New York, 295-305.

Chronwall, B. M., Chase, T. N., and O'Donohue, T. L. (1984). Coexistence of neuropeptide Y and somatostatin in rat and human cortical and rat hypothalamic neurons. *Neurosci. Lett.*, **52**, 213-17.

Constantinidis, J. (1979). Zinc metabolism in presenile dementias. In Glen, A. I. M., and Whalley, L. J. (eds.), *Alzheimer's Disease. Early recognition of potentially reversible deficits*. Churchill Livingstone, Edinburgh, London and New York, pp. 48-49.

Constantinidis, J. (1982). Neurotransmitter alterations in degenerative aging brain. *Third International Meeting of the International Society for Developmental Neuroscience*, Patra (Greece), Program and Abstract, p. 72.

Constantinidis, J. (1983). Neuromédiateurs et démences de l'âge avancé. *Confrontations psychiatriques (Paris), 16ème année, No 22 Les Neuromédiateurs*, pp. 403–46.

Constantinidis, J. (1984). Acetylcholine, glutamate, GABA and neuropeptides in senile dementia of Alzheimer type. In Wertheimer, J. and Marois, M. (eds.), *Senile Dementia: Outlook for the Future*. Alan Liss Inc., New York, pp. 55–68.

Constantinidis, J., and Tissot, R. (1979). Plaques séniles, dégénérescences neurofibrillaires et autres lésions cérébrales associées. *Arch. Suisses Neurol. Neurochirg. Psychiat.*, 124, (2), 317–33.

Constantinidis, J., and Tissot, R. (1981). Role of glutamate and zinc in the hippocampal lesions of Pick's disease. In Di Chiara, G. and Gessa, G. L. (eds.), *Glutamate as Neurotransmitter*, Advances in Biochemical Pharmacology, vol. 27. Raven Press, New York, pp. 413–22.

Constantinidis, J., Richard, J., and De Ajuriaguerra, J. (1978). Dementias with senile plaques and neurofibrillary tangles. In Isaaks, A. D., and Post, F. (eds.), *Studies in Geriatric Psychiatry*, John Wiley & Sons, London and New York, pp. 119–52.

Coons, A. H. (1958). Fluorescent antibody methods. In Danielli, J. G. F. (ed.), *General Cytochemical Methods*, Acad. Press, New York, pp. 399–422.

Cote, L. J., and Kremzner, L. T. (1974). Changes in neurotransmitter systems with increasing age in human brain. *Trans. Am. Soc. Neuroch.*, 5, 83.

Coyle, J. T., Price, D. L., and Delong, M. R. (1983). Alzheimer's disease: a disorder of cortical cholinergic innervation. *Science*, 219, 1184–90.

Cross, A. J., Crow, T. J., Ferrier, I. N., Johnson, J. A., Bloom, S. R., and Corsellis, J. A. N. (1984a). Serotonin receptor changes in dementia of the Alzheimer type. *J. Neurochem.*, 43, 1574–81.

Cross, A. J., Crow, T. J., Johnson, J. A., Perry, E. K., Perry, R. H., Blessed, G., and Tomlinson, B. E. (1984b). Studies on neurotransmitter receptor sytems in neocortex and hippocampus in senile dementia of the Alzheimer-type. *J. neurol. Sci.*, 64, 109–17.

Cross, A. J., Crow, T. J.. Johnson, J. A., Joseph, M. H., Perry, E. K., Perry, R. H., Blessed, G. and Tomlinson, B. E. (1983). Monoamine metabolism in senile dementia of Alzheimer type. *J. neurol. Sci.*, 60, 383–92.

Crystal, H. A. and Davies, P. (1982). Cortical substance P-like immunoreactivity in cases of Alzheimer's disease and senile dementia of the Alzheimer type. *J. Neurochem.*, 38, 1781–4.

Davies, P. (1979). Neurotransmitter-related enzymes on senile dementia of the Alzheimer type. *Brain Res.*, 171, 319–27.

Davies, P. and Terry, R. D. (1981). Cortical somatostatin-like immunoreactivity in cases of Alzheimer's disease and senile dementia of the Alzheimer type. *Neurobiol. Ageing.*, 2, 9–14,

Davies, P., Katz, D. A., and Crystal, H. A. (1982). Choline acetyltransferase, somatostatin and substance P in selected cases of Alzheimer's disease. In Corkin, S., Davies, K. L., Growdon, J. H., Usdin, E., and Wurtman, R. J. (eds.), *Alzheimer's Disease: A Report of Progress in Research*, Aging Vol. 19, Raven Press, New York, pp. 9–14.

Davis, K. L., Mohs, R. C., Davis, B. M., Horvath, T. B., Greenwald, B. S., Rosen, W. G., Levy, M. I., and Johns, C. A. (1983). Oral physostigmine in Alzheimer's disease. *Psychopharmacol. Bull.*, 19, 451–3.

Eckenstein, F., and Baughman, R. W. (1984). Two types of cholinergic innervation in cortex, one co-localized with vasoactive intestinal polypeptide. *Nature*, 309, 153–5.

Emson, P. C. (1979). Peptides as neurotransmitter candidates in the mammalian CNS. *Progr. Neurobiol.*, 13, 61–116.

Epelbaum, J., Ruberg, M., Moyse, E., Javoy-Agid, F., Dubois, B. and Agid, Y. (1983). Somatostatin and dementia in Parkinson's disease. *Brain Res.*, 278, 376–9.

Fahrenkrug, Y., and Schaffalittky de Muckadell, O. B. (1978). Radio-immunoassay of vasoactive intestinal polypeptide (VIP) in plasma. *J. Lab. clin. Med.*, 89, 1379–88.

Ferrier, I. N., Cross, A. J., Johnson, J. A., Roberts, G. W., Crow, T. J., Corsellis, J. A. N., Lee, Y. C., O'Shaughnessy, D., Adrian, T. E., McGregor, G. P., Baracese-Hamilton, A. J., and Bloom, S. R. (1983). Neuropeptides in Alzheimer type dementia. *J. neurol. Sci.*, 62, 159–70.

Feuerstein, C. (1984). Aspects biologiques: l'atteinte des grands systèmes, les systèmes peptidergiques. In *Maladie de Type Alzheimer et Autres Démences Séniles*. Actes du Colloque des 30 et 31.1.84, Paris, Fondation Nationale de Gérontologie, Groupe d'Etudes et de Recherches sur la démence sénile. pp. 47–56.

Flood, J. F., Smith, G. E., and Cherkin, A. (1985). Memory enhancement: supra–additive effect of subcutaneous cholinergic drug combinations in mice. *Psychopharmacology*, 86, 61–7.

Gottfries, C. G., Gottfries, I., and Roos, B. E. (1969). Homovanillic acid and 5-hydroxy-indoleacetic acid in the cerebrospinal fluid of patients with senile dementia, presenile dementia and parkinsonism. *J. Neurochem.*, 16, 1341–9.

Grafe, M. R., Forno, L. S., and Eng, L. F. (1985). Immunocytochemical studies of substance P and Met-Enkephalin in the basal ganglia and substantia nigra in Huntington's Parkinson's and Alzheimer's diseases. *J. Neuropath. exp. Neurol.*, 44, 47–59.

Iversen, L. L., Rossor, M. N., Reynolds, G. P., Huis, R., Roth, M., Mountjoy, C. Q., Foote, S. L., Morrison, J. H., and Bloom, F. E. (1983). Loss of pigmented dopamine-β-hydroxylase positive cells from locus coeruleus in senile dementia of Alzheimer's type. *Neurosci. Lett.*, 39, 95–100.

Javoy-Agid, F., Taquet, H., Gesselin, F., Epelbaum, J., Grouselle, G., Mauborgne, A., Studler, J. M., and Agid, Y. (1984). Neuropeptides in Parkinson's disease. In Usdin, E. (ed.), *Proceedings of the 5th International Catecholamine Symposium*, Göteborg, June 1983, Catecholamines, Alan R. Liss Inc., New York.

Larsson, L. I., and Rehfeld, Y. F. (1979). Localization and molecular heterogenicity of cholecystokinin in central and peripheral nervous system. *Brain Res.*, 165, 201–18.

Lundberg, J. M., Hökfelt, T., Schultzberg, M., Uväs-Wallenstein, K., Kohler, C., and Said, S. I. (1979). Occurrence of VIP-like immunoreactivity in certain cholinergic neurons of the cat: evidence from combined immunohistochemistry and acetylcholinesterase staining. *Neurosci.*, 4, 1539–45.

McGeer, E. G., and McGeer, P. L. (1976). Neurotransmitter metabolism in the aging brain. In Terry, R. D., and Gershon, S. (eds.), *Neurobiology of Aging*, Aging Vol. 3. Raven Press, New York, pp. 389–403.

Malthe-Sorenssen, D., Wood, P. L., Cheney, D. L., and Costa, E. (1978). Modulation of the turnover rate of acetylcholine in rat brain by intraventricular injections of thyrotropin-releasing hormone, somatostatin, neurotensin and angiotensin II. *J. Neurochem.*, 31, 685–91.

Mann, D. M. A., and Yates, P. O. (1983). Serotonin nerve cells in Alzheimer's disease. *J. Neurol. Neurosurg. Psychiat.*, 46, 96–8.

Mann, D. M. A., Yates, P. O., and Hawkes, J. (1982). The noradrenergic system in Alzheimer and multiinfarct dementias. *J. Neurol. Neurosurg. Psychiat.*, 45, 113–19.

Marcusson, J., Oreland, L., and Winblad, B. (1984). Effect of age on human brain serotonin (S-1) binding sites. *J. Neurochem.*, 43, 1699–705.

Morrison, J. H., Benoit, R., Magistretti, P. J., and Bloom, F. E. (1983). Immunohisto-chemical distribution of pro-somatostatin-related peptides in cerebral cortex. *Brain Res.*, 262, 344–51.

Morrison, J. H., Rogers, J., Scherr, S., Benoit, R., and Bloom, F. E. (1985). Somatostatin immunoreactivity in neuritic plaques of Alzheimer's patients. *Nature*, 314, 90–2.

Pearce, B. R., Palmer, A. M., Bowen, D. M., Wilcock, G. K., Esiri, M. M., and Davison, A. N. (1984). Neurotransmitter dysfunction and atrophy of the caudate nucleus in Alzheimer's disease. *Neurochem. Pathol.*, 2, 221–32.

Perry, R. H., Dockray, G. J., Dimaline, R., Perry, E. K., Blessed, G., and Tomlinson, B. E. (1981). Neuropeptides in Alzheimer's Disease – Depression and Schizophrenia. *J. neurol. Sci.*, 51, 465–72.

Perry, R. H., Candy, J. M., Perry, E. K., Irving, D., Blessed, G., Fairbairn, A. F., and Tomlinson, B. E. (1982). Extensive loss of choline acetyltransferase activity is not reflected by neuronal loss in the nucleus of Meynert in Alzheimer's disease. *Neurosci. Lett.*, 33, 311–15.

Reisine, T. D., Yamamura, H. I., Bird, E. D., Spokes, E., and Enna, S. J. (1978). Pre- and post-synaptic neurochemical alterations in Alzheimer's disease. *Brain Res.*, 159, 477–82.

Roberts, E., Chase, T. N., and Tower, D. B. (eds.) (1975). *GABA in Nervous System Function*. Raven Press, New York.

Rossor, M. N., and Emson, P. C. (1982). Neuropeptides in degenerative disease of the central nervous system. *Trends in Neurosci.*, 11, 399–401.

Rossor, M. N., Emson, P. C., Mountjoy, C. Q., Roth, M., and Iversen, L. L. (1980a). Reduced amounts of immunoreactive somatostatin in the temporal cortex in senile dementia of Alzheimer type. *Neurosci. Lett.*, 20, 373–7.

Rossor, M. N., Fahrenkrug, J., Emson, P. C., Mountjoy, C. W., Iversen, L. L., and Roth, M. (1980b). Reduced cortical choline acetyltransferase activity in senile dementia of Alzheimer's type is not accompanied by changes in vasoactive intestinal polypeptide. *Brain Res.*, 201, 249–53.

Rossor, M. N., Garrett, N. J., Johnson, A. L., Mountjoy, C. Q., Roth, M., and Iversen, J. L. (1982a). A post-mortem study of the cholinergic and GABA systems in senile dementia. *Brain*, 105, 313–30.

Rossor, M. N., Svendsen, S., Hunt, S. P., Mountjoy, C. Q., Roth, M., and Iversen, L. L. (1982b). The substantia innominata in Alzheimer's disease: an histochemical and biochemical study of cholinergic marker enzymes. *Neurosci. Lett.*, 28, 217–22.

Sagar, S. M., Flintbeal, M., Marshall, P. E., Landis, D., and Martin, J. (1984). Implications of neuropeptides in neurological diseases, *Peptides*, 5, pp. 255–62.

Sakamoto, N., Takatsuji, K., Shiosaka, S., Tateishi, K., Hashimura, E., Miura, S., Hamaoka, T., and Tohyama, M. (1984). Cholecystokinin-8-like immunoreactivity in the pre- and post-central gyri of the human cerebral cortex. *Brain Res.*, 307, 77–83.

Schmechel, D. E., Vickrey, B. G., Fitzpatrick, D., and Elde, R. P. (1984). Gabaergic neurons of mammalian cerebral cortex: widespread subclass defined by somatostatin content. *Neurosci. Lett.*, 47, 227–32.

Serby, M., Angrist, B., Corwin, J., Funari, D., Sudilovsky, A., Siekierski, J., Peselow, E. and Rotrosen, J. (1984). Cholecystokinin octapeptide in dementia. *Psychopharmacol. Bull.*, 20 (3), 546–7.

Sims, N. R., Bowen, D. M., Allen, S. J., Smith, C. C. T., Neary, D., Thomas, D. J., and Davison, A. M. (1983). Presynaptic cholinergic dysfunction in patients with dementia. *J. Neurochem.*, 40, 503–9.

Smith, C. C. T., Bowen, D. M., Sims, N. R., Neary, D., and Davison, A. (1983). Amino-acid release from biopsy samples of temporal neocortex from patients with Alzheimer's disease. *Brain Res.*, 264, 138–41.

Struble, R. G., Gork, L. C., Whitehouse, P. J., and Price, D. L. (1982). Cholinergic innervation in neuritic plaques. *Science*, 216, 413–15.

Tagliavini, F., and Pilleri, G. (1983). Basal nucleus of Meynert. A neuropathological study in Alzheimer's disease, simple senile dementia, Pick's disease and Huntington's chorea. *J. neurol. Sci.*, 62, 243–60.

Tarbit, I., Perry, E. K., Perry, P. H., Blessed, G., and Tomlinson, B. E. (1980). Hippocampal free aminoacids in Alzheimer's disease. *J. Neurochem.*, 35, 1246.

Thal, L. J., Fuld, P. A., Masur, D. M., Sharpless, N. S., and Davies, P. (1983). Oral physostigmine and lecithin improve memory in Alzheimer's disease. *Psychopharmacol. Bull.*, 19 (3), 454–6.

Tomlinson, B. E., Irving, D., and Blessed, G. (1981). Cell loss in the locus coeruleus in senile dementia of Alzheimer type. *J. neurol. Sci.*, 49, 419–28.

Whitehouse, P. J., Price, D. L., Clark, A. W., Coyle, J. T., and DeLong, M. R. (1981). Alzheimer disease: Evidence for selective loss of cholinergic neurons in the nucleus basalis. *Ann. Neurol.*, 10 (1), 122–6.

Whitehouse, P. J., Price, D. L., Clark, A. W., Coyle, J. T., and DeLong, M. R. (1982). Alzheimer's disease and senile dementia: loss of neurons in the basal forebrain. *Science*, 215, 1237–9.

Wikkelso, C., Fahrenkrug, J., Blomstrand, C., and Johansson, B. B. (1985). Dementia of different etiologies: vasoactive intestinal polypeptide in CSF. *Neurology*, 35, 592–5.

Wisniewsky, H. M., and Terry, R. D. (1976). Neuropathology of the aging brain. In Terry, R. D., and Gershon, S. (eds.), *Neurobiology of Aging*. Raven Press, New York, pp. 265–80.

Yates, C. M., Simpson, J., Maloney, A. J. F., Gordon, A., and Reid, A. H. (1980). Alzheimer-like cholinergic deficiency in Down syndrome. *Lancet*, ii, 979.

Yates, C. M., Simpson, J., Gordon, A., Maloney, A. J. F., Allison, V., Ritche, I. M., and

Urguhjart, A. (1983a). Catecholamines and cholinergic enzymes in the presenile and senile Alzheimer-type dementia and Down's syndrome. *Brain Res.*, **280**, 119–26.

Yates, C. M., Harmar, A. J., Rosie, R., Sheward, J., Sanchez de Levy, G., Simpson, J., Maloney, A. F. J., Gordow, A., and Fink, G. (1983b). Thyrotropin-releasing hormone, luteinizing hormone-releasing hormone and substance P immunoreactivity in post-mortem brain from cases of Alzheimer type dementia and Down's syndrome. *Brain Res.*, **258**, 45–52.

8

Serotonin Neurones and Receptors in Alzheimer's Disease

D. N. Middlemiss, D. M. Bowen and A. M. Palmer

8.1 Introduction

Recent research into the senile and presenile dementias (collectively termed Alzheimer's disease) has concentrated on deficits in the cholinergic system (*see*, for example, Perry and Perry, 1980; Rossor, 1982; Sims and Bowen, 1983), and there is much circumstantial and direct evidence to link the cholinergic deficit with the cognitive deterioration seen in this disease (Perry *et al.*, 1978; Drachman, 1981; Francis *et al.*, 1985). Nevertheless, there are selective deficits in other neurotransmitter pathways in Alzheimer's disease and, in particular, losses of somatostatin-containing cells and ascending aminergic pathways have been reported (for a recent review *see* Hardy *et al.*, 1985). The relationship of these changes in non-cholinergic neurones to the cognitive and behavioural deterioration seen in Alzheimer's disease is not yet understood but it would be surprising if the changes seen in aminergic pathways were not in some way related to aspects of the personality changes manifested in this disease (Semple *et al.*, 1982).

The purpose of this review is to examine the evidence for changes in one facet of the aminergic system, that of serotonin (5-hydroxytryptamine, 5-HT), in Alzheimer's disease. In addition, we report on new radioligand binding studies in Alzheimer brain which confirm and extend previous studies of the 5-HT$_1$ recognition site in this disease to the recently delineated subtypes of this site.

8.2 5-HT Neurones in Alzheimer's Disease

Studies of the cholinergic system in Alzheimer's disease have been markedly advanced by the possibility of studying the enzymes of synthesis and breakdown of acetylcholine in post-mortem tissue. In the serotonergic system, work has been hampered by an inability to demonstrate tryptophan hydroxylase in postmortem samples (McGeer and McGeer, 1981). Studies of the neurochemical aspects of the serotonergic system have, therefore, concentrated on the measurement of the amount of 5-HT and its principal metabolite 5-hydroxyindoleacetic acid (5-HIAA). A number of recent post-mortem studies have been published which, in general, confirm studies (Adolfsson *et al.*, 1979; Bowen *et al.*, 1979) which indicate a drop in either 5-HT or 5-HIAA levels in Alzheimer's disease (Table 8.1). These reductions in markers of serotonergic neurones have been demonstrated in both clinically diagnosed and histologically verified Alzheimer's disease. The losses appear to be widespread in both cortical and subcortical regions but are smaller in magnitude and less consistent than those seen in the cholinergic system as indicated by changes in choline acetyltransferase activity (Table 8.1). These post-mortem studies are complemented by a number of reports of lowered 5-HIAA in the CSF of patients with histologically diagnosed

Table 8.1 Changes in 5-HT neurochemistry in selected brain areas in Alzheimer's disease

Brain region	ChAT activity	5-HT levels	5-HIAA levels	References
Temporal cortex	–	–	46	Cross *et al.* (1983)
	47	–	49	Cross *et al.* (1984a)
	41	52	82	Francis *et al.* (1985)
	–	–	46	Crow *et al.* (1984)
	34	51	87 (NS)	Middlemiss *et al.* (1986)
Frontal cortex	58	–	55	Cross *et al.* (1984a)
	–	81 (NS)	85 (NS)	Reynolds *et al.* (1984)
	–	–	67	Crow *et al.* (1984)
	47	75 (NS)	99 (NS)	Middlemiss *et al.* (1986)
Hippocampus	–	–	70	Cross *et al.* (1983)
	–	83 (NS)	71	Adolfsson *et al.* (1979)
	53	22	64	Carlsson *et al.* (1980)
	58	21	110 (NS)	Gottfries *et al.* (1983)
	–	44 (NS)	56 (NS)	Arai *et al.* (1984)
	53	–	51	Cross *et al.* (1984a)
	–	–	70	Crow *et al.* (1984)
Caudate nucleus	55	49	87 (NS)	Carlsson *et al.* (1980)
	62	62	115 (NS)	Gottfries *et al.* (1983)
	–	44 (NS)	54	Arai *et al.* (1984)
	–	–	117 (NS)	Cross *et al.* (1984a)

Results are expressed as % of corresponding control levels.
– = Not determined. NS = Not significantly different from corresponding controls.

Alzheimer's disease (Palmer *et al.*, 1984) as well as in clinically suspected samples (Gottfries *et al.*, 1969; Gottfries and Roos, 1973; Gottfries *et al.*, 1974; Soininen *et al.*, 1981), although this reduction is not a universal finding (Bareggi *et al.*, 1982; Wood *et al.*, 1982; Kay *et al.*, 1984).

The tendency towards reductions in both 5-HT and 5-HIAA in Alzheimer's disease suggests that the 5-HT nerve terminal undergoes degeneration in this disease. This interpretation is strengthened by studies which show a drop in another index of presynaptic 5-HT function, that is in the energy-dependent 5-HT uptake system. Thus, in neurosurgical specimens from the temporal cortex, 5-HT uptake was reduced to 28 % of control levels (Bowen *et al.*, 1983). In the same study, utilising autopsy material, the binding of (^{3}H)imipramine to the 5-HT carrier (Rehavi *et al.*, 1980) was reduced to an average of 77 % of control. Cell loss and neurofibrillary tangle formation within the raphé nucleus (Ishii, 1966; Yamada and Mehraein, 1977; Mann and Yates, 1983; Mann *et al.*, 1984; Curcio and Kemper, 1984) support the idea that the 5-HT neuroterminal has degenerated in Alzheimer's disease. The cell loss in the raphe nuclei is not as great as in the nucleus basalis or in the locus coeruleus (Mann *et al.*, 1984).

8.3 5-HT Receptor Sites in Alzheimer's Disease

In addition to the neurochemical approaches alluded to above there have been a number of studies in Alzheimer's disease of the various 5-HT receptor subtypes present in the brain. These have been considerably aided by the advent of the technique of receptor binding and the availability of selective radioligands for the detection of these receptors. Receptor binding studies utilising rat cortical membranes led to a classification of central 5-HT receptors which recognises two main subclasses of receptor, defined as 5-HT$_1$ (labelled by (^{3}H)5-HT) and 5-HT$_2$ (labelled by (^{3}H)spiperone and, more recently (^{3}H)ketanserin) (Peroutka and Snyder, 1979). The published studies in Alzheimer's disease utilising these ligands are summarised in Table 8.2 and extend and confirm data from an earlier study (Bowen *et al.*, 1979) which shows reduced cortical binding of (^{3}H)lysergic acid diethylamide. The losses seen in the binding of these radioligands to their recognition sites in Alzheimer brain are more consistent and widespread than those seen in the neurochemical markers discussed above and are probably related to a change in receptor number rather than in affinity (Cross *et al.*, 1984a,b; Cross *et al.*, 1986; Reynolds *et al.*, 1984). The potencies of a range of serotonergic drugs in displacing these ligands from binding sites in rat and human cortex are closely similar (Cross *et al.*, 1984a), which is consistent with the interpretation that the recognition sites in both species are the same. Since animal studies indicate that both the 5-HT$_1$ and 5-HT$_2$ recognition sites are located predominantly postsynaptically (Middlemiss, 1982), these receptor binding studies in Alzheimer's disease may indicate that losses in postsynaptic 5-HT function accompany the changes in presynaptic function discussed above.

Table 8.2   Changes in 5-HT$_1$ and 5-HT$_2$ recognition sites in Alzheimer's disease

Brain region	ChAT activity	5-HT$_1$ binding	5-HT$_2$ binding	References
Temporal cortex	48	69	–	Bowen et al. (1983)
	–	54	36	Cross et al. (1984a)
	–	70	66	Cross et al. (1984b)
	–	87 (NS)	57	Cross et al. (1986)
	34	68	–	This study
Frontal cortex	–	53	–	Bowen et al. (1983)
	–	85 (NS)	54	Cross et al. (1984a)
	–	77	71	Cross et al. (1984b)
	–	–	58	Reynolds et al. (1984)
	47	64	–	This study
Hippocampus	–	60	67 (NS)	Cross et al. (1984a)
	–	56	38	Cross et al. (1984b)
Entorhinal cortex	19	–	42	Perry et al. (1984)
Parietal cortex	–	74	65 (NS)	Perry et al. (1984)

Results are expressed as % of corresponding control levels.
– = Not determined. NS = Not significantly different from corresponding controls.

8.4   Subtypes of 5-HT$_1$ Receptors in Alzheimer's Disease

Although the original hypothesis by Peroutka and Snyder (1979), that central 5-HT receptors can be divided into two main classes, has received much experimental support, it is now recognised that this classification is an oversimplification and that there are likely to be at least three, and probably more, 5-HT receptor types in the brain (Middlemiss, 1982). Several of these receptors can now be identified by radioligand binding studies and, in particular, it has become evident that the 5-HT$_1$ recognition site has at least two components, denoted 5-HT$_{1A}$ and 5-HT$_{1B}$ respectively (Pedigo et al., 1981; Engel et al., 1983; Schnellmann et al., 1984). The 5-HT$_{1A}$ site can be selectively labelled with the 5-HT$_{1A}$ agonist 8-hydroxy-2-(di-n-propylamino)tetralin (8-OH-DPAT) (Gozlan et al., 1983; Middlemiss and Fozard, 1983; Marcinkiewicz et al., 1984; Middlemiss, 1985). The high affinity and selectivity of the neuroleptic drug spiperone for the 5-HT$_{1A}$ site allows the identification of the 5-HT$_{1B}$ site if (^{3}H)5-HT receptor binding studies are carried out in the presence of a concentration of spiperone sufficient to saturate the 5-HT$_{1A}$ sites (Middlemiss and Fozard, 1983). Since the subtypes of the 5-HT$_1$ recognition site have not been examined in Alzheimer's disease we have carried out radioligand binding studies on post-mortem tissue utilising (^{3}H)8-OH-DPAT and (^{3}H)5-HT to label the 5-HT$_{1A}$ sites and (3H)5-HT in the presence of spiperone to label the 5-HT$_{1B}$ sites.

Brain tissue for the study was taken post-mortem from patients with a clinical and histologically verified diagnosis of Alzheimer's disease. Tissue for neurochemical investigations was frozen, dissected and stored as described by Bowen *et al.* (1983). Tissue from Brodmann area 21 pooled with 22 (temporal cortex) and 9 pooled with 46 (frontal cortex) were used in these investigations.

Radioligand binding studies on membranes prepared from both human and rat cortex were carried out as described in detail by Middlemiss and Fozard (1983) and Middlemiss *et al.* (1986). Tissue was homogenised in Tris-HCl buffer, centrifuged to pellet down the membranes, and the pellet washed twice and then incubated at 37 °C to remove endogenous 5-HT. The final pellet was suspended in Tris-HCl buffer containing 10 μmol/l pargyline, 5.7 mmol/l $CaCl_2$ and 0.1 % ascorbic acid, and radioligand binding studies were carried out in this buffer. Incubations (37 °C, 15 min) were terminated by rapid filtration through GF/B filters. The concentrations of radioligands used in the determination of the affinity of various drugs for the (^{3}H)8-OH-DPAT and 5-HT$_{1B}$ recognition sites were 1 and 2 nmol/l, respectively. In order to process the large number of samples investigated in Alzheimer patients and to use the minimum amount of tissue, a full kinetic analysis was not, in general, undertaken but binding at two concentrations of radioligand was performed. This permitted assessment of whether the total number of binding sites changed, while controlling for any variation in binding density brought about by changes in the apparent K_d of the receptor. This would be reflected by a perturbation in the ratio between ligand binding at the two concentrations (Reynolds *et al.*, 1984). The radio-ligand concentrations used for 5-HT$_1$, 5-HT$_{1A}$ and 5-HT$_{1B}$ receptors were 2 and 8 nmol/l (^{3}H)5-HT; 8-OH-DPAT binding was performed with 1 and 4 nmol/l (^{3}H)8-OH-DPAT. 5-HT$_{1A}$ binding was defined as the difference between total binding and that displaced by 1 μmol/l spiperone (Pedigo *et al.*, 1981). 5-HT$_{1B}$ binding was the residual specific binding in the presence of 1 μmol/l spiperone. Non-specific binding was defined using 10 μmol/l 5-HT. Protein was measured by the method of Lowry *et al.* (1951).

(^{3}H)8-OH-DPAT bound to a saturable site in the neocortex from control patients (Fig. 8.1). The K_d value in three subjects was 2.1 ± 1.2 nmol/l, which is close to the value found in rat frontal cortex for this ligand (1.7 ± 1.3 nmol/l (Middlemiss, 1985)). The potency of a number of serotonergic agonists and antagonists of widely differing structure was determined for both the (^{3}H)8-OH-DPAT and the 5-HT$_{1B}$ recognition sites in rat and human cortex. The data, which are given in Table 8.3, indicate that these sites have the expected pharmacological profile of these two putative 5-HT receptors and that there are essentially no differences between the two species.

Figures 8.2 and 8.3 show the changes which were found in the various 5-HT recognition sites in the two brain areas examined. The 5-HT$_1$ recognition site was reduced in both temporal (to 64 % of control) and frontal cortex (to 60 % of control). When total 5-HT$_1$ binding was broken down into the two subtypes of this site, both the 5-HT$_{1A}$ and 5-HT$_{1B}$ recognition sites were significantly reduced in the frontal cortex but a statistically significant fall was confined to the 5-HT$_{1B}$ site in the temporal cortex.

The reduction in 5-HT$_{1A}$ binding in the frontal cortex was confirmed by a

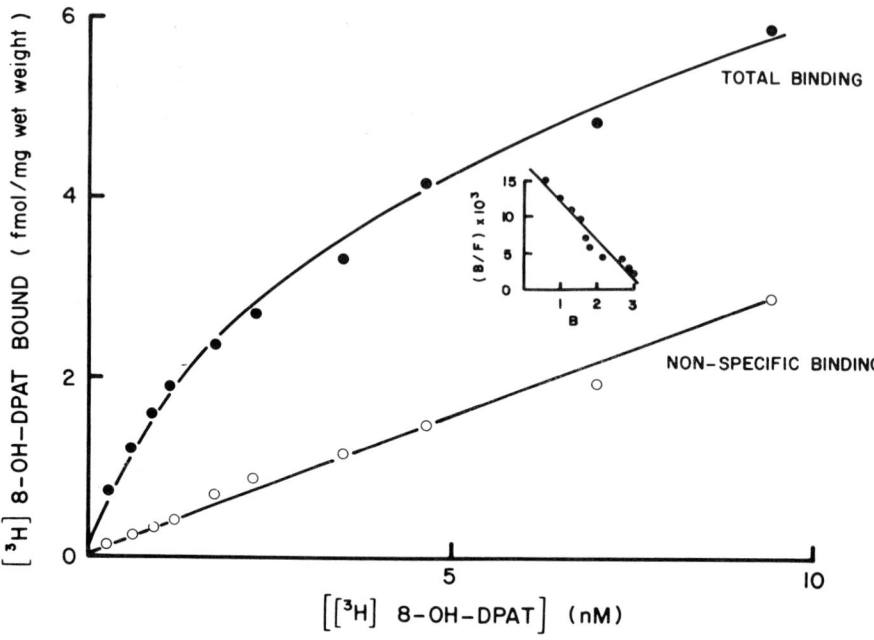

Fig. 8.1 The binding of (^{3}H)8-OH-DPAT to membranes from human neocortex. Receptor binding studies were carried out using human neocortex membranes as described in the text. The figure, taken from a typical experiment, represents total and non-specifically bound (^{3}H)8-OH-DPAT as a function of the free concentration of the radioligand. The inset shows a Scatchard transformation of the data.

Table 8.3   The pharmacological profile of human and rat cortex (^{3}H)8-OH-DPAT and 5-HT$_{1B}$ recognition sites

Drug	(^{3}H)8-OH-DPAT pIC$_{50}$		5-HT$_{1B}$ pIC$_{50}$	
	Human	Rat	Human	Rat
5-HT	8.29 ± 0.03	8.15 ± 0.02	8.27 ± 0.09	7.78 ± 0.14
8-OH-DPAT	8.65 ± 0.07	8.52 ± 0.06	6.59 ± 0.19	5.42 ± 0.08
Spiperone	6.84 ± 0.03	6.90 ± 0.11	5.19 ± 0.27	4.82 ± 0.12
Methiothepin	7.19 ± 0.05	7.06 ± 0.04	6.29 ± 0.28	6.49 ± 0.02
Ketanserin	5.35 ± 0.03	5.20 ± 0.06	4.92 ± 0.23	4.66 ± 0.14
(−)-propranolol	6.76 ± 0.19	6.84 ± 0.05	−	6.31 ± 0.10
(+)-propranolol	5.51 ± 0.10	5.45 ± 0.06	−	5.38 ± 0.08
Buspirone	7.44 ± 0.10	7.52 ± 0.10	<5	<5
MDL 72222	<5	<5	<5	<5

Results are expressed as pIC$_{50}$ values (which is $-\log_{10}$ of the concentration of drug needed to inhibit specific binding by 50 %). Results are the mean ± S.E.M. of 3–5 independent experiments.

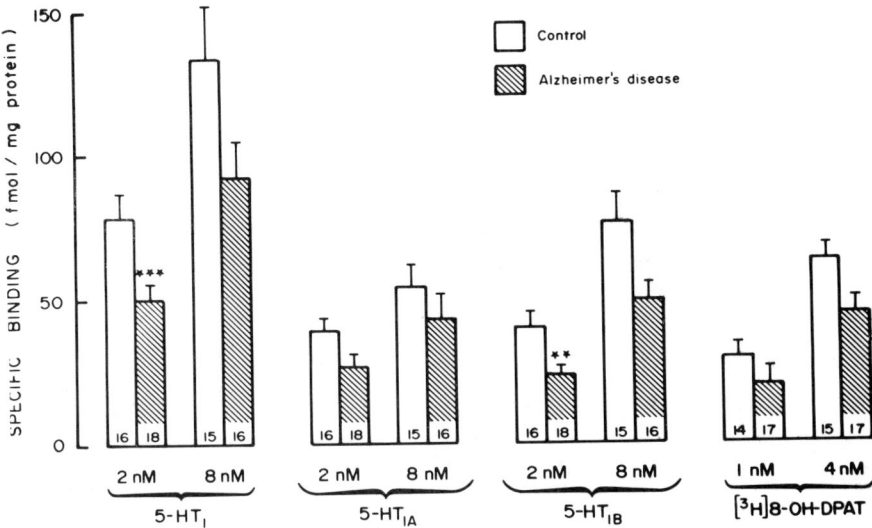

Fig. 8.2 The binding of (^{3}H)5-HT and (^{3}H)8-OH-DPAT to subtypes of the 5-HT$_1$ recognition site in the temporal cortex of control and Alzheimer's disease patients. The binding studies were carried out as described in the text. The results are expressed as specifically bound ligand in fmol/mg protein at the two concentrations of ligand examined. The number inside each histogram represents the number of individual samples assayed. $\star = p < 0.04$, $\star\star = p < 0.01$, $\star\star\star = p < 0.001$ (Krusal–Wallis statistic followed by a Mann–Whitney U test).

substantial (to 56 % of control) drop in (^{3}H)8-OH-DPAT binding. (^{3}H)8-OH-DPAT binding was reduced in the temporal cortex to 68 % of control, but this drop did not reach statistical significance. However, (^{3}H)8-OH-DPAT binding in the temporal cortex of controls showed a highly significant correlation with age ($R_s = -0.78$ and -0.83 for 1 and 4 nmol/l respectively, $p < 0.001$). This was not shown in the frontal cortex or in either region of the Alzheimer patients. The age distributions of controls and Alzheimer patients were similar, so the absence of an age effect in Alzheimer disease temporal cortex and an effect in controls suggests that a disease-related change does occur in this region.

The changes seen in any of the 5-HT recognition sites are unlikely to be due to epiphenomena, as mean values for post-mortem delay and duration of tissue storage at $-70\,^\circ$C were similar in control and Alzheimer's disease, and patient age did not correlate with these variables. Although most Alzheimer's disease patients died following prolonged terminal illness and/or had received drugs affecting monoamine neurotransmitter systems, we found no evidence from small groups of patients without these variables that the differences observed in (^{3}H)8-OD-DPAT binding could be explained by these factors. In all recognition sites examined a similar reduction was seen at the two concentrations

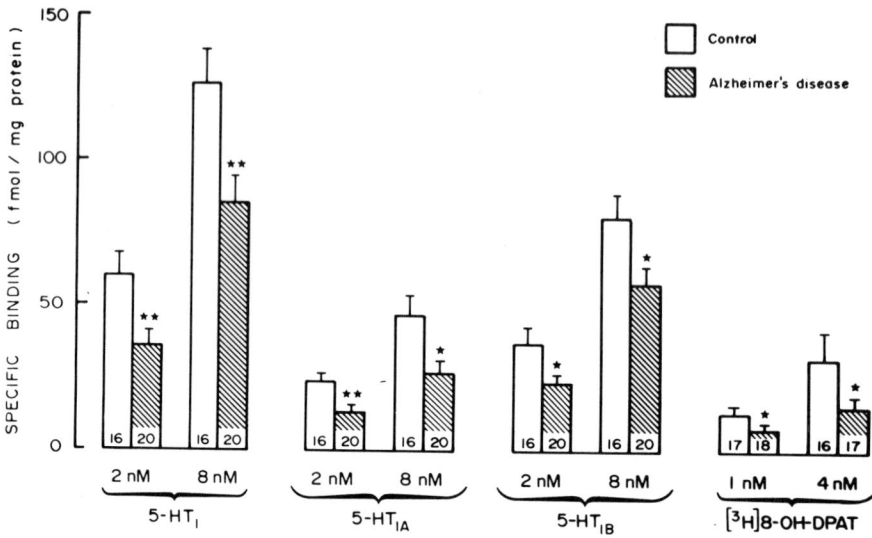

Fig. 8.3   The binding of (^{3}H)5-HT and (^{3}H)8-OH-DPAT to subtypes of the 5-HT$_1$ recognition site in the frontal cortex of control and Alzheimer's disease patients. The symbols and statistical methods are as shown in the caption to Fig. 8.2.

of (^{3}H) ligand used and, together with the similarity of the ratio of the bound ligand in normal and disease tissue (data not shown), this suggests that the losses do not reflect an alteration in binding affinity (Reynolds *et al.*, 1984).

In both brain regions choline acetyltransferase activity was reduced but the effect was more marked in the temporal cortex (to 34 % of control) than in the frontal cortex (down to 47 % of control). In contrast, 5-HT concentrations (measured by HPLC with electrochemical detection) were significantly reduced only in the temporal cortex (to 51 % of control, data not shown). 5-HIAA concentrations were not altered in either brain region.

8.5   Discussion and Conclusions

The present study has confirmed and extended previous work on the serotonergic 'synapse' in Alzheimer's disease, which suggests that all aspects of 5-HT function, be it pre- or postsynaptic, are reduced in this disease. Of the variables which have been studied, however, the most consistent reports have been concerned with reductions in the number of 5-HT receptors identified by radioligand binding techniques. Thus it is likely that the 5-HT$_1$, 5-HT$_{1A}$, 5-HT$_{1B}$ and 5-HT$_2$ sites are reduced in Alzheimer's disease (Table 8.2 and Figs. 8.2 and 8.3). These losses suggest a special role for 5-HT receptors in the pathology of Alzheimer's disease since, in general, other receptor types are not reduced (Cross *et al.*, 1984b; Bowen and Davison, 1985; Cross *et al.*, 1986).

The origin of these alterations in 5-HT receptors could be caused either by a receptor down-regulation due to elevated 5-HT function or by a loss in both pre- and postsynaptic aspects of the 5-HT neurones. Of these two options we favour the latter because the probable loss in presynaptic function noted in the 5-HT system, in particular the evidence of reduced 5-HT uptake and release (Bowen *et al.*, 1983; Bowen and Davison, 1985), is incompatible with down-regulation of postsynaptic 5-HT receptors by an excess of 5-HT. A working hypothesis (Bowen, 1983; Bowen *et al.*, 1985; Bowen and Davison, 1985) is that many 5-HT receptors are associated with tangle-forming glutamatergic neurones in the cerebral cortex as well as with the glutamatergic pyramidal cells that are lost both in Alzheimer's disease and in normal ageing, but direct evidence for this possibility is lacking. Recent research suggests that the loss of fibres running between pyramidal cells in the cortex and from the cortex to other structures correlates with the severity of the dementia at least as well as measures of cholinergic activity (Bowen and Davison, 1985; Neary *et al.*, 1985). It is evident, therefore, that the identification of the affected cells in the cortex as well as the precise cellular localisation of 5-HT receptors is critical for the further under- standing of the origins of this disease (Fig. 8.4).

The relationship of the reduction in 5-HT function in Alzheimer's disease discussed here to the clinical symptoms of the disease are not at present clear since it would appear that the reductions in 5-HT transmitter receptors and function do not seem to relate to clinical assessment of the degree of dementia (Cross *et al.*, 1983; Cross *et al.*, 1984b; Francis *et al.*, 1985). Nevertheless, there is evidence which suggests that central 5-HT pathways play a significant role in acquisition, retention and extinction of a variety of learning tasks in animals (Hunter *et al.*, 1977; Ogren *et al.*, 1981; Ogren, 1982), and that selective 5-HT uptake blockers also seem to have beneficial effects in learning and memory tasks in man (Weingartner *et al.*, 1983a,b). It has been suggested that decreased 5-HT function underlies the symptoms of some depressed patients (for a recent review of this area see Byerley and Risch (1985)) and therefore the decreased serotonergic activity may be responsible for this behavioural consequence of Alzheimer's disease. It is, however, clear that the therapeutic strategies in this disease must now encompass the facilitation of not only cholinergic but also serotonergic function in the brain.

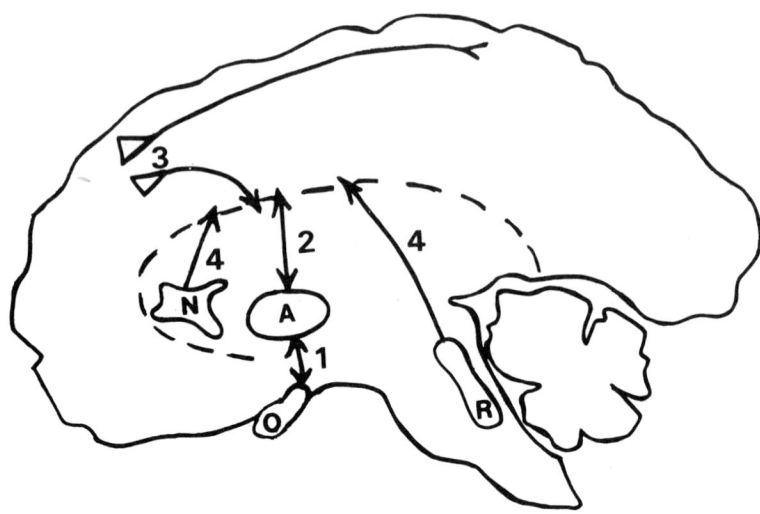

Fig. 8.4 Diagrammatic representation of a possible sequence of events (1–4) in Alzheimer's disease leading to the loss of 5-HT neurones from the raphe nucleus (R), and cortical 5-HT receptors and cholinergic neurones from the nucleus basalis of Meynert (N). Retrograde degeneration of ascending fibres (4) may be due to reduced output of neuronotrophic factors (Hefti, 1983; Rudge *et al.*, 1985) by the cortex, secondary to loss of pyramidal (? 5-HT receptor-bearing glutamatergic) cells in the cortex (3) (Bowen and Davison, 1985). Small cells (interneurones) are spared (Francis *et al.*, 1985) and bear muscarinic receptors. Increased glucose oxidation (Sims *et al.*, 1983), possibly in glutamatergic cells (Bowen and Davison, 1985) and secondary to partial uncoupling of mitochondria (Sims *et al.*, 1985), may be associated with senile plaque formation (Terry, 1978). The metabolic disturbance may also lead to the utilisation of glutamine/glutamate as an alternative energy source (Butterworth, 1983), resulting in decreased glutamine concentration (Smith *et al.*, 1985) and elevated aspartic acid (inferred from the post-mortem increase in a substrate of the urea cycle (Tarbit *et al.*, 1980), tangle formation (DeBoni and Crapper McLachlan, 1985), pyramidal cell loss and astrocytosis. There is evidence that these changes begin in olfactory areas of the brain (1, 2; O, olfactory bulb; A, amygdala; Bowen and Davison, 1985; Pearson *et al.*, 1985). R and N also have direct anatomical connections with olfactory areas so another possible pathogenic mechanism related to glutamatergic neurone dysfunction exists (Bowen, 1984).

References

Adolfsson, R., Gottfries, C. G., Roos, B. E., and Winblad, B. (1979). Changes in the brain catecholamines in patients with dementia of Alzheimer type. *Brit. J. Psychiat.*, **135**, 216–23.

Arai, H., Kosaka, K., and Iizuka, R. (1984). Changes of biogenic amines and their metabolites in postmortem brains from patients with Alzheimer-type dementia. *J. Neurochem.*, **43**, 388–93.

Bareggi, S. R., Franceschi, M., Bonini, L., Zecca, L., and Smirne, S. (1982). Decreased CSF concentrations of homovanillic acid and γ-aminobutyric acid in Alzheimer's disease. *Arch. Neurol.*, **39**, 709–12.

Bowen, D. M. (1983). Biochemical assessment of neurotransmitter and metabolic dysfunction and cerebral atrophy in Alzheimer's disease. In Katzman, R. (ed.), *Biological Aspects of Alzheimer's Disease*, Banbury Report, 15, Cold Spring Harbor, 219–31.

Bowen, D. M. (1984). Cellular Ageing: Selective vulnerability of cholinergic neurones in human brain. In Sauer, H. W. (ed.), *Monographs in Developing Biology*, Karger, Basel, pp. 42–59.

Bowen, D. M., and Davison, A. N. (1985). Biochemical studies of nerve cells and energy metabolism in Alzheimer's disease. *Brit. Med. Bull.*, 42, 75–80.

Bowen, D. M., White, P., Spillane, J. A., Goodhardt, M. J., Curzon, G., Iwangoff, P., Meier-Ruge, W., and Davison, A. N. (1979). Accelerated ageing or selective neuronal loss an important cause of dementia? *Lancet*, i, 11–14.

Bowen, D. M., Allen, S. J., Benton, J. S., Goodhardt, M. J., Haan, E. A., Palmer, A. M., Sims, N. R., Smith, C. C. T., Spillane, J. A., Esiri, M. M., Neary, D., Snowdon, J. S., Wilcock, G. K., and Davison, A. N. (1983). Biochemical assessment of serotonergic and cholinergic dysfunction and cerebral atrophy in Alzheimer's disease. *J. Neurochem.*, 41, 266–72.

Bowen, D. M., Davison, A. N., Francis, P. T., *et al.* (1985). Neurotransmitter and metabolic dysfunction in Alzheimer's dementia: Relationship to histopathological features. In Rose, F. C. (ed.), *Modern Approaches to the Dementias*, Karger, Basel, pp. 156–74.

Butterworth, R. F. (1983). Metabolism of glutamate and related amino acids in insulin hypoglycaemia. In Hertz, L., Kvamme, E., McGeer, E. G., and Schoushoe, A. (eds), *Glutamine, Glutamate, and GABA in the Central Nervous System*, Alan R. Liss, New York, pp. 595–608.

Byerley, W. F., and Risch, S. C. (1985). Depression and serotonin metabolism: Rationale for neurotransmitter precursor treatment. *J. Clin. Psychopharm.*, 5, 191–206.

Carlsson, A., Adolfsson, R., Aquilonius, S-M., Gottfries, C-G., Oreland, L., Svennerholm, L., and Winblad, B. (1980). Biogenic amines in human brain in normal aging, senile dementia, and chronic alcoholism. *Adv. Biochem. Psychopharmac.*, 23, 295–304.

Cross, A. J., Crow, T. J., Ferrier, I. N., and Johnson, J. A. (1986). The selectivity of the reduction of serotonin S2 receptors in Alzheimer-type dementia. *Neurobiol. Aging* (In press).

Cross, A. J., Crow, T. J., Ferrier, I. N., Johnson, J. A., Bloom, S. R., and Corsellis, J. A. N. (1984a). Serotonin receptor changes in dementia of the Alzheimer type. *J. Neurochem.*, 43, 1574–81.

Cross, A. J., Crow, T. J., Johnson, J. A., Perry, E. K., Perry, R. H., Blessed, G., and Tomlinson, B. E. (1984b). Studies on neurotransmitter receptor systems in neocortex and hippocampus in senile dementia of the Alzheimer-type. *J. neurol. Sci.*, 64, 109–17.

Cross, A. J., Crow, T. J., Johnson, J. A., Joseph, M. H., Perry, E. K., Perry, R. H., Blessed, G., and Tomlinson, B. E. (1983). Monoamine metabolism in senile dementia of Alzheimer type. *J. neurol. Sci.*, 60, 383–92.

Crow, T. J., Cross, A. J., Cooper, S. J., Deakin, J. F. W., Ferrier, I. N., Johnson, J. A., Joseph, M. H., Owen, F., Poulter, M., Lofthouse, R., Corsellis, J. A. N., Chambers, D. R., Blessed, G., Perry, E. K., Perry, R. H., and Tomlinson, B. E. (1984). Neurotransmitter receptors and monoamine metabolites in the brains of patients with Alzheimer-type dementia and depression, and suicides. *Neuropharmac.*, 23, 1561–9.

Curcio, C. A., and Kemper, T. (1984). Nucleus raphe dorsalis in dementia of Alzheimer type: Neurofibrillary changes and neuronal packing density. *J. Neuropathol. exp. Neurol.*, 43, 359–68.

DeBoni, U., and Crapper McLachlan, D. R. (1985). Controlled induction of paired helical filaments of the Alzheimer type in cultured human neurones, by glutamate and aspartate. *J. neurol. Sci.*, 68, 105–18.

Drachman, D. A. (1981). The cholinergic system, memory, and aging. In Enna, S. J., Samorajski, T., and Beer, B. (eds.), *Brain Neurotransmitters and Receptors in Aging and Age-Related Disorders*, Aging, Vol. 17. Raven Press, New York, pp. 255–68.

Engel, G., Göthert, M., Müller-Schweinitzer, E., Schlicker, E., Sistonen, L., and Stadler, P. A. (1983). Evidence for common pharmacological properties of (^{3}H)5-hydroxy-tryptamine binding sites, presynaptic 5-hydroxytryptamine autoreceptors in CNS and inhibitory presynaptic 5-hydroxytryptamine receptors on sympathetic nerves. *Naunyn Schmiedeberg's Arch. Pharmac.*, 324, 116–24.

Francis, P. T., Palmer, A. M., Sims, N. R., Bowen, D. M., Davison, A. N., Esiri, M. M., Neary, D., Snowden, J. S., and Wilcock, G. K. (1985). Neurochemical studies in early-onset Alzheimer's disease: Possible influence on treatment. *New Eng. J. Med.*, **313**, 7–11.

Gibson, C. J., Logue, M., and Growdon, J. H. (1985). CSF monoamine metabolite levels in Alzheimer's and Parkinson's disease. *Arch. Neurol.*, **42**, 489–92.

Gottfries, C. G., and Roos, B. E. (1973). Acid monoamine metabolites in cerebrospinal fluid from patients with presenile dementia (Alzheimer's disease). *Acta Psychiat. Scand.*, **49**, 257–63.

Gottfries, C. G., Gottfries, I., and Roos, B. E. (1969). Homovanillic acid and 5-hydroxy-indoleacetic acid in the cerebrospinal fluid of patients with senile dementia, presenile dementia and Parkinsonism. *J. Neurochem.*, **16**, 1341–5.

Gottfries, C. G., Kjallquist, A., Pontén, U., Roos, B. E., and Sundbarg, G. (1974). Cerebrospinal fluid pH and monoamine and glucolytic metabolites in Alzheimer's disease. *Brit. J. Pharmac.*, **124**, 280–7.

Gottfries, C.-G., Adolfsson, R., Aquilonius, S.-M., Carlsson, A., Eckernäs, S.-A., Nordberg, A., Oreland, L., Svennerholm, L., Wiberg, A., and Winblad, B. (1983). Biochemical changes in dementia disorders of Alzheimer type (AD/SDAT). *Neurobiol. Aging*, **4**, 261–71.

Gozlan, H., El Mestikawy, S., Pichat, L., Glowinski, J., and Hamon, M. (1983). Identification of presynaptic serotonin autoreceptors using a new ligand: ^{3}H-PAT. *Nature*, **305**, 140–2.

Hardy, J., Adolfsson, R., Alafuzoff, I., Bucht, G., Marcusson, J., Nyberg, P., Perdahl, E., Wester, P., and Winblad, B. (1985). Transmitter deficits in Alzheimer's disease. *Neurochem. Int.*, **7**, 545–63.

Hefti, F. (1983). Is Alzheimer disease caused by lack of nerve growth factor? *Ann. Neurol.*, **13**, 109–10.

Hunter, B., Zornetzer, S. F., Jarvik, M. E., and McGaugh, J. L. (1977). Modulation of learning and memory: Effects of drugs influencing neurotransmitters. In Iversen, L. L., Iversen, S. D., and Snyder, S. H. (eds.), *Handbook of Psychopharmacology*, Vol. 8. Plenum Press, New York, pp. 531–77.

Ishii, T. (1966). Distribution of Alzheimer's neurofibrillary changes in the brain stem and hypothalamus of senile dementia. *Acta Neuropathologica*, **6**, 181–7.

Kay, A. D., Milstien, S., Kaufman, S., Rapoport, S. I., and Cutler, N. R. (1984). 5-HIAA and HVA in the CSF of patients with Alzheimer's disease. *Neurol.*, **34**, (Suppl. 1), 161.

Lowry, O. H., Rosebrough, N. J., Farr, A. L., and Randall, R. J. (1951). Protein measurement with the Folin phenol reagent. *J. Biol. Chem.*, **193**, 265–75.

McGeer, P. L., and McGeer, E. G. (1981). Neurotransmitters in the aging brain. In Thompson, R. H. S., and Davison, A. N. (eds.), *The Molecular Basis of Neuropathology*, Edward Arnold, London, pp. 631–48.

Mann, D. M. A., and Yates, P. O. (1983). Serotonin nerve cells in Alzheimer's disease. *J. Neurol. Neurosurg. Psychiat.*, **46**, 96.

Mann, D. M. A., Yates, P. O., and Marcyniuk, B. (1984). Alzheimer's presenile dementia, senile dementia of Alzheimer type and Down's syndrome in middle age form an age related continuum of pathological changes. *Neuropath. Appl. Neurobiol.*, **10**, 185–207.

Marcinkiewicz, M., Vergé, D., Gozlan, H., Pichat, L., and Hamon, M. (1984). Autoradiographic evidence for the heterogeneity of 5-HT$_1$ sites in the rat brain. *Brain Res.*, **291**, 159–63.

Middlemiss, D. N. (1982). Multiple 5-hydroxytryptamine receptors in the central nervous system of the rat. In De Belleroche, J. (ed.), *Presynaptic Receptors: Mechanisms and Functions*, Ellis Horwood, Chichester, pp. 46–74.

Middlemiss, D. N. (1985). Does 8-hydroxy (di-N-^{3}H-propylamino)tetralin ((³H)8-OH-DPAT) label the 5-HT$_{1A}$ recognition site in rat frontal cortex? *J. de Pharmacologie*, **16**, 495.

Middlemiss, D. N., and Fozard, J. R. (1983). 8-Hydroxy-2-(di-n-propylamino)-tetralin discriminates between subtypes of the 5-HT$_1$ recognition site. *Eur. J. Pharmac.*, **90**, 151–3.

Middlemiss, D. N., Palmer, A. M., Edel, N., and Bowen, D. M. (1986). Binding of the novel serotonin agonist 8-hydroxy-2-(di-n-propylamino)tetralin in normal and Alzheimer brain. *J. Neurochem.*, **46**, 993–6.

Neary, D., Snowdon, J. S., Mann, D. M. A., Bowen, D. M., Sims, N. R., Northern, B., Yates, P. O., and Davison, A. N. (1985). Alzheimer's disease: A correlative study. *J. Neurosurg. Psychiat.* (In press).

Ogren, S. O. (1982). Central serotonin neurones and learning in the rat. In Osborne, N. N. (ed.), *Biology of Serotonergic Transmission.* John Wiley, Chichester, pp. 317-35.

Ogren, S. O., Fuxe, K., Archer, T., Hall, H., Holm, A. C., and Kohler, C. (1981). Studies on the role of central 5-HT neurones in avoidance learning: A behavioral and biochemical analysis. In Haber, B., Gabay, S., Issidorides, M. R., and Alivisatos, S. G. A. (eds.), *Serotonin: Current Aspects of Neurochemistry and Function,* Adv. Exp. Med. Biol. Vol. 133. Plenum Press, New York, pp. 681-705.

Palmer, A. M., Sims, N. R., Bowen, D. M., Neary, D., Palo, J., Wikstrom, J., and Davison, A. N. (1984). Monoamine metabolite concentrations in lumbar cerebrospinal fluid of patients with histologically verified Alzheimer's dementia.*J. Neurol. Neurosurg. Psychiat.,* 47, 481-4.

Pearson, R. C. A., Esiri, M. M., Hiorns, R. W., Wilcock, G. K., and Powell, T. P. S. (1985). Anatomical correlates of the distribution of the pathological changes in the neocortex in Alzheimer's disease. *Proc. Nat. Acad. Sci. USA,* 82, 4531-5.

Pedigo, N. W., Yamamura, H. I., and Nelson, D. L. (1981). Discrimination of multiple (^{3}H)5-hydroxytryptamine binding sites by the neuroleptic spiperone in rat brain. *J. Neurochem..* 36. 220-6.

Peroutka, S. J., and Snyder, S. H. (1979). Multiple serotonin receptors: Differential binding of (^{3}H)5-hydroxytryptamine, (^{3}H)lysergic acid diethylamide and (^{3}H)spiroperidol. *Mol. Pharmac.,* 16, 687-99.

Perry, E. K., and Perry, R. H. (1980). The cholinergic system in Alzheimer's disease. In Roberts, P. J. (ed.), *Biochemistry of Dementia.* John Wiley, Chichester, pp. 135-83.

Perry, E. K., Tomlinson, B. E., Blessed, G., Bergman, K., Gibson, P. H., and Perry, R. H. (1978). Correlation of cholinergic abnormalities with senile plaques and mental test scores in senile dementia. *Br. Med. J.,* 2, 1457-9.

Perry, E. K., Perry, R. H., Candy, J. M., Fairbairn, A. F., Blessed, G., Dick, D. J., and Tomlinson, B. E. (1984). Cortical serotonin-S_2 receptor binding abnormalities in patients with Alzheimer's disease: Comparisons with Parkinson's disease. *Neurosci. Letts.,* 51, 353-7.

Rehavi, M., Paul, S. M., Skolnick, P., and Goodwin, F. K. (1980). Demonstration of specific high affinity binding sites for (^{3}H)imipramine in human brain. *Life Sci.,* 26, 2273-9.

Reynolds, G. P., Arnold, L., Rossor, M. N., Iversen, L. L., Mountjoy, C. Q., and Roth, M. (1984). Reducing binding of (^{3}H)ketanserin to cortical 5-HT$_2$ receptors in senile dementia of the Alzheimer type. *Neurosci. Lett.,* 44, 47-51.

Rossor, M. N. (1982). Dementia. *Lancet,* i, 1200-4.

Rudge, J. S., Manthorpe, M. and Varon, S. (1985). The output of neuronotrophic and neurite-promoting agents from rat brain astoglial cells: A microculture method for screening potential regulatory molecules. *Develop. Brain Res.,* 19, 161-72.

Semple, S. A., Smith, C. M., and Swash, M. (1982). The Alzheimer disease syndrome. In Corkin, S., Davis, K. L., Growdon, J. H., Usdin, E., and Wurtman, R. J. (eds.), *Alzheimer's Disease: A Report of Progress in Research,* Raven Press, New York, 93-108.

Schnellmann, R. G., Waters, S. J., and Nelson, D. L. (1984). (^{3}H)5-Hydroxytryptamine binding sites: Species and tissue variation. *J. Neurochem.,* 42, 65-70.

Sims, N. R., and Bowen, D. M. (1983). Changes in choline acetyltransferase and acetyl-choline synthesis. In Reisberg, B. (ed.), *Alzheimer's Disease. The Standard Reference.* Macmillan, New York, pp. 88-92.

Sims, N. R., Bowen, D. M., Neary, D., and Davison, A. N. (1983). Metabolic processes in Alzheimer's disease: Adenine nucleotide content and product of $^{14}CO_2$ from (U-^{14}C) glucose in vitro in human neocortex. *J. Neurochem.,* 41, 1329-4.

Sims, N. R., Finegan, J. M., Bowen, D. M., and Blass, J. P. (1985). Mitochondrial function in Alzheimer's disease measured in vitro using neocortical tissue homogenates. *J. Neurochem.,* 44, (Suppl.), S192A.

Smith, C. G. T., Bowen, D. M., Francis, P. T., Snowden, J. S., and Neary, D. (1985). Putative amino acid transmitters in lumbar cerebrospinal fluid of patients with histologically verified Alzheimer's dementia. *J. Neurol. Neurosurg. Psychiat.,* 48, 469-71.

Soininen, H., MacDonald, E., Rekonen, M., and Riekkinen, P. J. (1981). Homovanillic acid and 5-hydroxyindoleacetic acid levels in cerebrospinal fluid of patients with senile dementia of Alzheimer type. *Acta. Neurol. Scand.*, **64**, 101–7.

Tarbit, I., Perry, E. K., Perry, R. H., Blessed, G., and Tomlinson, B. E. (1980). Hippocampal free amino acids in Alzheimer's disease. *J. Neurochem.*, **35**, 1246–9.

Terry, R. D. (1978). Ultrastructural alterations in senile dementia. In Katzman, R., Terry, R. D., and Bick, K. L. (eds.), *Alzheimer's Disease, Senile Dementia and Related Disorders*. Raven Press, New York, pp. 375–82.

Weingartner, H., Buchsbaum, M. S., and Linnoila, M. (1983a). Zimelidine effects on memory impairments produced by ethanol. *Life Sci.*, **33**, 2159–63.

Weingartner, H., Rudorfer, M. V., Buchsbaum, M. S., and Linnoila, M. (1983b). Effects of serotonin on memory impairments produced by ethanol. *Science*, **221**, 472–4.

Wood, P. L., Etienne, P., Lal, S., Gauthier, S., Cajal, S., and Nair, N. P. V. (1982). Reduced lumbar CSF somatostatin levels in Alzheimer's disease. *Life Sci.*, **31**, 2073–9.

Yamada, M., and Mehraein, P. (1977). Verteilungsmuster der senilen Veränderungen in den Hirnstammkernen. *Folia Psychiat. Neurol.*, **31**, 219–24.

9

Two Drug Binding Sites on Muscarinic Receptors

N. J. M. Birdsall, E. C. Hulme, W. Kromer, B. S. Peck, J. M. Stockton and
M. J. Zigmond

9.1 Introduction

Neuropathological and biochemical examinations of the brains of patients suffering from senile dementia of the Alzheimer type (SDAT) reveal characterstic abnormalities. These include neurite plaques and neurofibrillary tangles which tend to be localised to the cerebral cortex and hippocampus. In these areas there are also decreased levels of the enzymes and uptake systems present in the nerve terminals which are involved in the synthesis of acetylcholine (for reviews see Bartus et al., 1982; Rossor, 1982; Coyle et al., 1983, 1984; Davies, 1984). In particular, there has been found to be a large reduction in cholineacetyltransferase activity. There is also in SDAT a considerable cell loss in the nucleus basalis of Meynert (Whitehouse et al., 1982; Henke and Lang, 1983). As neurones from this nucleus project to the cerebral cortex and account for an estimated 70 % of the cortical content of acetylcholine, it is not surprising that the degeneration of these neurones in SDAT has been assumed to make a contribution to the progression of the disease. It is still not clear whether the primary site of the lesion is in the cell bodies in the basal forebrain or at the cholinergic nerve terminals in the cerebral cortex (Perry et al., 1982; Whitehouse et al., 1982). More importantly, it is not known whether the cholinergic deficit is the primary lesion, as changes in adrenergic, 5-hydroxytryptamine and somatostatin systems have also been observed (for a review, see Rossor and Iversen, 1986).

The predominant receptors for acetylcholine in the central nervous system are muscarinic receptors, and these are present in high concentrations in the cerebral cortex and hippocampus. It is thought that the muscarinic cholinergic system is involved in the storage and retrieval of newly acquired information (Deutsch, 1981) and that a deficiency of this faculty is a hallmark of SDAT. Low doses of the muscarinic antagonist scopolamine, when administered to human volunteers, cause selective deficits in recent memory without affecting immediate registration or long term memory (Drachman and Leavitt, 1976; Drachman, 1977). Conversely, the agonist arecoline has been shown to increase recall of recently learned verbal material in young volunteers (Sitaram et al., 1978).

In view of the cholinergic deficit, it is important to know whether muscarinic receptors are altered in SDAT. Most of the studies have shown either no change or small decreases (10-15 %) in the cerebral cortex but these changes were not statistically significant (see, for example, White et al., 1977; Davies and Verth, 1978; Perry et al., 1978; Bowen et al., 1979; Caulfield et al., 1982; Lang and Henke, 1983). However, small significant differences in receptor number are very difficult to detect in heterogeneous populations. Two studies have in fact shown significant decreases in muscarinic receptors in SDAT but these decreases were found in the hippocampus and other limbic areas (Reisine et al., 1978; Rinne et al., 1984) and not in the cortex. However, in the last two years, there have been reports of a 20-25 % decrease in muscarinic receptor binding sites in the cortex of patients with SDAT (Wood et al., 1983; Mash et al., 1985).

The conclusion from these studies is that the changes, if any, in the number of muscarinic receptor binding sites in SDAT are relatively small. If the receptor binding sites represent functional receptors then the predominant deficit is in the levels of acetylcholine. Following this hypothesis, any treatment which restores normal cholinergic (muscarinic) function in the cerebral cortex may alleviate the memory deficits in SDAT.

Many attempts have been made to compensate pharmacologically for low levels of acetylcholine. The administration of large quantities of the precursor choline, or of lecithin (which generates choline), have not in general produced positive results (for a review see Growdon et al., 1985) although one recent study has suggested that some elderly patients may benefit from such therapy (Levy, 1985). Treatment with physostigmine, which blocks acetylcholinesterase and thereby prolongs the lifetime and duration of action of neuronally released acetylcholine, has resulted in transient improvements of cognitive function. However, the doses of physostigmine and of exogenously administered agonists such as arecoline and RS 86 (Wettstein and Spiegel, 1984) which can be used have been limited by additional effects produced by the activation of muscarinic receptors in other tissues (e.g. increased salivation, sweating, flushing, hypotension, nausea and vomiting). The most encouraging positive result is that of Harbaugh et al. (1984), who succeeded in improving cognitive and social functions in a small number of Alzheimer patients by controlled intracranial infusions of bethanechol. These findings suggest that a muscarinic therapy may be of relevance in the treatment of SDAT and that research should be aimed at minimising the occurrence of the unwanted muscarinic side effects.

There are two findings which are important to such an approach. First, there is an increasing realisation of the existence of muscarinic receptor subclasses and, second, there has been the discovery of a second drug binding site on muscarinic receptors (Birdsall *et al.*, 1981; Stockton *et al.*, 1983). In this chapter we will discuss some of the ramifications of these findings which may be pertinent to the treatment of SDAT.

9.2 Muscarinic Receptor Subclasses

There is now a strong body of evidence from both functional and biochemical studies on muscarinic receptors for the existence of receptor subclasses. Several recent reviews provide a comprehensive picture of this area of research (Birdsall and Hulme, 1983, 1985; Caulfield and Straughan, 1983; Hammer and Giachetti, 1984; Hirschowitz *et al.*, 1984; Kilbinger, 1984b; Sokolovsky, 1984).

9.3 Selective Competitive Antagonists

In 1976 there was a report by Barlow and coworkers that muscarinic receptors in smooth muscle and heart were not identical, and that several antagonists were up to ten times more potent on the smooth muscle receptors. The most selective agent was 4-diphenylacetoxy-N-methylpiperidine methiodide (4-DAMP, Fig. 9.1). No selectivity of the antagonists for ileal, bronchial muscle or iris muscarinic receptors has been reported (Barlow *et al.*, 1972). More recently, a smooth muscle/cardiac selectivity similar to that shown by 4-DAMP has been demonstrated for analogues of procyclidine and difenidol (Mutschler and Lambrecht, 1984), with hexahydrosiladifenidol (Fig. 9.1) exhibiting the greatest functional selectivity (27-fold).

The drug which has had the greatest impact on research into muscarinic receptor subclasses is pirenzepine (Fig. 9.1). This is perhaps due to the fact that it is in clinical use, in the treatment of peptic ulcer disease. Low doses of pirenzepine inhibit gastric acid secretion in animals and in man by an antimuscarinic mechanism, and considerably higher doses are required to block the muscarinic receptors involved in smooth muscle contraction, salivation and cardiac function. Pirenzepine exhibits a selectivity not shown by 'classical' non-selective antagonists such as atropine (see, for example, Blum and Hammer, 1979; Baron and Londong, 1980; Doteval *et al.*, 1982; Hammer and Giachetti, 1984; Hirschowitz *et al.*, 1984).

The selectivity shown by pirenzepine *in vivo* is also found in *in vitro* functional studies. For example, pirenzepine antagonises with high affinity (pA_2 8) the muscarinic depolarisation in sympathetic ganglia (Brown *et al.*, 1980; Barlow *et al.*, 1981; Ashe and Yarosh, 1984) and the muscarinic stimulation of resting release of acetylcholine from myenteric neurones (Kilbinger, 1984b; Kilbinger and Nafziger, 1985), as well as certain electrophysiological muscarinic responses

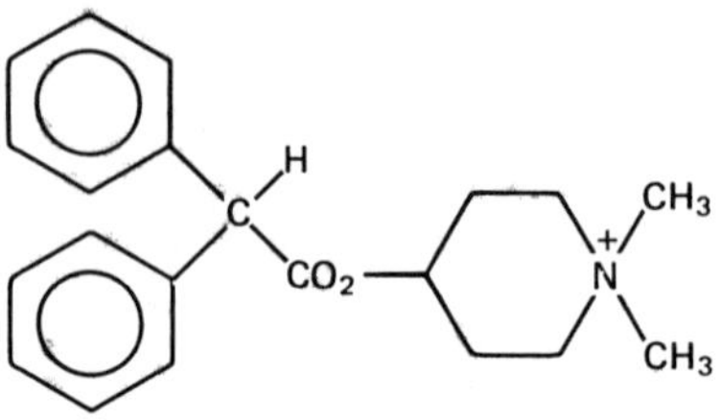

4-DAMP

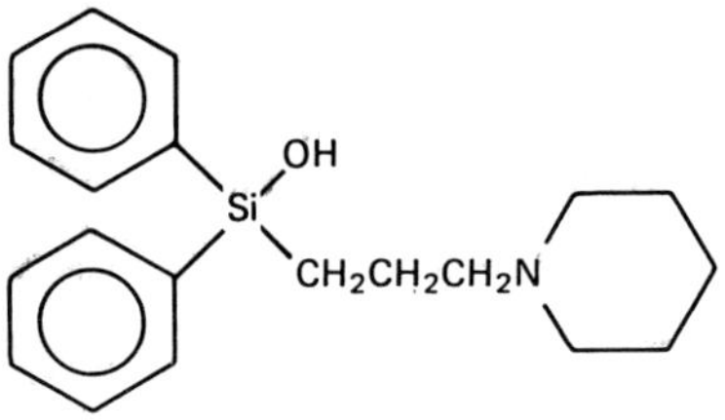

Hexahydrosiladifenidol

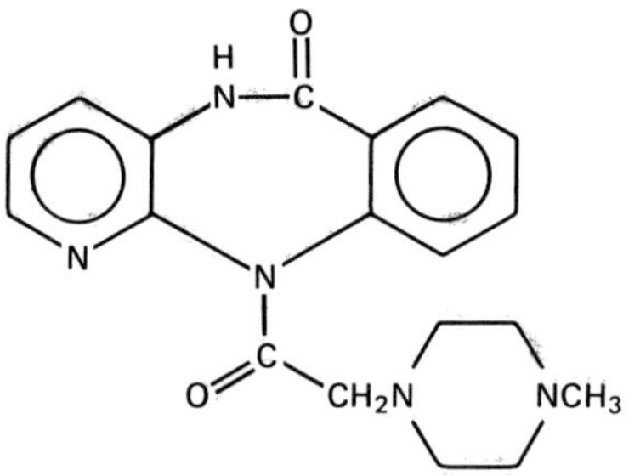

Pirenzepine

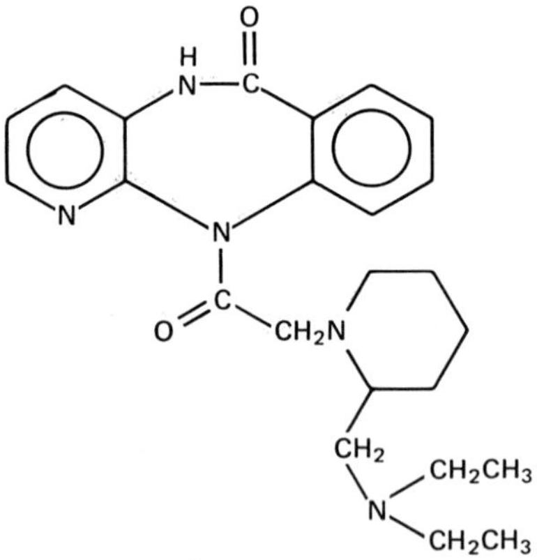

AFDX-116

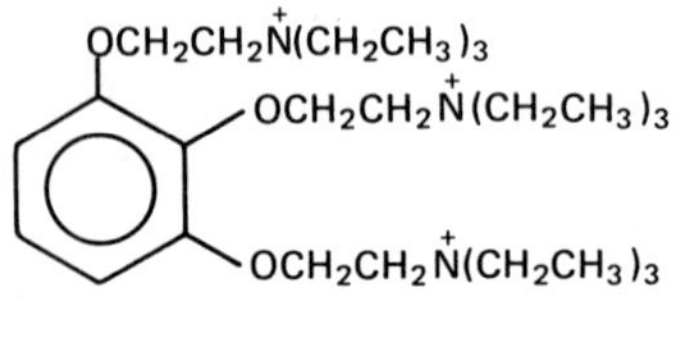

Gallamine

Fig. 9.1 Selective muscarinic antagonists.

in enteric neurones and in the cerebral cortex (North, 1986). Furthermore, in some studies of the muscarinic receptor stimulated turnover of polyphospho-inositides in the cerebral cortex, it has been found that this response is antago-nised by pirenzepine with high affinity (Fisher and Bartus, 1985; Gil and Wolfe, 1985; Smith and Yamamura, 1985; Fisher, 1986; but see Jacobson et al., 1985 and Lazareno et al., 1985). However, there appear to be regional and species differences in the coupling characteristics of muscarinic receptors in the CNS (Fisher and Bartus, 1985), and it cannot be concluded that in all tissues the breakdown of phosphoinositides is exclusively a characteristic of muscarinic receptors having a high affinity for pirenzepine.

Considerably lower pA_2 values for pirenzepine (6.2-6.7) are found in atrial and ileal smooth muscle (see, for example, Parsons et al., 1979, Barlow et al., 1981; Fuder et al., 1981, 1982; Chassaing et al., 1984), in single neurones of the rat nucleus parabrachialis (North, 1986), in the locus coeruleus (Egan and North, 1985), and on the muscarinic presynaptic inhibition of neurotransmitter release (Fuder et al., 1981, 1982; Kilbinger et al., 1984a,b). Interestingly, pirenzepine has a low affinity for blocking muscarinic stimulation of acid secretion from parietal cells (see, for example, Daly et al., 1982; Szelenyi, 1982; Rosenfeld, 1983; Soll, 1984). This is in apparent contrast to the ability of pirenzepine to block selectively vagal stimulated gastric secretion in vivo (see, for example, Jaup et al., 1982). However, in rodents, acid secretion promoted by vagal stimulation in vivo or by electrical stimulation in vitro is blocked with high affinity by pirenzepine (Hammer and Giachetti, 1982; Pagani et al., 1984). It would therefore seem that there may be two ways of stimulating gastric acid secretion, by vagal stimulation or by exogenous agonist, and that these are regulated by different muscarinic receptor subpopulations (but see Black et al., 1985 for a different interpretation). The conclusion has been drawn that mus-carinic receptors having a high affinity for pirenzepine are located in neuronal tissue, whereas the receptors with a low affinity for pirenzepine are located on peripheral effector organs (Hammer and Giachetti, 1982) but this is probably an oversimplification.

The selectivity of pirenzepine, which has been found in functional studies, can be demonstrated in receptor binding studies, as first reported by Hammer et al. (1980). Pirenzepine binds with high potency to muscarinic receptors in the cerebral cortex, hippocampus and sympathetic ganglia, with intermediate potency to the receptors in the sublingual, parotid and lacrimal gland, and with low affinity to the receptors in the heart and smooth muscle of the urinary bladder and ileum (Hammer et al., 1980; Hammer, 1982; Hammer and Giachetti, 1982). The binding studies indicate that within most tissues there is a hetero-geneous population of binding sites. In fact, the binding data can be explained by the presence of a population of binding sites with an affinity of 5×10^7 M^{-1}, the remaining sites having affinities of $1-5 \times 10^6$ M^{-1} (Birdsall et al., 1980). The membrane-bound sites with a high affinity for pirenzepine could be labelled directly with [^{3}H]-pirenzepine (Watson et al., 1982, 1983, 1984; Birdsall et al.,

1983b, 1984; Yamamura *et al.*, 1983; Luthin and Wolfe, 1984a,b) and be shown to have characteristic agonist binding properties (Birdsall *et al.*, 1984). We also suggested tentatively that the sites with a low affinity for pirenzepine were heterogeneous and consisted of populations with affinities of $4-6 \times 10^6$ M^{-1} (lacrimal, parotid) and 1×10^6 M^{-1} (heart, hindbrain) (Birdsall *et al.*, 1980). In general, the results of the binding and the pharmacological data are in excellent agreement.

Although most of the functional and binding studies relating to muscarinic receptor subtypes have used pirenzepine, there is evidence that other drugs such as dicyclomine (Potter *et al.*, 1984), telenzepine (Eltze *et al.*, 1985; and Birdsall *et al.* (unpublished results)) and trihexyphenidyl (Tien and Wallace, 1985; Stockton *et al.* (unpublished results)) exhibit a similar selectivity to that shown by pirenzepine.

So far, the selective agents considered have all had a low affinity for cardiac muscarinic receptors. However, a cardioselective muscarinic antagonist AFDX-116 (Fig. 9.1) has very recently been described (Giachetti *et al.*, 1986; Hammer *et al.*, 1986). This agent has some structural features in common with pirenzepine but its pharmacological and binding profiles are completely different. It has a forty-fold higher affinity for cardiac receptors than for those in exocrine glands. The neuronal muscarinic receptors which have a high affinity for pirenzepine have an intermediate affinity for AFDX-116. It appears that, from the binding profile, the three receptor subtypes as defined by AFDX and pirenzepine are all present in the brain, and each subtype has a distinctive regional localisation (Hammer *et al.*, 1986).

Assuming that the receptor binding sites found in the CNS represent *functional* muscarinic receptor subtypes, there is now a tremendous scope for the design of and investigation of the action of selective centrally acting antagonists.

9.4 A Second Drug Binding Site on Muscarinic Receptors

There is a cardioselective antagonist, reports of whose selectivity predate those of other antagonists by twenty-five years. This drug is the neuromuscular blocking drug gallamine (Fig. 9.1), which in 1951 was reported by Riker and Wescoe to have potent vagolytic side effects which were confined to the cardiac vagus. No effects on salivation or gut motility were observed. Other neuromuscular blockers, such as pancuronium (Marshall *et al.*, 1980; Leung and Mitchelson, 1982), stercuronium (Li and Mitchelson, 1980) and anatruxonium (Kharkevitch and Shorr, 1980) exhibit a cardiac selectivity in their muscarinic side effects.

The action of gallamine was investigated in detail by Clark and Mitchelson (1976) who concluded that gallamine did not act competitively with carbachol at atrial muscarinic receptors. They could not, however, determine the site of action of gallamine, that is whether it was interacting directly with the receptor or with a component of a 'downstream' effector system. We have examined the binding of gallamine to membrane-bound (Stockton *et al.*, 1983), soluble (Keen *et al.* (unpublished results)) are purified (Hulme *et al.* (unpublished results)) muscarinic receptors from several rat tissues. These studies confirmed the pharmacological studies both in terms of the cardioselective action of gallamine and the fact that it does not act competitively with acetylcholine and a considerable number of other muscarinic agonists and antagonists. The evidence that the same interaction persists in soluble and purified (Berrie *et al.*, 1985) receptor preparations suggests that gallamine is interacting directly with the receptor. However, the non-competitive nature of the interaction implies that gallamine is binding to a site different from that to which acetylcholine and atropine bind.

The evidence for the existence of a second drug binding site (the 'gallamine' or the allosteric site) on muscarinic receptors is detailed elsewhere (Stockton *et al.*, 1983; Birdsall *et al.*, 1986) and is hence only summarised briefly here. When gallamine binds to muscarinic receptors it changes the binding of ligands to the conventional (acetylcholine) binding site, but at high concentrations of gallamine a maximum effect on ligand binding is observed. This is manifested in a $[^3H]$-ligand–gallamine competition experiment by the inability of gallamine to completely inhibit the receptor-specific binding of the $[^3H]$-ligand, that is the inhibition curve reaches a plateau of less than 100 % at high concentrations of gallamine. The allosteric interaction of gallamine is also manifested by the ability of gallamine to strongly affect the off- (and on-) rate kinetics of $[^3H]$-muscarinic ligands. It should be noted that other authors have confirmed some, but not always all, of our findings (Dunlap and Brown, 1983; Mitchelson, 1984; Ellis and Lenox, 1985; Nedoma *et al.*, 1985). The reasons for the discrepancies may be due to proteolysis of smooth muscle receptor and/or the very slow kinetics of the binding processes. These are discussed in some detail in Birdsall *et al.* (1986).

By using the equilibrium and kinetic protocols delineated in the previous paragraph together with the observation that the binding of agents to the allosteric site is very sensitive to ionic strength (Birdsall *et al.*, 1981; Ellis and Lenox, 1985; Nedoma *et al.*, 1985), it has been possible to begin to elucidate the structure–binding relationships of the allosteric site (Birdsall *et al.*, 1986; Stockton *et al.* (unpublished results)). Some agents which appear to bind to the allosteric site are shown in Table 9.1. We have included some drugs which, from the data presented in the original papers, appear to be binding to an allosteric site on muscarinic receptors, but the authors did not necessarily draw this conclusion. This list must be considered to be tentative in that although the drugs have been shown to affect allosterically the binding of ligands to the acetylcholine binding site, they have not been shown to bind competitively with each other at the allosteric site. It should also be noted that some of the drugs listed in Table 9.1 are capable of binding to both the acetylcholine binding site and the allosteric site. This implies that there could be certain elements of similarity between the two binding sites. In this context, it is of interest that two other

Table 9.1 Some drugs which appear to bind to the allosteric site

Neuromuscular blockers and related compounds	Antidysrhythmic drugs	Channel blockers	Muscarinic agonist	Nicotinic agonist	Other drugs
Gallamine[1-4]	*(+) and (−) disopyramide[5]	Verapamil[7]	McN-A-343[10]	Lobeline[5]	*Clomiphen[9]
*Pancuronium[4,5]	*Quinidine[5,6]	4-aminopyridine (?)[8]			
ORG-NC-45[5]					Quinacrine
*Cyclobutonium[5]					
*Benzoquinonium[5]					
Bis- and mono-analogues of gallamine[5]					

* Appears to bind to both the conventional and the allosteric sites.

[1] Stockton et al. (1983); [2] Nedoma et al. (1985); [3] Jagadeesh and Sulakhe (1985); [4] Dunlap and Brown (1983); [5] Birdsall, Hulme, Kromer, Peck and Stockton (unpublished results); [6] Cohen-Armon et al. (1985); [7] Waelbroeck et al. (1984); [8] Lai et al. (1985); [9] Ben-Baruch et al. (1982); [10] Birdsall et al. (1983a).

acetylcholine recognition molecules, the nicotinic acetylcholine receptor and acetylcholinesterase, both bind gallamine with relatively high affinity, the latter interaction being via its binding to an allosteric site! (Changeux, 1966).

A most interesting compound is the selective agonist McN-A-343 (Roszkowski, 1961; Fig. 9.2(a)), which interacts allosterically with the cardiac receptor although its binding to the cortical receptors cannot be distinguished from that of a competitive agonist (Birdsall et al., 1983a). In the heart, the binding of McN-A-343, like that of conventional agonists but unlike gallamine, is sensitive

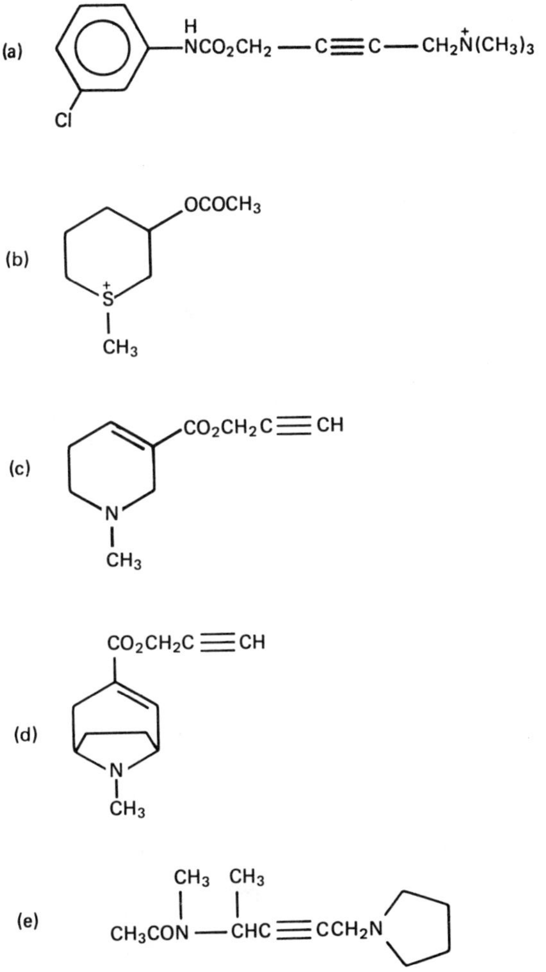

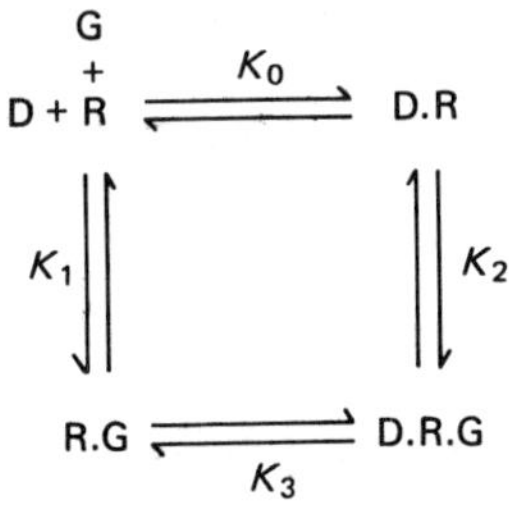

(a)

$$D + R \underset{}{\overset{\displaystyle G \atop +}{}} \xrightarrow{K_0} D.R$$

$$K_1 \big\updownarrow \qquad \qquad \big\updownarrow K_2$$

$$R.G \underset{K_3}{\rightleftharpoons} D.R.G$$

Scheme I

(b)

(c)

(d)

(e)

Fig. 9.2 (left, above) Selective muscarinic agonists: (a) McN-A-343; (b) cis-3-acetoxy-S-methylthiane; (c) arecaidine propargyl ester; (d) a bridge arecoline analogue; and (e) an oxotremorine analogue.

to GTP and it may thus be possible to activate cardiac (and perhaps other) muscarinic receptors by the binding of a drug to the allosteric site.

The simple binding process which fits the binding processes at muscarinic receptors is shown in Scheme I (p. 111). A conventional drug D and an allosteric drug G are both capable of binding to the receptor R. The allosteric interaction between D and G (and vice versa) results from the formation of the ternary complex D.R.G. The binding of G is characterised by two parameters, K_1 the affinity of G for the allosteric site and K_1/K_2, the cooperativity or the maximum change in affinity of G produced by the binding of D to the receptor. Parameter K_1 is dependent on the nature of G and R, whereas K_1/K_2 depends on G, R and D.

9.5 Selective agonists

The first evidence of a selective muscarinic agonist was that of Roskowski (1961), who reported that McN-A-343 appeared to be a selective stimulant of ganglionic muscarinic receptors. The pressor response of McN-A-343 has been shown to be selectively blocked *in vivo* by pirenzepine (Hammer and Giachetti, 1982), and in the cortex we have noted that McN-A-343 exhibits an anomalously high affinity for binding to high affinity pirenzepine sites (Birdsall *et al.*, 1984). Hence the ability of pirenzepine and McN-A-343 to discriminate between muscarinic receptor subtypes may be correlated. Agonists which have been reported to mimic the pressor actions of McN-A-343 include AHR-602 (Franko *et al.*, 1963), a spiroquinuclidine (Fisher *et al.*, 1976), a dihydroisoarecaidine ester (Porsius *et al.*, 1981) and pilocarpine (Caulfield and Stubley, 1982).

Barlow *et al.* (1980) were the first to suggest that agonists might differ in their actions on ileal muscarinic receptors and on the cardiac receptors mediating the rate and force of contraction. (All of these receptors have a low affinity for pirenzepine, but not for other selective antagonists.) The differences in potency were relatively small, but Mutschler and Lambrecht (1984) have recently reported that both enantiomers of cis-3-acetoxy-S-methylthiane (Fig. 9.2(b)) were 11–15 times more potent on the ileum than on the inotropic atrial response. Conversely, arecaidine propargyl ester (Fig. 9.2(c)) was 2–3 times more potent on the atrial receptors. Several agonists have been reported to be more potent on force than rate in the heart (Clague *et al.*, 1985). However, all these agonists contained acetoxy functions and 'lost' their selectivity when the assays were carried out in the presence of cholinesterase inhibitors. Presumably these agonists were being selectively hydrolysed by acetylcholinesterase present in high concentrations in conduction tissue. A most interesting compound is a bridged arecoline analogue (the enantiomeric mixture, Fig. 9.2(d)) which is forty-fold more potent on force than rate in the atria (probably too large a factor to be ascribed to cholinesterase susceptibility), whereas it is a pure antagonist on smooth muscle (Mutschler and Lambrecht, 1984). The simplest conclusion from these data is that the muscarinic receptors mediating the inotropic and chronotropic responses are different, as is suggested from the evidence that the receptor in nodal tissue appears to be coupled to a K^+ channel (Soejima and Noma, 1984), whereas that in the myocardium is linked to a GTP binding protein Ni which can inhibit adenylate cyclase (e.g. Murad *et al.*, 1962; Hulme *et al.*, 1981; Kurose *et al.*, 1983; but see Pfaffinger *et al.*, 1985; and Breitwieser and Szabo, 1985). Another potentially interesting finding is that of Nordstrom *et al.* (1983), who reported that an oxotremorine analogue (Fig. 9.2(e)) acted as a presynaptic antagonist and a postsynaptic agonist. As these responses were made in different tissues (hippocampus and ileum respectively) it is not certain, however, whether the selectivity resulted in differing efficiencies of receptor–response coupling.

Little evidence has come from binding studies for the existence of selective agonists. This has in part been due to the complex nature of agonist binding curves (Birdsall *et al.*, 1978) and the ability of divalent ions and guanine nucleotides, such as GTP, to modulate agonist binding (see, for example, Birdsall and Hulme, 1983; Hulme *et al.*, 1983). It has, however, been possible to demonstrate small differences in the structure–binding relationships of agonists for the highest affinity binding site of the myocardial receptor and the two subtypes present in the rat cerebral cortex (Birdsall and Hulme, 1986). In addition, an anomalously high affinity of McN-A-343 for cortical receptor binding sites which have a high affinity for pirenzepine has been noted (Birdsall *et al.*, 1984).

9.6 Proposed Receptor Subtypes

The evidence for the existence of muscarinic receptor subtypes comes from: (1) studies of the actions of selective drugs *in vivo* and *in vitro*; (2) studies of receptor mechanisms; and (3) receptor binding studies. There is, however, little agreement on the nomenclature of the subtypes (for a discussion, see Birdsall and Hulme, 1983, 1985). The most common terminology defines the M_1 subtype by its high affinity for pirenzepine and the M_2 by its low affinity for pirenzepine, that is, as all the receptors which are not M_1 (see preface to Hirschowitz *et al.*, 1984). This seems to be an oversimplification.

We have suggested that there may be three, and possibly four, muscarinic receptor subtypes (Birdsall and Hulme, 1983, 1985). The properties of these putative subtypes are shown in Table 9.2, using a nomenclature which is deliberately chosen to avoid the suggestion that it may be a permanent subclassification. The classification is based primarily on functional studies but evidence from binding studies is considered, especially in the central nervous system where there are at present limited pharmacological data. The tissue location of the receptor subtypes is not meant to imply that only one receptor subtype is present in that tissue. Binding studies would suggest that, in most tissues, the binding sites of several receptor subtypes are present. Equally there is growing evidence that one receptor subtype may not be exclusively linked to a specific effector mechanism. It may be that a receptor subtype can couple to, for example, different GTP

Table 9.2 Properties of proposed subtypes

	Subtype			
	I	II	III	IV
Selective antagonists	Pirenzepine	AF-DX-116 gallamine	4-DAMP, Hexahydrosiladifenidol	AF-DX-116 gallamine
Selective agonists	McN-A-343 pilocarpine	'Bridged' propargyl ester of arecaidine	cis-3-Acetoxy-S-methylthiane	—
Effector mechanism*	phosphoinositide hydrolysis. M-channels (?)	Inhibition of adenylate cyclase	phosphoinositide hydrolysis (?)	K^+ channel
Location†	Sympathetic ganglia (slow EPSP), cerebral cortex, hippocampus	Myocardium, sympathetic ganglia (slow IPSP), medulla-pons, cerebellum	Smooth muscle, exocrine glands, hypothalamus	Conduction tissue, nucleus parabrachialis (?)

†Other muscarinic receptor subtypes may be (and probably are) located in the tissues specified.
*It may not be possible in all instances to ascribe a unique effector mechanism to a pharmacological subtype.

binding proteins which mediate different biochemical events (e.g. inhibition of adenylate cyclase, or stimulation of the phospholipase C which hydrolyses phosphoinositides). The effector mechanism could depend on the nature and concentration of the GTP binding protein(s) in the vicinity of the receptor, and the relative coupling efficiency of the receptor subtype to the different effector proteins.

9.7 Prospects for the Design of a Muscarinic Drug for Use in the Treatment of Alzheimer's Disease

The evidence at the present time suggests the existence of at least three muscarinic receptor subtypes in the central nervous system (Table 9.2). This immediately gives the potential for developing selective agents. However, confirmation of the existence of the receptor subtypes (as defined pharmacologically) is required from functional studies in the central nervous system, and the distribution of receptor subtypes needs to be mapped in detail at the light microscope, and preferably electron microscope, level. As the Type I (M_1) binding sites are located primarily in the cerebral cortex and hippocampus and these sites are unchanged in Alzheimer's brains, it is possible that an agonist acting selectively at these receptor sites could be useful in alleviating the cholinergic deficit and could produce fewer side effects. A further possibility is to regulate the feedback inhibition of acetylcholine release caused by the binding of acetylcholine to presynaptic autoreceptors. A selective antagonist directed against the presynaptic autoreceptors, which appear to have a low affinity for pirenzepine (Raiteri et al., 1984), could increase the neuronal release of acetylcholine and hence be of therapeutic benefit, especially in conjunction with a selective inhibitor of brain acetylcholinesterase. Equally, a selective presynaptic antagonist and postsynaptic agonist could be useful in providing a dual stimulation (Nordstrom et al., 1983).

The allosteric binding site on muscarinic receptors provides an opportunity to design novel muscarinic drugs. A drug which binds to the allosteric site and enhances the binding and actions of acetylcholine would have the effect of 'tuning up' the muscarinic response. This would be useful in alleviating the cholinergic deficit in Alzheimer's disease and perhaps providing some therapeutic benefit. Such an approach, analogous to the ability of some benzodiazepines to enhance $GABA_A$-receptor function, has certain advantages. First, the drug would have a defined maximal effect on the actions of acetylcholine and the possibility of overdosing and overstimulating the muscarinic system would be minimised. Second, the drug would only act under neuronal control. That is, the chronic stimulation and possible resultant desensitisation of the receptors by exogenous agonist would be eliminated. Third, the muscarinic receptor subtypes exhibit a selectivity in their binding profile for allosteric agents, and it may hence be possible to selectively 'tune up' muscarinic responses.

At the moment this approach is somewhat theoretical as no compound has, to our knowledge, been described as enhancing muscarinic function by binding to the allosteric site. Furthermore, this approach, together with those of the cholinesterase inhibitor and the presynaptic antagonist described earlier, do rely for their efficacy on a residuum of cholinergic input to the cerebral cortex. Nevertheless, there may be a guarded optimism that one of the strategies described in this section may be of use in alleviating the confusional states and memory deficits in Alzheimer's disease, at least in the earlier stages of the progression of the disease.

References

Ashe, J. H., and Yarosh, C. A. (1984). Differential and selective antagonism of the slow-inhibitory postsynaptic potential and slow-excitatory postsynaptic potential by gallamine and pirenzepine in the superior cervical ganglion of the rabbit. *Neuropharmacol.*, **23**, 1321-9.

Barlow, R. B., Burston, K. M., and Vis, A. (1980). Three types of muscarinic receptors? *Brit. J. Pharmacol.*, **68**, 141P.

Barlow, R. B., Franks, F. M., and Pearson, J. D. M. (1972). A comparison of the affinities of antagonists for acetylcholine receptors in the ileum, bronchial muscle and iris of the guinea-pig. *Br. J. Pharmacol.*, **46**, 300-12.

Barlow, R. B., Berry, K. J., Glenton, P. A. N., Nikolau, N. M., and Soh, K. S. (1976). A comparison of affinity constants for muscarine-sensitive acetylcholine receptors in guinea-pig atrial pacemaker cells at 29 °C and in ileum at 29 °C and 37 °C. *Br. J. Pharmacol.*, **58**, 613-20.

Barlow, R. B., Caulfield, M. P., Kitchen, R., Roberts, P. M., and Stubley, J. K. (1981). The affinities of pirenzepine and atropine for functional muscarinic receptors in guinea-pig atria and ileum. *Br. J. Pharmacol.*, **73**, 183P-4P.

Baron, J. H., and Londong, W. (eds.). (1980). Advances in basic and clinical pharmacology of Pirenzepine. *Scand. J. Gastroenterol.*, **15**, Suppl. 66, 1-114.

Bartus, R. T., Dean, R. L., Beer, B., and Lippa, A. S. (1982). The cholinergic hypothesis of geriatric memory dysfunction. *Science*, **217**, 408-17.

Ben-Baruch, G., Schreiber, G., and Sokolovsky, M. (1982). Cooperativity pattern in the interaction of the antiestrogen drug clomiphene with the muscarinic receptors. *Mol. Pharmacol.*, **21**, 287-93.

Berrie, C. P., Birdsall, N. J. M., Dadi, H. K., Hulme, E. C., Morris, R. J., Stockton, J. M., and Wheatley, M. (1985). Purification of the muscarinic acetylcholine receptor from rat forebrain. *Trans. Biochem. Soc.*, **13**, 1101-3.

Birdsall, N. J. M., and Hulme, E. C. (1983). Muscarinic receptor subclasses. *Trends Pharmacol. Sci.*, **4**, 459-63.

Birdsall, N. J. M., and Hulme, E. C. (1985). Multiple muscarinic receptors: further problems in receptor classification. *Trends Autonom. Pharmacol.*, **3**, 17-34.

Birdsall, N. J. M., Burgen, A. S. V., and Hulme, E. C. (1978). The binding of agonists to brain muscarinic receptors. *Molec. Pharmacol.*, **14**, 723-36.

Birdsall, N. J. M., Hulme, E. C., and Stockton, J. M. (1984). Muscarinic receptor heterogeneity. *Trends Pharmacol. Sci. Suppl.*, 4-8.

Birdsall, N. J. M., Burgen, A. S. V., Hulme, E. C., and Stockton, J. M. (1981). Gallamine regulates muscarinic receptors in the heart and cerebral cortex. *Br. J. Pharmacol.*, **74**, 798P.

Birdsall, N. J. M., Burgen, A. S. V., Hammer, R., Hulme, E. C., and Stockton, J. M. (1980). Pirenzepine — a ligand with original binding properties to muscarinic receptors. *Scand. J. Gastroenterol.*, **15**, Suppl. 66, 1-4.

Birdsall, N. J. M., Burgen, A. S. V., Hulme, E. C., Stockton, J. M., and Zigmond, M. J. (1983a). The effect of McN-A-343 on muscarinic receptors in the cerebral cortex and heart. *Br. J. Pharmac.*, 78, 257-9.

Birdsall, N. J. M., Hulme, E. C., Kromer, W., Stockton, J. M., and Zigmond, M. J. (1986). A second drug binding site on muscarinic receptors. *Fed. Proc.* (in press).

Birdsall, N. J. M., Hulme, E. C., Stockton, J. M., Burgen, A. S. V., Berrie, C. P., Hammer, R., Wong, E. H. F., and Zigmond, M. J. (1983b). Muscarinic receptor subclasses: evidence from binding studies. In De Feudis, F. V., and Mandel, P. (eds.), *CNS Receptors: From Molecular Pharmacology to Behaviour*, Raven Press, New York, pp. 323-9.

Black, J. W., Leff, P., and Shankley, N. P. (1985). Further analysis of anomalous pK_B values for muscarinic antagonists on the mouse stomach assay. *Br. J. Pharmacol.*, 85, 212P.

Blum, A. L., and Hammer, R. (eds.) (1979). *Die Behandlung des Ulcus pepticum mit Pirenzepin*. Demeter Verlag, Munich.

Bowen, D. M., Spillane, J. A., Curzon, G., Meier-Ruge, W., White, P., Goodhardt, M. J., Iwangoff, P., and Davison, A. N. (1979). Accelerated aging on selective neuron loss as an important cause of dementia. *Lancet*, i, 11-14.

Breitwieser, G. E., and Szabo, G. (1985). Uncoupling of cardiac muscarinic and adrenergic receptors from ion channels by a guanine nucleotide analogue. *Nature*, 317, 538-40.

Brown, D. A., Forward, A., and Marsh, S. (1980). Antagonist discrimination between ganglionic and ileal muscarinic receptors. *Br. J. Pharmac.*, 71, 362-4.

Caulfield, M., and Straughan, D. (1983). Muscarinic receptors revisited. *Trends Neurosci.*, 6, 73-5.

Caulfield, M. P., and Stubley, J. K. (1982). Pilocarpine selectively stimulates muscarinic receptors in rat sympathetic ganglia. *Br. J. Pharmacol.*, 76, 216P.

Caulfield, M. P., Straughan, D. W., Cross, A. J., Crow, T. J., and Birdsall, N. J. M. (1982). Cortical muscarinic receptor subtypes and Alzheimer's disease. *Lancet*, ii, 1279-80.

Changeux, J. P. (1966). Responses of acetylcholinesterase from *Torpedo* marmorata to salts and curarising agents. *Mol. Pharmacol.*, 2, 369-92.

Chassaing, C., Dureng, G., Baissat, J., and Duchene-Marullaz, P. (1984). Pharmacological evidence for cardiac muscarinic receptor subtypes. *Life Sci.*, 35, 1739-45.

Clague, R. U., Eglen, R. M., Strachan, A. C., and Whiting, R. L. (1985). Action of agonists and antagonists at muscarinic receptors present on ileum and atria *in vitro*. *Brit. J. Pharmacol.*, 86, 163-70.

Clark, A. L., and Mitchelson, F. (1976). The inhibitory effect of gallamine on muscarinic receptors. *Br. J. Pharmac.*, 58, 323-31.

Cohen-Armon, M., Henis, Y. I., Kloog, Y., and Sokolovsky, M. (1985). Interactions of quinidine and lidocaine with rat brain and heart muscarinic receptors. *Biochem. Biophys. Res. Commun.*, 127, 326-32.

Coyle, J. T., Price, D. L., and DeLong, M. R. (1983). Alzheimer's disease: a disorder of cortical cholinergic innervation. *Science*, 219, 1184-90.

Coyle, J. T., Price, D. L., and DeLong, M. R. (1984). Anatomy of cholinergic projections to cerebral cortex: implications for the pathophysiology of senile dementia of the Alzheimer's type. *Trends Pharmacol. Sci. Suppl.*, 90-3.

Daly, M. J., Humphrey, J. M., and Stables, R. (1982). Effects of H_2-receptor antagonists and anticholinoceptor drugs on gastric and salivary secretion induced by bethanechol in the anaesthetised dog. *Br. J. Pharmacol.*, 76, 361-5.

Davies, P. (1984). Neurochemical aspects of Alzheimer's disease. *Trends Pharmacol. Sci. Suppl.*, 98-9.

Davies, P., and Verth, A. H. (1978). Regional distribution of muscarinic acetylcholine receptor in normal and Alzheimer's type dementia brains. *Brain Res.*, 138, 385-92.

Deutsch, J. A. (1971). The cholinergic synapse and the site of memory. *Science*, 174. 788-93.

Doteval, G., Jaup, B. H., and Stockbrugger, R. W. (eds.) (1982). On the selectivity of anti-muscarinic compounds. *Scand. J. Gastroenterol.*, 17, Suppl. 72, 1-273.

Drachman, D. A. (1977). Memory and cognitive function in man: does the cholinergic system have a specific role? *Neurology*, 27, 783-90.

Drachman, D., and Leavitt, J. (1974). Human memory and the cholinergic system: a relationship to aging? *Arch. Neurol.*, 30, 113-20.

Dunlap, J., and Brown, J. H. (1983). Heterogeneity of binding sites on cardiac muscarinic receptors induced by the neuromuscular blocking agents gallamine and pancuronium. *Molec. Pharmacol.*, **24**, 15–22.

Egan, T. M., and North, R. A. (1985). Acetylcholine acts on m_2-muscarinic receptors to excite rat locus coeruleus neurones. *Br. J. Pharmacol.*, **85**, 733–5.

Ellis, J., and Lenox, R. H. (1985). Characterisation of the interactions of gallamine with muscaric receptors from brain. *Biochem. Pharmacol.*, **34**, 2214–17.

Eltze, M., Gonne, S., Riedel, R., Schlotke, B., Schudt, C., and Simon, W. A. (1985). Pharmacological evidence for selective inhibition of gastric acid secretion by telenzepine, a new antimuscarinic drug. *Eur. J. Pharmacol.*, **112**, 211–24.

Fisher, S. K. (1986). Inositol lipids and signal transduction at CNS muscarinic receptors. *Trends Pharmacol. Sci. Suppl.* 61–5.

Fisher, S. K., and Bartus, R. T. (1985). Regional differences in the coupling of muscarinic receptors to inositol phospholipid hydrolysis in guinea-pig brain. *J. Neurochem.*, **45**, 1085–95.

Fisher, A., Weinstock, M., Glitter, S., and Cohen, S. (1976). A new probe for heterogeneity in muscarinic receptors: 2-methyl-spiro(1,3-dioxolane-4,3')-quinuclidine. *Eur. J. Pharmacol.*, **37**, 329–38.

Franko, B. V., Ward, J. W., and Alphin, R. S. (1963). Pharmacologic studies of N-benzyl-3-pyrrolidinyl acetate methobromide (AHR-602), a ganglion stimulating agent. *J. Pharmacol. exp. Ther.*, **139**, 25–30.

Fuder, H., Rink, D., and Muscholl, E. (1982). Sympathetic nerve stimulation on the perfused rat heart. Affinities of N-methylatropine and pirenzepine at pre- and postsynaptic muscarine receptors. *Naunyn Schmiedeberg's Arch Pharmacol.*, **318**, 210–19.

Fuder, H., Meiser, C., Wormstall, H., and Muscholl, E. (1981). The effects of several muscarinic antagonists on pre- and postsynaptic receptors in the isolated heart. *Naunyn Schmiedeberg's Arch. Pharmacol.*, **316**, 31–7.

Giachetti, A., Micheletti, R., and Montagna, E. (1986). Cardioselective profile of AF-DX 116, a muscarine M_2 receptor antagonist. *Fed. Proc.* (in press).

Gil, D. W., and Wolfe, B. B. (1985). Pirenzepine distinguishes between muscarinic receptor-mediated phosphoinositide breakdown and inhibition of adenylate cyclase. *J. Pharm. exptl Ther.*, **232**, 608–16.

Growdon, J. H., Corkin, S., and Huff, F. J. (1985). Clinical evaluation of compounds for the treatment of memory dysfunction. *Ann. N.Y. Acad. Sci.*, **444**, 437–49.

Hammer, R. (1982). Subclasses of muscarinic receptors and pirenzepine. Further experimental evidence. *Scand. J. Gastroenterol.*, **17**, Suppl. 72, 59–67.

Hammer, R., and Giachetti, A. (1982). Muscarinic receptor subtypes: M1 and M2 biochemical and functional characterization. *Life Sci.*, **31**, 2991–8.

Hammer, R., and Giachetti, A. (1984). Selective muscarinic receptor antagonists. *Trends Pharmacol. Sci.*, **5**, 18–20.

Hammer, R., Berrie, C. P., Birdsall, N. J. M., Burgen, A. S. V., and Hulme, E. C. (1980). Pirenzepine distinguishes between subclasses of muscarinic receptor. *Nature (Lond.)*, **283**, 90–2.

Hammer, R., Giraldo, E., Schiavi, G. B., Monferini, E., and Ladinsky, H. (1986). Binding profile of a novel cardioselective muscarine receptor antagonist. AF-DX 116 to membranes of peripheral tissues and brain in the rat. *Life Sci.*, **38**, 1653–62.

Harbaugh, R. E., Roberts, D. W., Coombs, D. W., Sauders, R. L., and Reeder, T. M. Intracranial cholinergic drug infusion in patients with Alzheimer's disease. *Neurosurgery*, **15**, 514–18.

Henke, H., and Lang, W. (1983). Cholinergic enzymes in neocortex, hippocampus and basal forebrain of non-neurological and senile dementia of Alzheimer-type patients. *Brain Res.*, **267**, 281–91.

Hirschowitz, B. I., Hammer, R., Giachetti, A., Kierns, J. J., and Levine, R. R. (eds.). (1984). Subtypes of muscarinic receptors. *Trends Pharmacol. Sci. Suppl.*, 1–103.

Hulme, E. C., Berrie, C. P., Birdsall, N. J. M., and Burgen, A. S. V. (1981). Interactions of muscarinic receptors with guanine nucleotides and adenylate cyclase. In Birdsall, N. J. M. (ed.), *Drug Receptors and their Effectors*. Macmillan, London, 23–4.

Hulme, E. C., Berrie, C. P., Birdsall, N. J. M., Jameson, M., and Stockton, J. M. (1983), Regulation of muscarinic agonist binding by cations and guanine nucleotides. *Eur. J. Pharmacol.*, 94, 59–72.

Jacobson, M. D., Wusternan, M., and Downes, C. P. (1985). Muscarinic receptors and hydrolysis of inositol phospholipids in rat cerebral cortex and parotid gland. *J. Neurochem.*, 44, 465–72.

Jagadeesh, G., and Sulakhe, P. V. (1985). Gallamine binding to heart M_2 cholinergic receptors does not antagonize cholinergic inhibition of adenylate cyclase in isolated plasma membrane. *Eur. J. Pharmacol.*, 109, 311–13.

Jaup, B. H., Stockbrugger, R. W., and Doteval, G. (1982). Comparison between the effects of pirenzepine and 1-hyoscyamine in man. *Scand. J. Gastroenterol.*, 17, Suppl. 72, 119–22.

Kharkevich, D. A. and Shorr, V. A. (1980). Cardiotropic antimuscarinic action of some curare-like agents. *Arch. Int. Pharmacodyn. Ther.*, 248, 238–50.

Kilbinger, H. (1984a). Presynaptic muscarine receptors modulating acetylcholine release. *Trends Pharmacol. Sci.*, 5, 103–5.

Kilbinger, H. (1984b). Facilitation and inhibition by muscarinic agonists of acetylcholine release from guinea-pig myenteric neurones: mediation through different types of neuronal muscarinic receptors. *Trends Pharmacol. Sci. Suppl.*, 49–52.

Kilbinger, H., and Nafziger, M. (1985). Two types of neuronal muscarinic receptors modulating acetylcholine release from guinea-pig myenteric plexus. *Naunyn-Schmiedeberg's Arch. Pharmacol.*, 328, 304–9.

Kurose, H., Katada, T., Amano, T., and Ui, M. (1983). Specific uncoupling by islet-activating protein, pertussis toxin, of negative signal transduction via α_2-adrenergic, cholinergic and opiate receptors in neuroblastoma X glioma hybrid cells. *J. Biol. Chem.*, 258, 4870–5.

Lai, W. S., Ramkumar, V., and El-Fakahany, E. E. (1985). Possible allosteric interaction of 4-aminopyridine with rat brain muscarinic acetylcholine receptors. *J. Neurochem.*, 44, 1936–42.

Lang, W., and Henke, H. (1983). Cholinergic receptor binding and autoradiography in brains of non-neurological and senile dementia of Alzheimer-type patients. *Brain Res.*, 267, 271–80.

Lazareno, S., Kendall, D. A., and Nahorski, S. R. (1985). Pirenzepine indicates heterogeneity of muscarinic receptors linked to cerebral inositol phospholipid metabolism. *Neuropharmacol.*, 24, 593–5.

Li, C. K., and Mitchelson, F. (1980). The selective antimuscarinic action of stercuronium. *Br. J. Pharmacol.*, 70, 313–21.

Leung, E., and Mitchelson, F. (1982). The interaction of pancuronium with cardiac and ileal muscarinic receptors. *Eur. J. Pharmacol.*, 80, 1–9.

Levy, R. (1985). Rational drug treatment of dementia? *Br. Med. J.*, 291, 139.

Luthin, G. R., and Wolfe, B. B. (1984a). Comparison of [^{3}H]-pirenzepine and [^{3}H]-quinuclidinyl benzilate binding to muscarinic cholinergic receptors in rat brain. *J. Pharmacol. Expl. Ther.*, 228, 648–55.

Luthin, G. R., and Wolfe, B. B. (1984b). [^{3}H]quinuclidinyl benzilate binding to brain muscarinic cholinergic receptors. Differences in measured receptor density are not explained by differences in receptor isomerization. *Molec. Pharmacol.*, 26, 164–9.

Marshall, R. J., McGrath, J. C., Miller, R. D., Docherty, J. R., and Lamar, J.-C. (1980). Comparison of the cardiovascular actions of ORG NC 45 with those produced by other non-depolarising neuromuscular blocking agents in experimental animals. *Br. J. Anaesth.*, 52, 215–325.

Mash, D. C., Flynn, D. D., and Potter, L. T. (1985). Loss of M2 muscarine receptors in the cerebral cortex in Alzheimer's disease and experimental cholinergic denervation. *Science*, 288, 115–17.

Mitchelson, F. (1984). Heterogeneity of muscarinic receptors: evidence from pharmacologic studies with antagonists. *Trends Pharmacol. Sci. Suppl.*, 12–16.

Murad, F., Chi, Y.-M., Rall, T. W., and Sutherland, E. W. (1962). Adenyl cyclase III. The effect of catecholamines and choline esters on the formation of adenosine 3',5'-phosphate by preparations from cardiac muscle and liver. *J. Biol. Chem.*, 237, 1233–8.

Mutschler, E., and Lambrecht, G. (1984). Selective muscarinic agonists and antagonists in functional tests. *Trends Pharmacol. Sci. Suppl.*, 39–44.

Nedoma, J., Dorofeeva, N. A., Tucek, S., Shelkovnikov, S. A., and Danilov, A. F. (1985). Interaction of the neuromuscular blocking drugs alcuronium, decamethonium, gallamine, pancuronium, ritebronium, tercuronium and d-tubocurarine with muscarinic acetylcholine receptors in the heart and ileum. *Naunyn Schmiedeberg's Arch. Pharmacol.*, **329**, 176–81.

Nordstrom, O., Alberts, P., Westlind, A., Unden, A., and Bartfai, T. (1983). Presynaptic antagonist–postsynaptic agonist at muscarinic cholinergic synapses. *Mol. Pharmacol.*, **24**, 1–5.

North, R. A. (1986). Muscarinic receptors and membrane ion conductances. *Trends Pharmacol. Sci. Suppl.*, 19–22.

Pagani, F., Schiavone, E., Monferini, E., Hammer, R., and Giachetti, A. (1984). Distinct muscarinic receptor subtypes (M_1 and M_2) controlling acid secretion in rodents. *Trends Pharmacol. Sci. Suppl.*, 66–8.

Parsons, M. E., Bunce, T., Blakemore, C., and Rasmussen, C. (1979). Pharmacological studies on the gastric antisecretory agent, pirenzepine. In Blum, A. L., and Hammer, R. (eds.), *Die Behandlung des Ulcus pepticum mit Pirenzepin*. Demeter Verlag, Munich, pp. 26–34.

Perry, E. K., Tomlinson, B. E., Blessed, G., Bergmann, K., Gibson, P. H., and Perry, R. H. (1978). Correlation of cholinergic abnormalities with senile plaques and mental test scores in senile dementia. *Brit. Med. J.*, **25**, 1457–9.

Perry, R. H., Candy, J. M., Perry, E. K., Irving, D., Blessed, G., Fairbairn, A. F., and Tomlinson, B. E. (1982). Extensive loss of choline acetyltransferase activity is not reflected by neuronal loss in the nucleus of Meynert in Alzheimer's disease. *Neurosci. Lett.*, **33**, 311–15.

Pfaffinger, P. J., Martin, J. M., Hunter, D. D., Nathanson, N. M., and Hille, B. (1985). GTP-binding proteins couple cardiac muscarinic receptors to a K channel. *Nature*, **317**, 536–8.

Porsius, A. J., Wilffert, B., Lambrecht, G., Moser, U., and Mutschler, E. (1981). Muscarinic effects of various isoarecaidine esters in sympathetic ganglia. *J. Auton. Pharmacol.*, **1**, 119–26.

Potter, L. T., Flynn, D. D., Hanchett, H. E., Kalinoski, D. L., Luber-Narod, J., and Mash, D. C. (1984). Independent M_1 and M_2 receptors: ligands, autoradiography and functions. *Trends Pharmacol. Sci. Suppl.*, 22–31.

Raiteri, M., Leardi, R., and Marchi, M. (1984). Heterogeneity of presynaptic muscarinic receptors regulating neurotransmitter release in the rat brain. *J. Pharm. expl Therap.*, **228**, 209–14.

Reisine, T. D., Yamamura, H. I., Bird, E. D., Spokes, E., and Enna, S. J. (1978). Pre- and post-synaptic neurochemical alterations in Alzheimer's disease. *Brain Res.*, **159**, 477–80.

Riker, W. F., and Wescoe, W. C. (1951). The pharmacology of flaxedil with observations on certain analogs. *Ann. N.Y. Acad. Sci.*, **54**, 373–94.

Rinne, J. O., Rinne, J. K., Laakso, K., Paljarvi, L., and Rinne, U. K. (1984). Reduction in muscarinic receptor binding in limbic areas of Alzheimer brain. *J. Neurol. Neurosurg. Psychiat.*, **47**, 651–3.

Rosenfeld, E. C. (1983). Pirenzepine (LS 519): A weak inhibitor of acid secretion in isolated rat parietal cells. *Eur. J. Pharmacol.*, **86**, 99–101.

Rossor, M. N. (1982). Dementia. *Lancet*, **ii**, 1200–4.

Rossor, M. N., and Iversen, L. L. (1986). Non-cholinergic neurotransmission abnormalities in Alzheimer's disease. *Br. Med. Bull.*, **42**, 1–114.

Roszkowski, A. P. (1961) An unusual type of sympathetic ganglionic stimulant. *J. Pharmacol. Exp. Ther.*, **132**, 156–70.

Sitaram, N., Weingartner, H., and Gillin, J. C. (1978). Human serial learning: enhancement with arecoline and choline and impairment with scopolamine. *Science*, **201**, 274–6.

Smith, T. L., and Yamamura, H. I. (1985). Carbachol stimulation of phosphatidic acid synthesis: competitive inhibition by pirenzepine in synaptosomes from rat cerebral cortex. *Biochem. Biophys. Res. Commun.*, **130**, 282–5.

Soejima, M., and Noma, A. (1984). Mode of regulation of the ACh-sensitive K-channel by the muscarinic receptor in rabbit atrial cells. *Pflugers Arch.*, **400**, 424.

Sokolovsky, M. (1984). Muscarinic receptors in the central nervous system. *Int. Rev. Neurobiol.*, **25**, 139-83.

Soll, A. H. (1984). Fundic mucosal muscarinic receptors modulating acid secretion. *Trends Pharmacol. Sci. Suppl.*, 60-2.

Stockton, J., Birdsall, N. J. M., Burgen, A. S. V., and Hulme, E. C. (1983). Modification of the binding properties of muscarinic receptors by gallamine. *Mol. Pharmacol.*, **23**, 551-7.

Szelenyi, I. (1982). Does pirenzepine distinguish between 'subtypes' of muscarinic receptors. *Br. J. Pharmacol.*, **77**, 567-9.

Tien, X.-Y., and Wallace, L. J. (1985). Trihexyphenidyl – further evidence for muscarinic receptor subclassification. *Biochem. Pharmacol.*, **34**, 588-90.

Waelbroeck, M., Robberecht, P., De Neff, P., and Christophe, J. (1984). Effects of verapamil on the binding properties of rat heart muscarinic receptors: evidence for an allosteric site. *Biochem. Biophys. Res. Commun.*, **121**, 340-5.

Watson, M., Roeske, W. R., and Yamamura, H. I. (1982). [^{3}H] pirenzepine selectively identifies a high affinity population of muscarinic cholinergic receptors in the rat cerebral cortex. *Life Sci.*, **31**, 2019-23.

Watson, M., Yamamura, H. I., and Roeske, W. R. (1983). A unique regulatory profile and regional distribution of [^{3}H] pirenzepine binding in the rat provide evidence for distinct M_1 and M_2 muscarinic receptor subtypes. *Life Sci.*, **32**, 3001-11.

Watson, M., Vickroy, T. W., Roeske, W. R., and Yamamura, H. I. (1984). Subclassification of muscarinic receptors based upon the selective antagonist pirenzepine. *Trends Pharmacol. Sci. Suppl.*, 9-11.

Wettstein, A., and Spiegel, R. (1984). Clinical trials with the cholinergic drug RS 86 in Alzheimer's disease (AD) and senile dementia of the Alzheimer type (SDAT). *Psychopharmacol.*, **84**, 572-3.

White, P., Hiley, C. R., Goodhart, M. J., Carrasco, L. H., Keet, J. P., Williams, I. E. I., and Bowen, D. M. (1977). Neocortical cholinergic neurons in elderly people. *Lancet*, i, 668-71.

Whitehouse, P. J., Price, D. L., Struble, R. G., Clark, A. W., Coyle, J. T., and De Long, M. R. (1982). Alzheimer's disease and senile dementia: loss of neurons in the basal forebrain. *Science*, **215**, 1237-9.

Wood, P. L., Etienne, P., Lai, S., Nair, N. P., Finlayson, M. H., Gauthier, S., Palo, J., Haltia, M., Paetau, A., and Bird, E. D. (1983). A post-mortem comparison of the cortical cholinergic system in Alzheimer's disease and Pick's disease. *J. neurol. Sci.*, **62**, 211-17.

Yamamura, H. I., Wamsley, J. K., Deshmukh, P., and Roeske, W. R. (1983). Differential light microscopic autoradiographic localisation of muscarinic cholinergic receptors in the brainstem and spinal cord of the rat using [^{3}H] pirenzepine. *Eur. J. Pharmacol.*, **91**, 147-9.

10

Soluble and Membrane-bound Forms of Choline-o-Acetyltransferase Activity in the Purely Cholinergic Neurons of *Torpedo*

L. Eder-Colli, S. Amato and Y. Froment

10.1 Introduction

The enzyme choline-o-acetyltransferase (EC 2.3.1.6; ChAT), which catalyses the biosynthesis of the neurotransmitter acetylcholine (ACh) from choline and acetylcoenzyme A (AcCoA), was traditionally thought to exist solely in a soluble form in the cytoplasm of cholinergic nerve endings. In the present study we describe the biochemical and immunological identification of a membrane-bound form of ChAT in the plasma membrane of cholinergic nerve endings; this form differs from the soluble ChAT activity in some of its biochemical and physical properties. Our investigation was carried out on the plasma membrane purified from cholinergic synaptosomes isolated from the electric organ of the fish *Torpedo*. This tissue, which presents homology to vertebrate neuromuscular junction, receives a profuse and purely cholinergic innervation.

ChAT is synthetised in the perikarya of cholinergic neurons from whence it is transported into the nerve endings by slow axonal transport (Dahlström, 1983). Subfractionation of brain tissue produced the highest specific activity (SA) for ChAT in the fractions enriched in isolated nerve endings (synaptosomes) (Hebb and Whittaker, 1958; Whittaker, 1965; Tucek, 1967). Disruption of synaptosomes occurs after suspension in hypotonic media. In this condition ChAT activity was found to distribute into soluble and particulate activity; the proportion of particulate activity varying according to the animal species used, this being attributed to differences in the isoelectric points displayed by the enzyme from one species to another (Fonnum, 1967; 1970). The membrane-bound activity was ionically associated with membranes, since it could be solubilised by high salt washings of the membrane fractions (Fonnum, 1968). These findings led to the conclusion that ChAT is freely soluble in the cytoplasm of the nerve terminal and that the ability of the enzyme to bind non-specifically to membranes through ionic interactions probably does not play a physiological role.

Carroll and co-workers (Smith and Carroll, 1980; Benishin and Carroll, 1981a,b; Benishin and Carroll, 1983, 1984), however, have described a specific form of membrane-bound ChAT which could not be solubilised in high salt solutions. They found this form of ChAT to be present in a crude mitochondrial fraction obtained after subfractionation of mammalian brain tissue and considered it to be non-ionically bound to membranes. This form, which could be solubilised by the detergent Triton DN-65 appeared to be more specifically associated with nerve terminals. However, it is not known if it is associated with synaptic vesicles, with plasma membrane of the nerve terminals, or both. The membrane-bound and soluble ChAT activities were reported to have different properties. The possibility was raised that this non-ionically membrane-bound ChAT is soluble ChAT occluded into synaptosomes which escaped hypotonic disruption (Tucek, 1984, 1985).

10.2 Material and Methods

10.2.1 Isolation of the Synaptosomal Plasma Membranes (SPM)

Membranes were isolated from *Torpedo* synaptosomes (Israël *et al.*, 1976), by applying procedures previously described by Stadler and Tashiro (1979) and Morel *et al.* (1982), which make use of subfractionation on discontinuous and continuous density gradients of sucrose. As shown in the flow chart of Fig. 10.1, the synaptic plasma membranes (SPMs) are purified from crude SPM obtained after hypoosmotic disruption of synaptosomes which are or are not washed with high salt solutions (0.5 M NaCl in 5 mM Tris HCl, 1 mM EDTA, pH 8.2).

10.2.2 Other Subfractionations

Isolation of axonal membranes of the electric nerves innervating the electric organ were performed as previously described by Eder-Colli and Amato (1985). Purification of synaptic vesicles was as described by Carlson *et al.* (1978). Preparation of rat brain synaptosomes was performed according to Dodd *et al.* (1981).

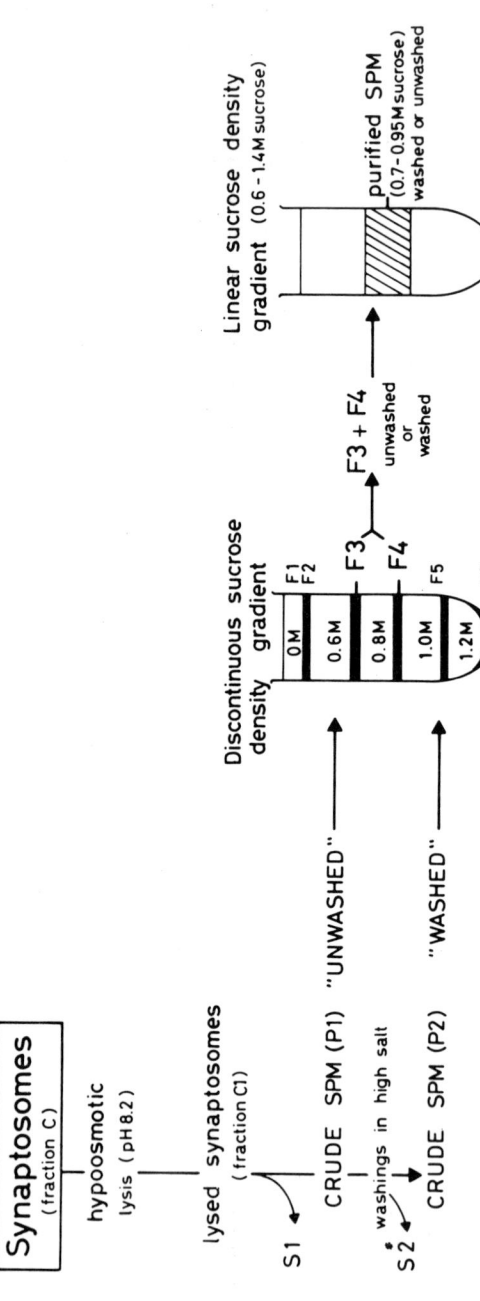

Fig. 10.1 Flow chart of the purification of *Torpedo* synaptosomal plasma membranes (SPMs). The *Torpedo* synaptosomes are hypotonically disrupted by suspension in 5 mM Tris HCl, 1 mm EDTA, pH 8.2 (buffer A). Centrifugation at 100 000g, 1 h at 4 °C, provides soluble (S1) and crude SPM (P1) fractions. To remove the ionically membrane-bound ChAT activity, the fraction P1 is washed three times by high speed centrifugation with 0.5 M NaCl in buffer A; this provides the fraction P2 of washed crude SPMs and the fraction S2* which corresponds to the pool of the supernatants of the three high salt washes. The crude SPM fraction (P1 or P2) is loaded on a discontinuous sucrose density gradient (2 mg protein/gradient; the gradient is composed from top to bottom of: 2 ml 0.6 M, 3 ml 0.8 M, 3 ml 1.0 M and 2 ml 1.2 M sucrose in buffer A). After centrifugation at 240 000g, 4 h at 4 °C, fractions F3 and F4, which are enriched in SPMs, are collected, pooled and concentrated by centrifugation; the pellet is resuspended in buffer A and 1 mg protein is further purified on a continuous density gradient of sucrose (0.6 to 1.4 M sucrose in buffer A, 11 ml). After centrifugation at 240 000g, 19 h at 4 °C, 0.5 ml fractions are collected.

10.2.3 Partition of Hydrophilic and Hydrophobic Synaptosomal Proteins by Triton X-114

The non-ionic detergent Triton X-114 was used successfully by Bordier (1981) to partition hydrophilic proteins from integral membrane (hydrophobic) proteins of cells. At $0\,^{\circ}C$ Triton X-114 forms a homogeneous solution in water but separates into an aqueous and a detergent phase above $20\,^{\circ}C$ (cloud point of Triton X-114), and the extent of this separation increases with temperature. A short (3 min) centrifugation of the mixture at room temperature allows complete separation into an aqueous (upper) and detergent (lower) phases. Triton X-114 solubilisation of *Torpedo* or rat brain synaptosomes was performed at $0\,^{\circ}C$; the solubilised material was first submitted to high speed centrifugation (30 min, $100\,000g$) at $4\,^{\circ}C$ to remove the detergent-insoluble material (structural proteins) and then brought to $37\,^{\circ}C$ (3 min). The solubilised proteins were finally separated into hydrophilic (aqueous phase) and hydrophobic (detergent phase) proteins by a brief centrifugation. ChAT activity was assayed in the solubilised synaptosomes (initial step), in the aqueous and detergent phases and in the detergent-insoluble residue.

10.2.4 Production of Monoclonal Antibodies to Torpedo SPM

Balb/c mice were immunised with the purified SPMs according to a protocol used previously by Eder-Colli *et al.* (1982). The most positive sera against this purified membrane were selected for the subsequent production of McAB. The fusion protocol was as described by Galfré *et al.* (1977). The PAI myeloma cell line, a non-secreting one, was used for the fusion. Immune responses were analysed by dot immunobinding assay (Hawkes *et al.*, 1981) and immunoblotting techniques (Burnette, 1981). When required McAB were affinity purified on protein-A Sepharose.

10.2.5 SDS-PAGE

SDS-PAGE were performed in 6–15 % polyacrylamide slab gels using the discontinuous buffer system of Laemmli (1970).

10.2.6 Biochemical Assays

ChAT activity was assayed as described by Fonnum (1969) and modified by Rossier *et al.* (1973). Acetylcholinesterase (AChE) activity was measured according to Ellmann *et al.* (1961). The nicotinic receptor to ACh (nAcChR), a marker for postsynaptic membranes, was determined according to Schmidt and Raftery (1973). Proteins were measured by the Amido-Black method (Schaffner and Weissman, 1973); when samples containing detergent (Triton X-114) were measured, standard curves were prepared in the presence of the detergent.

10.3 Results

10.3.1 Characterisation of the Purified SPMs

The purification of SPMs was monitored by assaying AChE activity and the presence of nAcChR in the different fractions (Fig. 10.2). In agreement with Morel *et al.* (1982), the purified SPMs exhibited an enrichment in AChE activity whereas the SA for the nAcChR is greatly decreased in this fraction. AChE activity is an integral protein of the plasma membrane of *Torpedo* nerve endings (Morel and Dreyfus, 1982; Li and Bon, 1983). AChE activity is, however, widely distributed in neuronal as well as in non-neuronal tissue and therefore cannot be considered a good marker for presynaptic plasma membrane. Morel *et al.* (1982) used morphological criteria to ascertain that the purified SPMs are presynaptic plasma membrane.

The distribution of ChAT activity was also measured during SPM purification (Fig. 10.2, bottom). Although a large proportion of ChAT appeared as soluble activity (supnt) after hypotonic lysis of the synaptosomes, the crude SPM fraction also contained significant amounts of ChAT (300 nmol/h/mg prot.). The membrane-bound activity became four times enriched in the final preparation of purified SPMs. A very similar distribution of ChAT activity was obtained when SPMs were purified from crude SPMs which were previously washed with high salt solutions in order to solubilise the ionically-bound ChAT. Although the SA for ChAT in the different fractions was decreased after the washing, significant levels of activity were still present as non-ionically membrane-bound activity and, again, a four-fold enrichment in ChAT activity was observed when purified and crude SPMs were compared.

The distribution and the SA values for AChE and nAcChR were similar whether the crude SPMs were unwashed or washed.

Thus, a non-ionically membrane-bound form of ChAT appears to copurify with the plasma membranes of cholinergic nerve endings. The specificity of the non-ionic association of ChAT with the SPMs was investigated. As shown in Fig. 10.3, very little ChAT activity remained non-ionically bound to axonal membranes isolated from the electric nerves innervating the *Torpedo* electric organ (SA: 2.4 nmol/h/mg prot.), and no activity was detectable in highly purified synaptic vesicles.

These results suggest that the non-ionically bound ChAT activity may be used as a marker for plasma membranes of cholinergic nerve endings.

10.3.2 Triton X-114 Solubilisation and Phase Partition: Hydrophilic and Hydrophobic ChAT

If the non-ionically membrane-bound ChAT is really a membrane protein, it should be distinguishable from soluble ChAT by using the Triton X-114 phase separation method, which allows partition of hydrophilic from integral membrane (hydrophobic) proteins of cells. The results obtained with *Torpedo* and

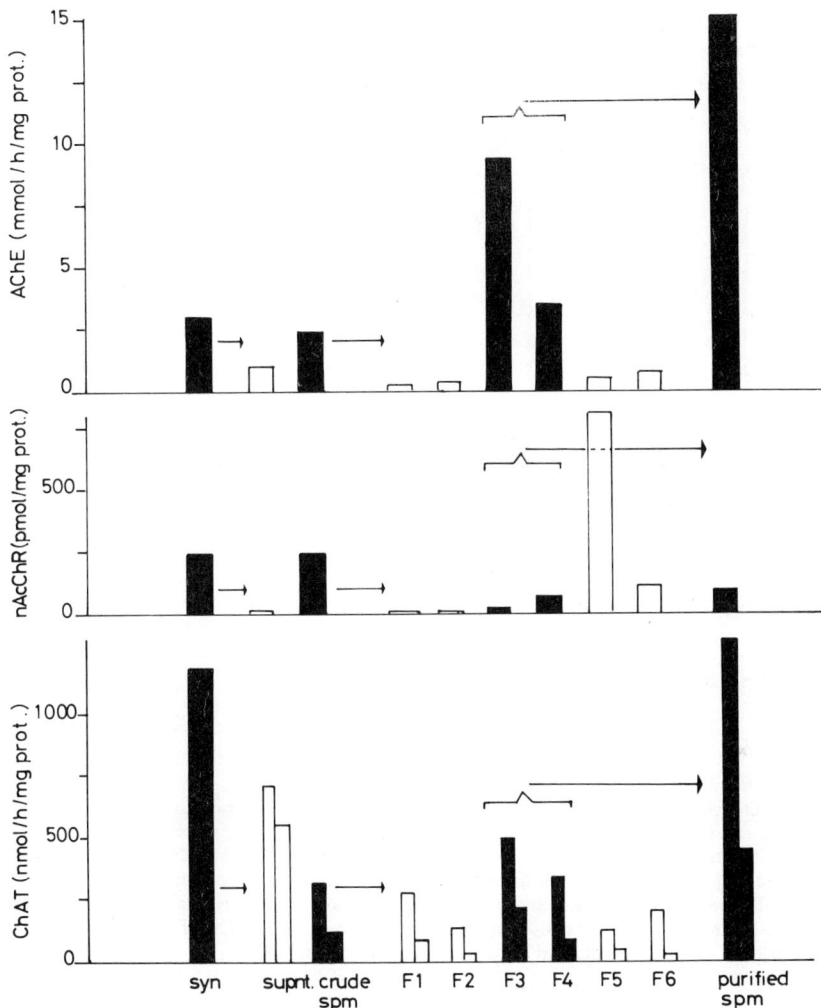

Fig. 10.2 Distribution of AChE, nAcChR and ChAT specific activities (SAs) during the purification of *Torpedo* SPMs. The SA for AChE (mmol/h/mg protein (top panel)), nAcChR (pmol/mg protein (middle panel)) and ChAT (nmol/h/mg protein (lower panel)) were determined in each fraction obtained during the purification of SPMs as described in Fig. 10.1 from unwashed or washed crude SPMs. For AChE and nAcChR no significant difference was observed in the distribution or in the SA, whether the SPMs were unwashed or washed with high salt solutions; therefore only the results obtained with the unwashed membranes are represented here for these two markers. With regard to the distribution of ChAT activity, the left-hand columns and the right-hand columns give the SA values obtained during the purification from unwashed and from washed crude SPMs, respectively. The high salt washings of the crude SPMs leave about 125 nmol/h/mg protein of ChAT non-ionically bound to membranes (crude SPMs, right-hand column), whilst 550 nmol/h/mg protein of activity are solubilised in high salt (supnt, right-hand column). (The SA of ChAT in the purified SPMs (left-hand column) corresponds to the SA which was present in the SPMs we used to develop McAB against *Torpedo* SPM.)

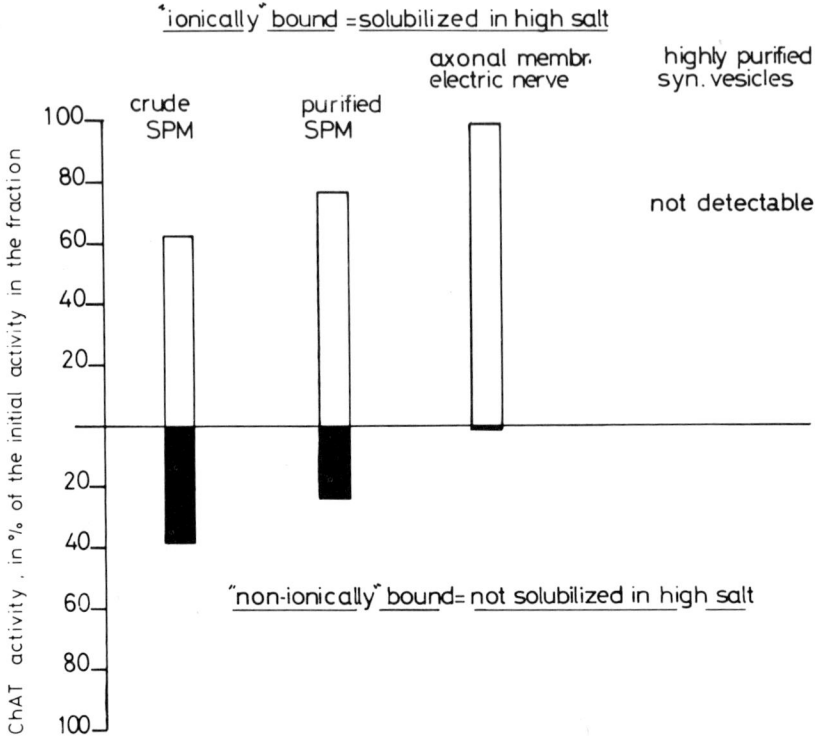

Fig. 10.3 Distribution of high salt soluble and non-ionically bound ChAT activity in particulate fractions isolated from *Torpedo*: specificity of the non-ionic association with SPMs. Each membrane fraction was washed three times with 0.5 M NaCl in 5 mM Tris-HCl, 1 mM EDTA, pH 8.2, and ChAT activity was determined in the washed membranes (i.e. non-ionically membrane-bound) and in the supernatants of the high salt washes (ionically membrane-bound). The results are expressed in per cent of the ChAT activity which was present in each membrane fraction before the washing.

rat brain synaptosomes are shown in Fig. 10.4 and 10.5. For *Torpedo* ChAT, the aqueous phase (hydrophilic activity), the detergent phase (hydrophobic activity) and the detergent-insoluble residue had activities of 850, 250 and 370 nmol/h/mg prot., respectively (Fig. 10.4). The presence of detergent-insoluble ChAT raises the question of a possible interaction of ChAT with cytoskeleton; this has to be further investigated. The ChAT activity defined above as non-ionically bound corresponds most probably to hydrophobic ChAT, and the hydrophilic ChAT represents most of the soluble ChAT (soluble in low and high ionic salt media).

ChAT from rat brain synaptosomes also partitioned into hydrophilic, hydro-phobic and detergent-resistant activity (Fig. 10.5). The hydrophobic ChAT

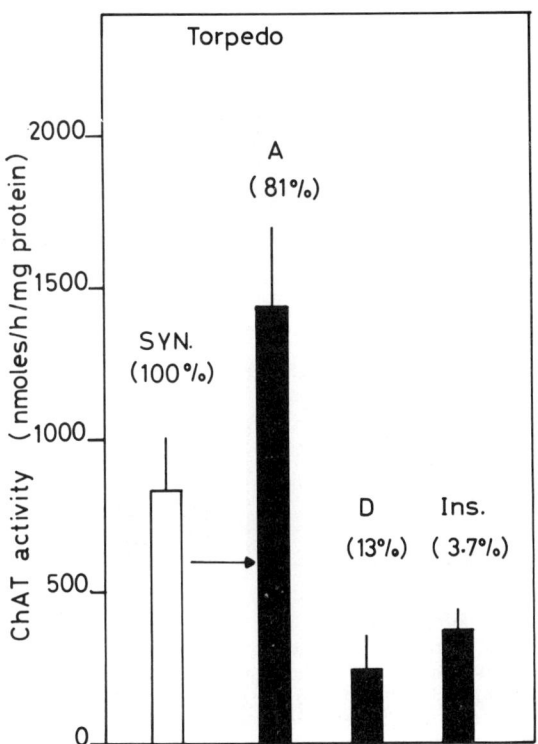

Fig. 10.4 Triton X-114 solubilisation of *Torpedo* synaptosomes: phase partition of hydrophilic and hydrophobic ChAT activities. *Torpedo* synaptosomes isolated as described by Israël *et al.* (1976), were obtained in 0.45 M sucrose; this preparation was diluted with an equal volume of isotonic solution containing no sucrose and was concentrated by centrifugation at 32 000*g*, 15 min at 4 °C; the pellet was then suspended at 0.5–0.7 mg protein/ml of 10 mM Tris-HCl, 0.15 M NaCl, 1 mM EDTA, pH 8.2 and extracted 3 min at 0 °C with 1 % (w/v) Triton X-114 (SYN); the sample was centrifuged at 100 000*g*, 30 min at 4 °C to remove the detergent-insoluble protein (Ins); the solution was then placed at 37 °C for 3 min, during which the mixed micelles of detergent-hydrophobic protein separate from the aqueous phase. Three minute centrifugation at 10 000*g* at room temperature completely separated the aqueous phase from the detergent phase. The aqueous phase (A) was extracted two additional times in the same way with 1 % Triton X-114 and the three detergent phases obtained at the end of the experiment were pooled (D). ChAT specific activity (nmol/h/mg protein; mean value ± SEM of four separate experiments) was determined in each fraction. ChAT activity as a percentage of the total activity present in solubilised synaptosomes is indicated in brackets.

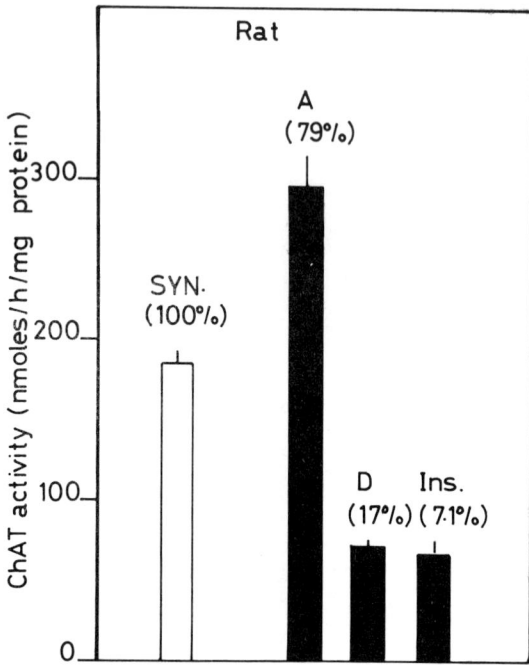

Fig. 10.5 Triton X-114 solubilisation of rat brain synaptosomes: phase partition of hydrophilic and hydrophobic ChAT activities. The experiments were conducted exactly as described in Fig. 10.4 for *Torpedo* synaptosomes. ChAT specific activity (nmol/h/mg protein;
mean value ± SEM of three determinations) was determined for the solubilised synaptosomes (SYN), in the aqueous (A) and in the detergent (D) phases and in the detergent-
resistant residue (Ins). ChAT activity as a percentage of the activity initially present (SYN)
is indicated in brackets.

amounted to 18 % of the synaptosomal activity, a value very close to that found
by Benishin and Carroll (1983) for the Triton DN-65 soluble ChAT in rat brain
synaptosomes.

In conclusion, two forms of ChAT exist in cholinergic nerve endings that
interact differently with non-ionic detergents: this may indicate a difference in
the hydrophobicity of the two forms but does not prove that hydrophobic
ChAT is an integral protein of the plasma membrane of cholinergic nerve endings.

10.3.3 *Characterisation of the Hydrophilic and Hydrophobic Forms of* Torpedo *ChAT*

10.3.3.1 *Inhibition by Bromoacetylcholine*

Bromoacetylcholine (BrACh) was used by Tuček (1982) to inhibit specifically
ChAT activity. This inhibitor (2 μM final concentration) was able to inhibit

85 % of synaptosomal ChAT, 85 % of hydrophilic and 90 % of hydrophobic ChAT. This indicates that the choline acetylating activity we were measuring is mainly due to ChAT and not to non-specific choline acetylating activity (Tuček, 1984, 1985).

10.3.3.2 Velocity of Choline Acetylation

The affinities for choline and for AcCoA were determined by measuring the velocity of choline acetylation as a function of increasing choline concentrations (0.155 to 5 mM) or AcCoA concentrations (4.5 to 72 μM). Acetylation by hydrophilic and hydrophobic ChAT was saturable and exhibited linearity with time when assayed between 5 and 20 minutes. The affinities for choline and AcCoA for both forms of ChAT are presented in Table 10.1. The two forms of ChAT exhibit very similar affinities for choline; this is also true for AcCoA. The mammalian brain enzyme (soluble and membrane-bound) has higher affinities for choline (0.3-4.0 mM; Benishin and Carroll, 1983).

Table 10.1   Affinities for choline and AcCoA of hydrophilic and hydrophobic ChAT activities

	app. K_m	
	Choline (mM)	AcCoA (μM)
Hydrophilic ChAT	0.87	12.5
Hydrophobic ChAT	0.99	11.2

The velocity of choline acetylation by the ChAT activity present in the aqueous phase (hydrophilic ChAT) and in the detergent phase (hydrophobic ChAT) obtained after Triton X-114 solubilisation of *Torpedo* synaptosomes was determined as a function of: (a) increasing concentrations of choline (from 0.0155 to 8.3 mM), the AcCoA concentration being kept constant at 50 μM; and (b) increasing concentrations of ^{14}C-AcCoA/AcCoA (from 4.3 to 72 μM), the choline concentration being kept constant at 5 mM. In each experiment the aqueous and the detergent phases were normalised for their Triton X-114 and buffer concentration. The acetylation of endogenous substrates obtained without choline addition was subtracted from each value. The app K_m values were obtained from Eadie-Hofstee plots of v (nmol/h/mg protein) as a function of v/S (concentration of the substrate).

10.3.3.3 Sensitivity of Choline Acetylation to Temperature and to pH Variations

For the ChAT assay we usually measure the ACh formed after 10 min incubation at 37 °C. When the incubation temperature is varied from 15 to 45 °C (Fig. 10.6(a)), a broad peak of activity is observed between 25 and 37 °C for both hydrophilic and hydrophobic ChAT. At 45 °C, both forms are inactivated, however preincubation at 45 °C for increasing periods of time (30 s to 5 min) showed a faster rate of inactivation of hydrophilic than hydrophobic ChAT (Fig. 10.6(b)).

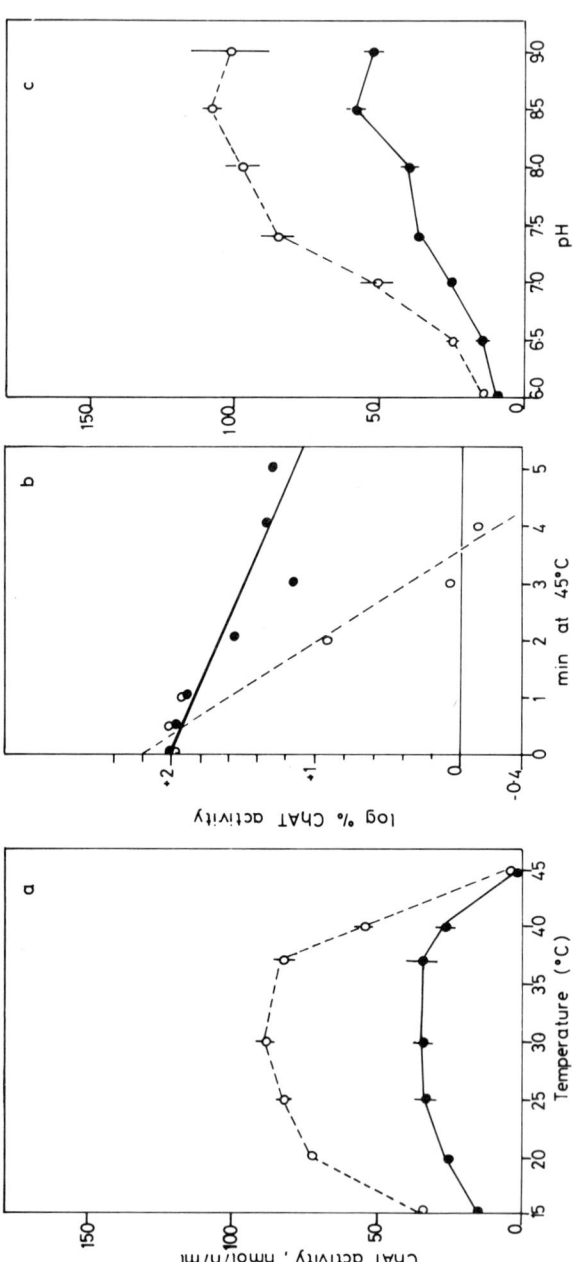

Fig. 10.6 Sensitivity of hydrophilic and hydrophobic ChAT to temperature and to pH variations. In all these experiments ChAT activity in the aqueous (dashed curve; hydrophilic) and the detergent (continuous curve; hydrophobic) phases obtained after Triton X-114 extraction of *Torpedo* synaptosomes was assayed. Both fractions were normalised for their Triton X-114 and buffer concentrations. ChAT activity was measured by its ability to synthesise radiolabelled ACh from choline (5 mM final concentration) and ^{14}C-AcCoA (50 μM, final concentration; specific activity 6.3 mCi/mmole); the incubation time for the reaction was 10 min. (a) Choline acetylation was assayed at the different temperatures indicated (between 15 and 45 °C). Values (nmol ACh formed per min and per ml of sample) are means ± SEM of three determinations. (b) The sensitivity to heat denaturation was analysed by preincubating hydrophilic or hydrophobic ChAT at 45 °C for different periods of time (30 s to 5 min). Values are expressed as the logarithm of the percentage of ChAT activity remaining and are means of six determinations. (c) The velocity of choline acetylation by hydrophilic or hydrophobic ChAT activity was determined at different pHs of the incubation buffer (sodium phosphate buffer) for the ChAT assay. ChAT activity is expressed in nmoles of ACh formed per hour and per ml of sample and the values are means ± SEM of three determinations.

For the ChAT assay pH 7.4 is used. When the pH of the reaction medium was varied from 6.0 to 9.0, hydrophilic and hydrophobic ChAT exhibited broad pH optima around 8.5. However, a more pronounced activation of hydrophilic than hydrophobic ChAT occurred between pH 7.0 and pH 8.5 (Fig. 10.6(c)).

10.3.3.4 Effect of Increasing Concentrations of ACh

The hydrophilic and hydrophobic activities were assayed in the presence of increasing concentrations of ACh. As shown in Fig. 10.7, inhibition of both

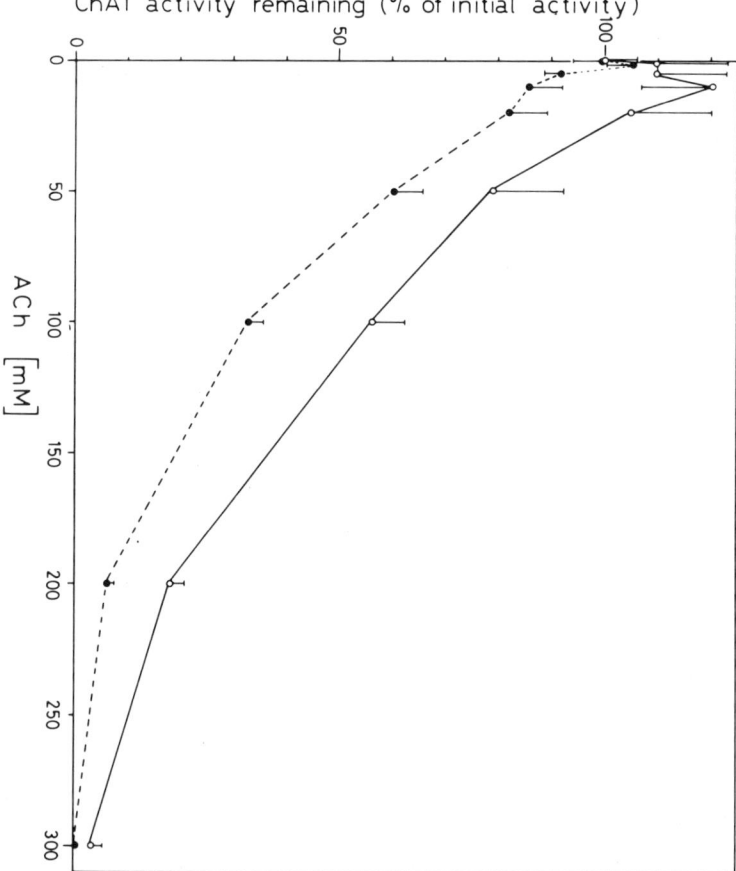

Fig. 10.7 Sensitivity of hydrophilic and hydrophobic ChAT to inhibition by ACh. Choline acetylation by ChAT present in the aqueous phase (dashed curve) or in the detergent phase (continuous curve) obtained after Triton X-114 solubilisation of *Torpedo* synaptosomes was measured in the presence of increasing concentrations of ACh added to the incubation mixture used for the ChAT assay. The assay was at 37 °C and the incubation time was 10 min. Values (means ± SEM, $n = 6$) are expressed as a percentage of the initial ChAT activity measured in the absence of ACh.

forms of ChAT increased as the ACh concentration was raised. ACh is known to be a competitive inhibitor of ChAT, however not only is hydrophobic ChAT less sensitive to ACh inhibition than hydrophilic ChAT, but this form is slightly activated by 5–20 mM ACh. In cholinergic nerve endings *in situ*, the ACh concentration is 20–50 mM (Dunant and Israel, 1975), therefore variations of ACh levels inside the nerve terminal may regulate differently hydrophilic and hydrophobic ChAT activity.

10.3.4 Monoclonal Antibodies against Torpedo *SPM Inhibit* Torpedo *ChAT*

Of the stable monoclonal antibodies we have selected as specifically recognising purified SPMs, two were able to inhibit ChAT activity. As shown in Fig. 10.8, both antibodies have similar inhibition curves for hydrophilic and hydrophobic ChAT. However, the antibody 8/38A is a more potent inhibitor than the 8/37 one.

The McAB 8/38A was used in immunoblotting experiments to determine the apparent molecular weight (app. MW) of hydrophilic and hydrophobic ChAT. As shown in Fig. 10.9, the antibody binds to two polypeptide bands of about 70 and 67 kilodaltons (kD) MW on 'western' blots of SDS-PAGE containing hydrophilic or hydrophobic ChAT. These two bands were also recognised on blots of whole synaptosomes which were solubilised in Triton X-114 (i.e. containing hydrophilic and hydrophobic ChAT). The same results were obtained by using the McAB 8/37. Therefore hydrophilic and hydrophobic ChAT appear to have similar MW.

10.4 Discussion

The results presented in this study show that at least two forms of ChAT activity exist in cholinergic nerve terminals of *Torpedo*: a soluble and a membrane form. The latter interacts non-ionically with the plasma membrane of the nerve terminal and appears to be hydrophobic from the strength of its interaction with the non-ionic detergent Triton X-114. Hydrophobic ChAT activity also appears to be present in nerve endings isolated from rat brain synaptosomes, and this form may correspond to the Triton DN-65 solubilised ChAT activity described by Benishin and Carroll (1983). The soluble and membrane forms of *Torpedo* ChAT do not have different affinities for choline or for AcCoA. This same observation was reported for both forms of the mammalian brain enzyme (Benishin and Carroll, 1983). The differences we present here concerning sensitiity to heat denaturation, to activation by alkaline pH or to inhibition by ACh, for soluble and membrane ChAT are very similar to those reported for soluble and membrane-bound ChAT of mammalian brain (Smith and Carroll, 1980; Benishin and Carroll, 1983), and may suggest that the two forms have some differences in their conformation and are differently regulated. Also, the

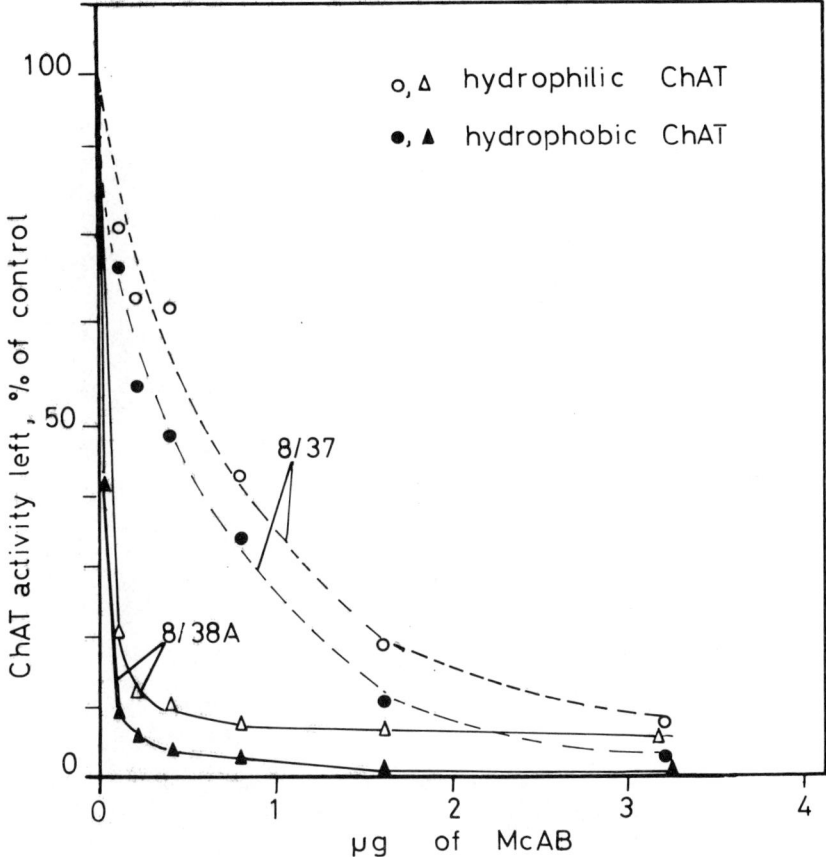

Fig. 10.8 Inhibition of hydrophilic and hydrophobic ChAT activity by anti-ChAT mono-clonal antibodies. 2 nmoles/h of ChAT activity contained in the aqueous or in the detergent phases obtained after Triton X-114 extraction of *Torpedo* synaptosomes were incubated for 24 h at 4 °C with increasing amounts of the anti-ChAT McAB 8/37 or 8/38A, the final volume of incubation being 100 μl. After incubation 20 μl aliquots of the mixture were assayed for ChAT activity remaining and the values are expressed as a percentage of the ChAT activity present in controls in which the McAB was replaced by naive mouse IgG. The two McAB, which have been developed against purified SPMs of *Torpedo*, were affinity-purified by chromatography on protein A Sepharose and are of the IgG1 subclass. The control mouse IgG used were also affinity-purified IgG1.

membrane form of ChAT may be widely present in animal species since it is present in two such unrelated species as *Torpedo* and mammals. Moreover, the membrane ChAT may be present in central (mammalian brain) as well as in peripheral cholinergic nerve endings (*Torpedo* electric organ is embryologically homologous to striated muscle). No data is yet available concerning which form of ChAT is synthetised in the perikarya of cholinergic neurons:

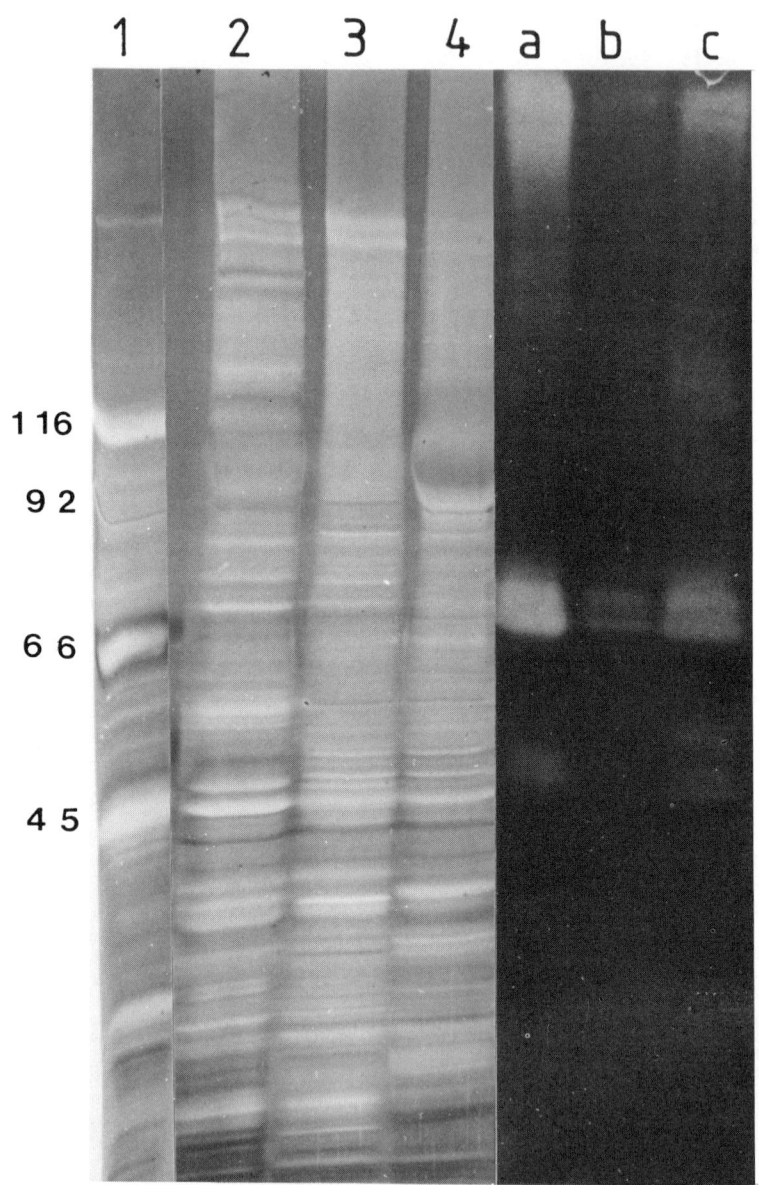

◀ Fig. 10.9   On the left-hand side is shown the protein pattern displayed on SDS-PAGE by *Torpedo* synaptosomes solubilised in Triton X-114 (lane 2), and by the aqueous phase (lane 3) and the detergent phase (lane 4) which were obtained after phase partition of the solubilised synaptosomes; lane 1 contains MW standards. Aliquots of each sample, containing about 100 to 200 μg of total protein, were precipitated by 5 % (final concentration) of trichloroacetic acid; the protein precipitate was washed twice in 95 % ethanol, twice in acetone, air dried and then solubilised in the sample buffer used for SDS-PAGE (2 % SDS, 10 % glycerol in 0.0625 M Tris-HCl, pH 6.8). About 15 to 20 μg of protein were loaded per lane. The gels were gradients of 6 to 15 % polyacrylamide and were silver nitrate stained. The samples contained in these gels were 'western' blotted to nitrocellulose filters, and hydrophobic ChAT (lane a), hydrophilic ChAT (lane b) and total ChAT activity present in Triton X-114 solubilised synaptosomes (lane c), were visualised immunochemically by using the affinity-purified anti-ChAT McAB 8/38A (results on the right-hand side). The immune complex formed on the blot was detected by incubating the nitrocellulose paper in rabbit anti-mouse IgG followed by ^{125}I protein A. Bands of MW lower than 66 kD are also labelled by the McAB 8/38A on 'western' blot of gels containing synaptosomes or hydrophobic ChAT; these polypeptides may have been generated by proteolytic clivage of ChAT during Triton X-114 extraction.

are the two forms coded by two different genes or are they produced by a post-translational modification of the same polypeptide? Synthesis of ChAT was found to occur in *Xenopus* oocytes injected with a crude preparation of mRNA extracted from the electric lobe of *Torpedo*, a central structure which is mainly composed of the cell bodies of the neurons innervating the electric organ: only soluble ChAT activity appeared to be synthetised (Gundersen *et al.*, 1985). It may be possible that membrane ChAT derives from a transformation of soluble ChAT which occurs post-translationally such as, for example, a covalent binding of a lipid or of a hydrophobic amino acid sequence that serves to anchor ChAT in the plasma membrane.

Another possible way in which membrane ChAT may interact with the plasma membrane of cholinergic nerve endings may be through specific binding with a lipid head group or with a protein of this membrane. This binding may be brought about by a change in the conformation of soluble ChAT.

No unequivocal mechanism has yet been proposed to explain the way in which ACh synthesis is regulated in a cholinergic nerve ending. It may be possible that the ratio of soluble to membrane ChAT activity plays a crucial role in maintaining ACh synthesis at rest and sustaining this synthesis during neuronal activity. The efficiency of ACh synthesis may be increased by the presence of membrane ChAT in close vicinity to choline supply systems, such as choline uptake and the enzymes involved in the breakdown of phospholipids. During neuronal activity one may imagine that the ratio of soluble to membrane ChAT is decreased in favour of membrane activity, thus improving the efficiency of ACh synthesis. In pathological conditions such as Alzheimer's disease, in which impairment of ACh synthesis occurs, the control of the ratio of soluble to membrane ChAT might be impaired. A better knowledge of the properties of soluble and membrane ChAT will certainly favour an understanding of the precise role ChAT plays in the regulation of ACh synthesis in health and in pathological conditions.

Acknowledgements

The authors wish to thank Dr G. Jones for useful suggestions and advice. We also thank S. Bonnet and F. Pillonel for manuscript preparation. This work was supported by the Fonds National Suisse de la Recherche Scientifique (Grant No 3.1581.0.84)₁and by a grant of 'La Société Académique de Genève' to L. E.-C. and by the 'Sir Jules Thorn Overseas Trust' Doctoral Fellowship to S.A.

References

Benishin, C. G., and Carroll, P. T. (1981a). Acetylation of choline and homocholine by membrane-bound choline-o-acetyltransferase in mouse forebrain nerve endings. *J. Neurochem.*, **36**, 732–40.

Benishin, C. G., and Carroll, P. T. (1981b). Differential sensitivity of soluble and membrane-bound forms of choline-o-acetyltransferase to inhibition by coenzyme A. *Biochem. Pharmacol.*, **30**, 2483–4.

Benishin, C. G., and Carroll, P. T. (1983). Multiple forms of choline-o-acetyltransferase in mouse and rat brain: solubilization and characterization. *J. Neurochem.*, **41**, 1030–9.

Benishin, C. G., and Carroll, P. T. (1984). Developmental differences between soluble and membrane-bound fractions of choline-o-acetyltransferase in neonatal mouse brain. *J. Neurochem.*, **43**, 885–7.

Bordier, C. (1981). Phase separation of integral membrane proteins in Triton X-114 solution. *J. Biol. Chem.*, **256**, 1604–7.

Brandon, C., and Wu, J.-Y. (1978). Purification and properties of choline acetyltransferase from *Torpedo californica*. *J. Neurochem.*, **30**, 791–7.

Burnette, W. N. (1981). 'Western blotting'. Electrophoretic transfer of proteins from SDS-polyacrylamide gels to unmodified nitrocellulose and radiographic detection with antibody and radioiodinated protein A. *Anal. Biochem.*, **112**, 195–203.

Carlson, S. S., Wagne, J. A., and Kelly, R. B. (1978). Purification of synaptic vesicles from elasmobranch electric organ and the use of biophysical criteria to demonstrate purity. *Biochemistry*, **17**, 1188–206.

Cozzari, C., and Hartman, B. K. (1980). Preparation of antibodies specific to choline acetyltransferase from bovine caudate nucleus and immunohistochemical localization of the enzyme. *Proc. Natl Acad. Sci. USA*, **77**, 7453–7.

Dahlström, A. (1983). Presence, metabolism and axonal transport of transmitters in peripheral mammalian axons. In Lajtha, A. (ed.) *Handbook of Neurochemistry*, Vol. 5. Plenum Press, New York, pp. 405–41.

Dodd, P. R., Hardy, J. A., Oakley, A. E., Edwardson, J. A., Perry, E. K., and Delaunoy, J.-P. (1981). A rapid method for preparing synaptosomes: comparison with alternative procedures. *Brain Res.*, **226**, 107–18.

Dunant, Y., and Israël, M. (1975). Acetylcholine tunover in the course of stimulation. In Waser, P. G. (ed.), *Cholinergic Mechanisms*, Raven Press, New York, pp. 161–7.

Eder-colli, L., and Amato, S. (1985). Membrane-bound choline acetyltransferase in *Torpedo* electric organ: a marker for synaptosomal plasma membranes? *Neuroscience*, **15**, 577–89.

Eder-Colli, L., Powell, J. F., Cuello, A. C., and Smith, A. D. (1982). Specific antibodies to bovine choline acetyltransferase raised in mice immunised with small amounts of partially purified enzyme. *Neurochem. Int.*, **4**, 383–8.

Ellmann, G. L., Courtney, K. D., Andres, V. Jr., and Featherstone, R. M. (1961). A new and rapid colorimetric determination of acetylcholinesterase activity. *Biochem. Pharmacol.*, **7**, 88–95.

Fonnum, F. (1967). The 'compartimentation' of choline-o-acetyltransferase within synaptosomes. *Biochem. J.*, **103**, 262–70.

Fonnum, F. (1968). Choline acetyltransferase binding to and release from membranes. *Biochem. J.*, **109**, 389-98.

Fonnum, F. (1969). Radiochemical microassays for the determination of choline acetyltransferase and acetylcholinesterase activities. *Biochem. J.*, **115**, 465-72.

Fonnum, F. (1970). Surface charge of choline acetyltransferase from different species. *J. Neurochem.*, **17**, 1095-100.

Galfre, G., Howe, S. C., Milstein, C., Butcher, G. W., and Howard, J. C. (1977). Antibodies to major histocompatibility antigens produced by hybrid cell lines. *Nature*, **266**, 550-2.

Gundersen, C. B., Jenden, D. J., and Miledi, R. (1985). Choline acetyltransferase and acetylcholine in *Xenopus* oocytes injected with mRNA from the electric lobe of *Torpedo*. *Proc. Natl Acad. Sci. USA*, **82**, 608-11.

Hawkes, R., Niday, E., and Gordon, J. (1982). A dot-immunobinding assay for monoclonal and other antibodies. *Anal. Biochem.*, **119**, 142-7.

Hebb, C. O. and Whittaker, V. P. (1958). Intracellular distribution of acetylcholine and choline acetylase. *J. Physiol.*, **142**, 187-96.

Hersh, L. B., Wainer, B. H., and Potter Andrews, L. (1984). Multiple isoelectric and molecular weight variants of choline acetyltransferase. Artifact or real? *J. Biol. Chem.*, **259**, 1253-8.

Israël, M., Manaranche, R., Mastour-Frachon, P., and Morel, N. (1976). Isolation of pure cholinergic nerve endings from the electric organ of *Torpedo marmorata*. *Biochem. J.*, **160**, 113-15.

Johnson, M. K. (1960). The intracellular distribution of glycolytic and other enzymes in rat brain homogenates and mitochondrial preparations. *Biochem. J.*, **77**, 610-18.

Laemmli, U. K. (1970). Cleavage of structural proteins during the assembly of the head of bacteriophage T_4. *Nature*, **227**, 680-5.

Li, Z.-Y., and Bon, C. (1983). Presence of a membrane-bound acetylcholinesterase form in a preparation of nerve endings from *Torpedo marmorata* electric organ. *J. Neurochem.*, **40**, 338-49.

Morel, N., and Dreyfus, P. (1982). Association of acetylcholinesterase with the external surface of presynaptic plasma membranes in *Torpedo* electric organ. *Neurochem. Int.*, **4**, 283-8.

Morel, N., Manaranche, R., Israël, M., and Gulik-Krzywicki, T. (1982). Isolation of a presynaptic plasma membrane fraction from *Torpedo* cholinergic synaptosomes: evidence for a specific protein. *J. Cell. Biol.*, **75**, 349-56.

Rossier, J., Bauman, A., and Benda, P. (1973). Improved purification of rat brain choline acetyltransferase by using an immunoadsorbent. *FEBS Lett.*, **32**, 231-4.

Schaffner, W., and Weissmann, C. (1973). A rapid, sensitive, and specific method for the determination of proteins in dilute solution. *Anal. Biochem.*, **56**, 502-14.

Schmidt, J., and Raftery, M. A. (1973). A simple assay for the study of solubilized acetylcholine receptors. *Anal. Biochem.*, **52**, 349-54.

Smith, C. P., and Carroll, P. T. (1980). A comparison of solubilized and membrane bound forms of choline-*o*-acetyltransferase (EC 2.3.1.6) in mouse brain nerve endings. *Brain Res.*, **185**, 363-71.

Stadler, H., and Tashiro, T. (1979). Isolation of synaptosomal plasma membranes from cholinergic nerve terminals and a comparison of their protein with those of synaptic vesicles. *Eur. J. Biochem.*, **101**, 171-8.

Tuček, S. (1967). Observations on the subcellular distribution of choline acetyltransferase in the brain tissue of mammals and comparisons of acetylcholine synthesis from acetate and citrate in homogenates and nerve-ending fractions. *J. Neurochem.*, **14**, 519-29.

Tuček, S. (1982). The synthesis of acetylcholine in skeletal muscles of the rat. *J. Physiol.*, **322**, 53-69.

Tuček, S. (1984). Problems in the organization and control of acetylcholine synthesis in brain neurons. *Prog. Biophys. Mol. Biol.*, **44**, 1-46.

Tuček, S. (1985). Regulation of acetylcholine synthesis in the brain. *J. Neurochem.*, **44**, 11-24.

Whittaker, V. P. (1965). The application of subcellular fractionation techniques to the study of brain function. *Prog. Biophys. Mol. Biol.*, **15**, 39-96.

11

Regulation and Biosynthesis of Cholinesterases in the Human Brain

H. Soreq and H. Zakut

11.1 Abstract

In the human brain, acetylcholinesterase (AChE) hydrolyses the neurotransmitter acetylcholine in cholinergic synapses. However, ample evidence suggests that a considerable part of the brain enzyme is involved in functions other than cholinergic transmission. In addition, human brain AChE is a highly polymorphic protein with an intricate regulation pattern. The tetrameric form of AChE was reported to be selectively depleted from the brain of patients suffering from senile dementia of the Alzheimer type, but it is unknown yet what level of the pathway for AChE biosynthesis and/or regulation is defective in the senile brain. To tackle this complicated research problem, it is important to distinguish between the different forms of AChE. It is, however, not yet clear whether these forms are produced from discrete genes or by post-transcriptional and post-translational processing. In addition, the amino acid sequence of the various AChE forms has not been revealed. This issue is being approached in our research group by simultaneous experiments at the levels of DNA, of mRNA and of the active brain enzyme. In the following report we present evidence suggesting that both post-transcriptional and post-translational regulation events contribute to the complex expression pattern of AChE in the developing and the mature human brain.

11.2 Introduction

11.2.1 Regulation and Properties of Human Brain Cholinesterases: Research Importance, Advantages and Difficulties

11.2.1.1 Acetylcholinesterase as a Major Cholinergic Constituent

Within cholinergic synapses in the human brain, the neurotransmitter acetylcholine is rapidly hydrolysed by the serine esterase acetylcholinesterase (acetylcholine acetyl hydrolase, EC 3.1.1.7, AChE). AChE appears in numerous cell types, tissues and organisms (Silver, 1984), albeit in extremely low concentrations and in multiple molecular forms (Massoulié and Bon, 1982). The various cholinesterase forms differ in their substrate specificity and sensitivity to selective inhibitors (Austin and Berry, 1953), in their glycosylation patterns (MeFlah et al., 1984), in their hydrophobicity (Rosenberry and Scoggin, 1984), and in their sedimentation properties (Zakut et al., 1985). Genetic linkage analysis suggests the existence of allelic polymorphism for the human genes coding for particular cholinesterases (Silver, 1984), and molecular cloning studies indicate that various human cholinesterases are produced from cross-homologous DNA and mRNA sequences (Soreq et al., 1985; Zevin-Sonkin et al., 1985; Soreq et al., 1986).

11.2.1.2 Problems to be Solved in the Study of Brain Cholinesterases

The route to the biosynthesis and regulation of brain cholinesterases is as yet unknown, which leaves open several questions of considerable importance. These include the following.

(a) Are the various cholinesterase forms produced from discrete genes, or is their biosynthesis regulated by post-transcriptional and/or post-translational processing?

(b) Are the multisubunit forms of brain AChE composed of similar polypeptides with identical amino acid sequences, or of different polypeptides with distinct domains which distinguish particular subunits from others?

(c) What is the biosynthetic origin of cholinesterases in different subcellular locations within the brain tissue? Was the soluble fraction of brain AChE originally destined to be cytoplasmic and/or secreted, or has it been produced from membrane-associated amphipathic form(s) of the enzyme via enzymatic cleavage of their hydrophobic domains?

(d) What is the biological role of AChE in non-cholinergic brain cells, and of butyrylcholinesterase (ψChE) in the brain in general?

(e) Is there an interrelationship between the regulation of AChE and of the muscarinic acetylcholine receptor in the mammalian brain?

11.2.2 Significance of Cholinesterase Research for Clinically-Oriented Issues

In addition to its importance as a subject for basic research, the study of cholinesterases bears several implications for clinical purposes.

(a) Genetic deficiencies in serum ψChE in humans (up to 0.05 % of homozygotes in the Caucasian population) result in prolonged apnoea following the use of succinylcholine during anaesthesia (Hodgkin et al., 1965). This clinical complication could be diagnosed by a rapid method to detect such deficiencies, or prevented by injecting, as a scavenger, active human ψChE which would degrade the excess of drug. Purified human cholinesterase can similarly be used to scavenge organophosphorous insecticides, which act by blocking AChE (Aldridge and Reiner, 1982), in cases of poisoning with these compounds (Klose and Gustensohn, 1986). Synthetic preparation of the pure enzyme from cloned human genes would considerably decrease the expenses involved, and promises to widen the use of this approach.

(b) Tetrameric AChE is secreted into the amniotic fluid in cases of neural tube closure defects (Brock and Beder, 1983), but its detection is rather laborious (Bonham and Atack, 1983). A simple radioimmunoassay, using specific antibodies for the tetrameric form of AChE, would be highly valuable for the routine detection of such defects.

(c) The tetrameric form of AChE is selectively lost from particular regions in the brain of patients suffering from senile dementia of the Alzheimer type (SDAT) (Atack et al., 1983; Fishman et al., 1985). Antibodies directed against this form of the enzyme could hence be employed to develop a method for the clinical diagnosis of this disease.

Thus, both for basic research and multiple clinical purposes, AChE is clearly an important protein to be studied extensively and, preferably, at all levels of the pathway for gene expression. In this manuscript, we describe the simultaneous use of in vitro and in ovo translation systems for the synthesis of cholinesterases from human brain mRNA. When combined with several biochemical and immunochemical approaches for the characterisation of the nascent cholinesterases produced, and with the use of molecularly cloned cholinesterase DNA sequences, these experiments strongly suggest that both post-transcriptional and post-translational processing events play important roles in the production of the polymorphic forms of AChE within the developing and the mature human brain.

11.3 The Experimental Approach

11.3.1 Human Brain Tissues and mRNA Preparations

The experiments covered in this report were carried out using tissue extracts and purified poly(A)-containing RNA from several tissue sources originating from human brain. These include primary brain tumours of glial and meningeal origin (for detailed descriptions of these tumour types see Libermann *et al.* (1984), Razon *et al.* (1984); and Soreq *et al.* (1984)), discrete regions from foetal human brain (Zakut *et al.*, 1985; *see* Fig. 11.1 for specific description) and dissected tissues from mature human brain (Razon *et al.*, 1984; Egozi *et al.*, 1985). Several precautions were taken to ensure the intactness of the cholinesterase mRNAs extracted from these tissues (Zevin-Sonkin *et al.*, 1985). To determine the migration properties of these mRNAs, poly(a)-containing RNA was denatured with dimethylsulphoxide and centrifuged in continuous sucrose gradients (Soreq *et al.*, 1984, 1985). Human epidermoid carcinoma, in which the levels of cholinesterases (Razon *et al.*, 1984) and of cholinesterase mRNA (Soreq *et al.*, 1984) are considerably lower than in the brain tissues, served as control.

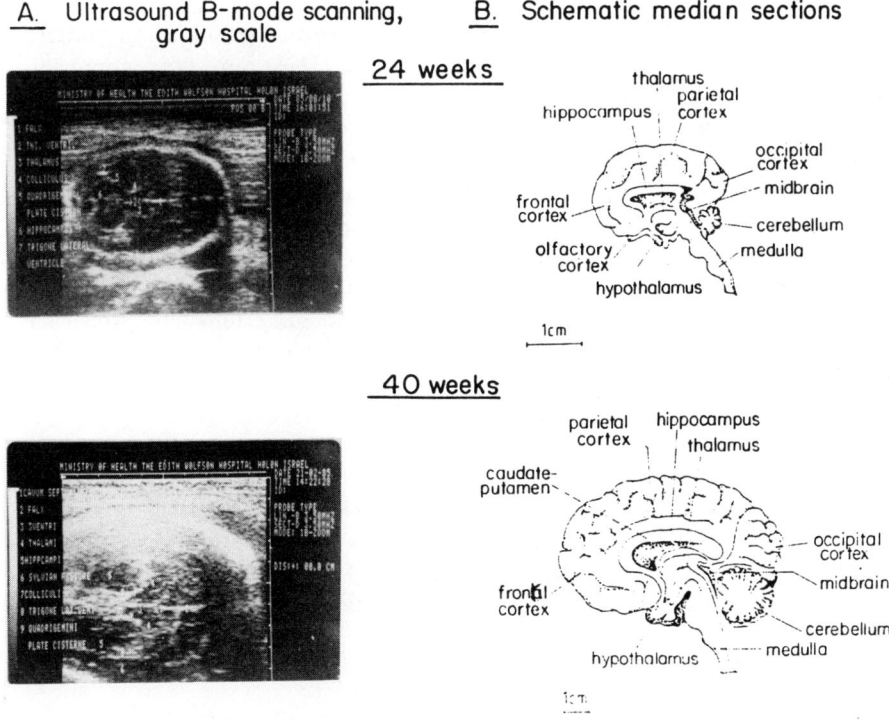

Fig. 11.1 Discrete regions of foetal brain as shown by ultrasound and in schematic median brain sections. (A) Ultrasound B-mode scanning, gray scale, was employed to determine whether the crown–rump length and biparietal diameter of the foetus corresponded to gestational age in weeks, calculated from the first day of the last menstrual period. (B) Areas marked by arrows were dissected out of the brain of aborted foetuses at the gestational ages noted in weeks. Amplification scale is marked by bars for brains of 24 weeks (upper) and 40 weeks old fetuses (Lower).

11.3.2 Translation Systems Employed for Cholinesterase Biosynthesis

The biosynthesis of human brain cholinesterases was examined using two different translation systems. In the *in vitro* system of rabbit reticulocyte lysate (Pelham and Jackson, 1976), poly(A)-containing cholinesterase mRNA from human brain directs the incorporation of (^{35}S)-methionine into newly synthesised nascent polypeptides which remain unprocessed and inactive (for detailed methodology, see Giveon and Soreq (1984)). In the *in ovo* system of micro-injected *Xenopus* oocytes (Gurdon *et al.*, 1971), the (^{35}S)-labelled cholinesterase polypeptides also undergo post-translational processing and correct compartmentalisation to yield the catalytically active enzyme in its natural subcellular localisation (Soreq, 1984, 1986).

11.3.3 Immunochemical Analyses of Newly Synthesised Cholinesterases

(^{35}S)-labelled, newly synthesised cholinesterases were purified and characterised by two independent immunochemical approaches. They were immunoprecipitated, following pre-adsorption of non-specific precipitates, with the aid of anti-AChE monoclonal antibodies elicited against human erythrocyte AChE (AE-2, Fambrough *et al.*, 1982; see Zevin-Sonkin *et al.* (1985) for further details). Alternatively, they were identified by crossed immunoelectrophoresis (Djiegielewska *et al.*, 1985) using rabbit antisera against human plasma proteins to precipitate ψChE, and against human erythrocyte membranes or against mammalian brain AChE to precipitate AChE (Djiegielewska *et al.* (1986)). In both cases, identification was performed by autoradiography and irrelevant antibodies served for controls.

11.3.4 Molecular Cloning Experiments

The origin and properties of the human brain-originated cholinesterase cDNA sequences described in this manuscript have been detailed elsewhere (Zevin-Sonkin *et al.*, 1985). DNA purification analyses, as well as hybridisation-selection experiments, were as described by Soreq *et al.* (1985). Hybrid-selected mRNA was translated *in vitro* or *in ovo* as above (*see* Section 11.3.2).

11.3.5 Cholinesterase Assays

Measurements of cholinesterase activity were performed by hydrolysis of (^{3}H)-acetylcholine, according to Johnson and Russell (1975), and in the presence of protease inhibitors, as detailed by Zakut *et al.* (1985). Alternatively, the hydrolysis of acetylthiocholine or butyrylthiocholine was measured spectrophotometrically, by the technique of Ellman *et al.* (1961) and as detailed by Razon *et al.* (1984). The selective inhibitors iso-OMPA and BW284C51 were used to specifically block the activities of ψChE and of AChE, respectively

(Austin and Berry, 1953). Extraction with low salt buffer, or with salt plus detergent, was employed to separate the hydrophylic fraction of active cholinesterases from the amphipathic part (Zakut *et al.*, 1985), and centrifugation in continuous sucrose gradients was used to separate the various molecular forms of the enzyme (Razon *et al.*, 1984).

11.4 Research Observations

11.4.1 Contribution of Post-transcriptional and of Post-translational Control to the Biosynthesis of Human Brain Cholinesterases

11.4.1.1 Polymorphism of Human Brain Cholinesterase mRNAs

Two independent approaches have indicated that human brain cholinesterases are produced from polymorphic mRNAs, with different sizes and distinct cross-homologous sequences. In the first approach, poly(A)-containing RNA from foetal human brain, glioblastomas and meningiomas was centrifuged in continuous sucrose gradients, the size-fractionated mRNA was microinjected into *Xenopus* oocytes and the catalytic activity of the newly synthesised cholinesterases was determined in oocyte homogenates and incubation medium in the presence of selective inhibitors. In this experiment it was found that several different mRNA fractions, of various sedimentation properties, induced the synthesis of AChE and of ψChE (Soreq *et al.*, 1984). In the other approach, human foetal brain mRNA was employed to derive cloned cDNA inserts with sequence homologies with a human AChE gene (see Soreq *et al.* (1985) for further details regarding this gene). These cDNAs were selected by colony hybridisation and were further characterised by enzymatic restriction and hybridisation-selection of human brain mRNA, followed by microinjection and cholinesterase measurements. The characterisation experiments proved that each of the examined cDNA inserts hybridised with translationally-active cholinesterase mRNAs from the human brain. Furthermore, these cDNAs were found to be derived from distinct, non-identical mRNA species (Zevin-Sonkin *et al.*, 1985). Since all of these cDNAs were selected by hybridisation with a single DNA probe, this also implied that the various mRNAs from which the cDNAs were reverse-transcribed were cross-homologous with each other.

The different cross-homologous cholinesterase mRNAs could have originated from distinct but closely related cholinesterase genes. Alternatively, or in addition, several promoters for a single cholinesterase gene could yield, under various conditions, different transcription products. A third possibility is the production of multiple mRNAs from a single transcription unit by differential splicing. Further experiments will be required to reveal the transcription mechanism(s) leading to the production of various cholinesterase mRNAs.

11.4.1.2 Human Brain mRNA is Translated into Multiple Nascent Cholinesterase Polypeptides

The different cholinesterase mRNAs could all be translated into a single polypeptide similarly to the mRNAs for kininogen (Nawa *et al.*, 1983) and glucagon (Lund *et al.*, 1981). Alternatively, they could each code for a distinct nascent cholinesterase polypeptide. To distinguish between these possibilities, we translated *in vitro* mRNA from foetal human brain and immunoprecipitated the (^{35}S)-labelled nascent cholinesterase polypeptides produced. Since the concentration of cholinesterase mRNA appears to be very low (Soreq *et al.*, 1982), we took special precautions to reduce to minimum the amount of immunoglobulins employed for the immunoprecipitation reaction and, thus, to prevent nonspecific background precipitation. Figure 11.2 presents schematically the various steps which were taken. Under these conditions, the anti-AChE AE-2 monoclonal antibodies (Fambrough *et al.*, 1982), but not an irrelevant monoclonal antibody, specifically immunoprecipitated several nascent polypeptides with clear differences in their electrophoretic migration properties in a gradient polyacrylamide gel (Fig. 11.3). Since size is the major criterion for separation in such gels (Giveon and Soreq, 1984), this implies that the various cholinesterase mRNAs in the foetal human brain give rise to several nascent polypeptides of different lengths, all of which contain the peptide domain which immunoreacts with anti-AChE antibodies. It should be noted that these may include polypeptides other than AChE ones, if these contain the same immunoreactive domain.

In order to reveal whether the nascent polypeptides leading to the production of AChE differ from those which eventually yield ψChE, we employed crossed immunoelectrophoresis in gels in which selective antibodies against either AChE or ψChE were encased. Our observations indicated the existence of non-crossreactive immunoprecipitates for AChE and ψChE (Soreq *et al.*, 1986), which further expands the variety of different polypeptides translated from cholinesterase mRNAs.

11.4.1.3 Post-translational Modifications Contribute to the Heterogeneity of Human Brain Cholinesterases

In order to examine the possibility that post-translational modifications also contribute to the heterogeneity of human brain cholinesterases, we employed the *in ovo* translation system of microinjected *Xenopus* oocytes, in which such modifications are performed. Oocytes were injected with poly-(A)-containing RNA from foetal human brain together with (^{35}S)-methionine, and the oocyte homogenates and incubation medium were subjected to cross immunoelectrophoresis and autoradiography, using rabbit antisera against AChE and ψChE, respectively. The electrophoretic separation in agarose gels is mainly based on charge differences (see Djiegielewska *et al.* (1985) for further details). Using this technique, we detected the appearance of polymorphic cholinesterase-

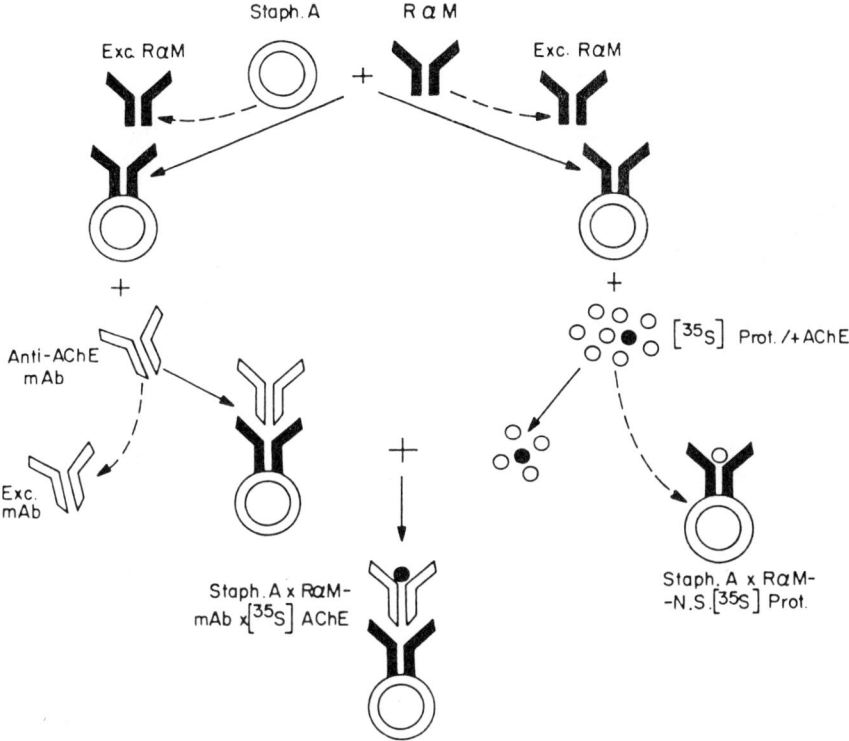

Fig. 11.2 Schematic drawing of the procedure employed for immunoprecipitation of nascent acetylcholinesterase polypeptides from foetal brain. Rabbit anti-mouse IgG (RαM; Miles Yeda) was bound to staphylococcus aureus ghosts (Staph. A; Calbiochem). AE-2 monoclonal antibodies against human acetylcholinesterase (mAb; Fambrough et al., 1982) were then bound to this complex. Excess RαM and mAb were removed by washing. The tertiary complex Staph. A × RαM-mAb was then used to bind nascent acetylcholinesterase polypeptides produced *in vitro* from foetal brain mRNA. Translation products ((^{35}S) Prot./+AChE) were preincubated with the Staph. A × RαM complex in order to remove proteins which bind non-specifically (N.S. (^{35}S) Prot.). Nascent AChE polypeptides which were bound to the immunocomplex (Staph. A × RαM-mAb × (^{35}S) AChE) were then analysed by gradient polyacrylamide gel electrophoresis followed by autoradiography (*see* Fig. 11.3).

immunoreactive polypeptides with distinguishable migration coordinates in both the oocyte homogenates and incubation medium. This indicates that in addition to the size and sequence differences inherent to the nascent cholinesterases, and which were observed in the *in vitro* immunoprecipitated polypeptides (Fig. 11.3), post-translational modifications alter the charge of the newly produced cholinesterases (Soreq et al., 1986). The cholinesterases observed in the incubation medium displayed limited heterogeneity and faster migration as compared with

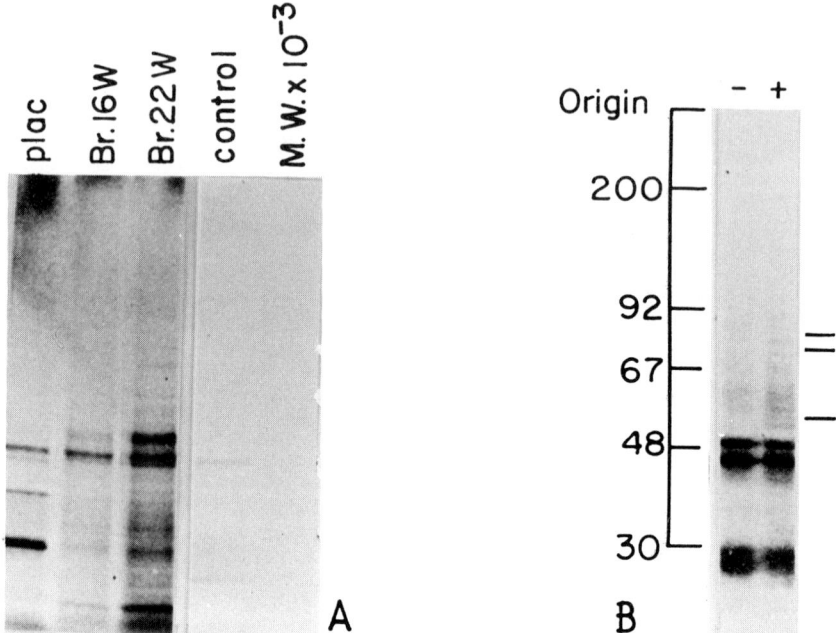

Fig. 11.3 *In vitro* translation of foetal brain mRNA and immunoprecipitation of nascent acetylcholinesterase polypeptides. (A) Poly-(A)-containing RNA was extracted from the brain of human foetuses of 16 and 22 weeks gestation, respectively (Br. 16W; Br. 22W) and from human placenta for control (plac). Translation *in vitro* was according to Pelham and Jackson (1976) and as previously detailed by Giveon and Soreq (1984). Translation in the absence of exogenous mRNA served as control (control). Electrophoresis was in a 5–15 % gradient polyacrylamide gel, with (^{14}C)-labelled molecular weight markers (M.W. $\times 10^{-3}$; Sigma). (B) Immunoprecipitation of nascent (^{35}S)-labelled acetylcholinesterase polypeptides was according to the binding procedure presented in Fig. 11.2. AE-2 monoclonal antibodies against human acetylcholinesterase (+) or an irrelevant monoclonal antibody for control (−) were employed. Gradient gel electrophoresis was as detailed in (A). The major immuno-precipitated bands are marked by lines.

the intracellular forms of the enzyme. This may indicate that a hydrophobic part of an intracellular nascent polypeptide had to be cleaved off to enable the release of the enzyme into the incubation medium in a soluble, hydrophylic form. A similar mechanism with the same effect on the electrophoretic migration of the enzyme has been demonstrated *in vitro* for purified human erythrocyte AChE (Weitz *et al.*, 1984).

It is not yet clear from our findings whether intracellular, amphipathic forms of the enzyme represent precursors of the secreted, soluble ones or whether each was produced from a different nascent polypeptide chain. Molecular cloning and DNA sequencing experiments will be necessary in order to reveal whether the secretory enzyme is formed in one step or whether it represents enzyme molecules which were released from their association with the membrane by natural enzymatic reactions.

Hybridisation-selection experiments were employed to confirm that the various cholinesterase mRNAs bear sequence homologies. Different cholinesterase cDNAs were used to hybrid-select foetal brain cholinesterase mRNAs; the hybrid-selected mRNAs were microinjected together with (^{35}S)-methionine into *Xenopus* oocytes, and oocyte extracts and incubation medium were subjected to cholinesterase assays and to crossed immunoelectrophoresis followed by auto-radiography. Multiple, polymorphic AChE and ψChE catalytically active (Zevin-Sonkin *et al.*, 1985) and immunoreactive (Soreq *et al.*, 1986) proteins were detected. This experiment revealed that although AChE and ψChE display distinct immunological domains, the mRNA species producing these enzymes both hybridise to several cholinesterase cDNA clones. Also, the various forms of AChE, which exhibit different migration coordinates on the crossed immuno-electrophoretic gels, were indicated by this experiment to be produced by cross-homologous mRNA sequences. Table 11.1 summarises the evidence we accumulated for the existence of various cross-homologous cholinesterase mRNAs which code for several distinct nascent polypeptides.

Table 11.1   Different cross-homologous cholinesterase mRNAs contribute to the polymorphism of foetal brain cholinesterases

Experimental indications	Reference
(a) Size separation of foetal brain mRNAs translatable into various cholinesterases in oocytes.	Soreq *et al.* (1984)
(b) Production of various foetal brain cDNAs, all homologous to a single acetylcholinesterase gene.	Zevin-Sonkin *et al.* (1985)
(c) *In vitro* translation of foetal brain mRNA into several polypeptides immunoprecipitable with anti-AChE monoclonal antibodies.	This chapter
(d) *In ovo* translation of foetal brain mRNA into distinguishable polypeptides, immunoreactive with anti-AChE or anti-ψChE polyclonal antibodies.	Soreq *et al.* (1986)

11.4.2 Polymorphism and Regulation of Cholinesterases in Adult, Foetal and Neoplastic Brain Tissues

The activities, molecular forms and membrane association of cholinesterases were studied in dissected regions of adult post-mortem human brain, in parallel regions of developing foetal brain and in a collection of primary brain tumours consisting primarily of gliomas and meningiomas. All of these tissue sources contained substantial amounts of cholinesterase activities, with several tissue samples expressing exceptionally high levels. In normal mature and foetal brain, and in meningiomas, AChE accounted for almost all the cholinesterase activity, but in almost all gliomas elevated levels of ψChE could be detected. Two major forms of AChE, sedimenting as 10-11S and 4-5S, respectively, were detected on sucrose gradients in most of the mature and foetal brain regions examined (Zakut et al., 1985) and in gliomas. In meningiomas a light (4-5S) form was the principal component (Razon et al., 1984). The 10S and the 4S forms of brain AChE appeared to possess similar catalytic properties, as judged by their individual K_m values towards (^{3}H)-acetylcholine ($\sim 4 \times 10^{-4}$ M) and their interaction with selective inhibitors. A representative K_m determination for the isolated 10S and 4S forms from 14 week thalamus is presented in Fig. 11.4.

Crossed immunoelectrophoresis of in vitro translation products revealed that cholinesterase biosynthesis proceeds even in the mature human brain, and takes place with different efficiencies in various brain regions and cell types (Djiegielewska et al., 1986). The ratio between the 10S and the 4S forms of AChE varied by up to four- to five-fold between discrete areas of foetal brain and within areas at various developmental stages, but reached similar values of about 5:2 in all areas of the mature brain and in gliomas. In contrast, the major component of ψChE activity was 10-11S in all areas of the developing foetal brain and in the mature brain. In gliomas a light, 4-5S form of ψChE could also be detected (Razon et al., 1984; Zakut et al., 1985).

In various regions of the foetal brain, AChE activity was $\sim$ 35-50 % low-salt-soluble and 45-65 % detergent-soluble, throughout brain development (Zakut et al., 1985). This implies, in agreement with Gennari and Brodbeck (1985), that a considerable part of foetal brain AChE contains a hydrophobic domain. This observation could explain the slow electrophoretic migration of part of the mRNA-directed brain AChE produced in microinjected oocytes and analysed by crossed-immunoelectrophoresis (see previous sections for details). Both the 10S and the 4S forms of the enzyme could be detected in the detergent-extractable fraction. Pseudocholinesterase, in contrast, was mostly low-salt soluble in all areas and developmental stages.

To examine whether AChE activity in the brain is co-regulated with other cholinoceptive properties, the muscarinic binding activity in these brain tissues was also examined, using the muscarinic antagonist (^{3}H)N-methyl-4-piperidyl benzilate ((^{3}H)-4NMPB). Individual data for cholinesterase activity were divided by the corresponding values for the density of (^{3}H)-4NMPB binding sites, and average values of these arbitrary ratios were calculated for the different tissue types. In most stages of brain development, the average arbitrary ratios expressed a tendency for decrease with maturation. The average values and variability ranges in the foetal brain were 83 ± 50 and 19 ± 19 at 14 and 24 weeks gestation, respectively. The parallel value calculated for the collection of brain tumours composed of undifferentiated brain cells was 86 ± 66, and in mature post-mortem brain samples it was as low as 11 ± 8. Figure 11.5 presents these findings

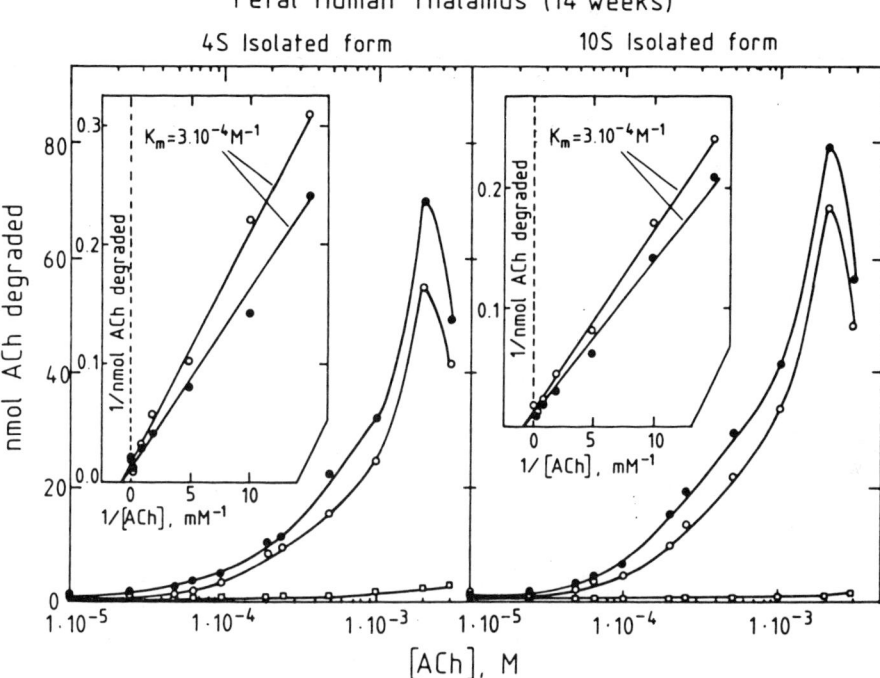

Fig. 11.4 Effect of selective inhibitors on (^{3}H)-acetylcholine hydrolysis by isolated forms of cholinesterase from foetal human thalamus. Cholinesterase molecular forms sedimenting as 10S and 4S were isolated from extracts of 14 week foetal thalamus by centrifugation in continuous sucrose gradients (Razon *et al.*, 1984). Activities were assayed by the Johnson and Russell (1975) technique, as detailed elsewhere and in the presence of protease and oxidase inhibitors (Zakut *et al.*, 1985). Each reaction mixture contained 30 μl of gradient-purified enzyme, the indicated concentrations of acetylcholine and, where noted, the appropriate inhibitor at a final concentration of 1×10^{-5} M. Incubation was for 24 h. Background hydrolysis in the absence of enzyme was subtracted. For iso-OMPA measurements, samples were preincubated for 30 min with the inhibitor. Activity was calculated in nmoles acetylcholine (ACh) degraded in the absence of inhibitors (full circles), or in the presence of iso-OMPA (empty circles) or BW284C51 (empty squares). The Lineweaver–Burk plot of cholinesterase activities yielded equal K_m values for both isolated forms in the presence or absence of iso-OMPA (see inserts).

as calculated from the data described by Gurwitz *et al.* (1984) and Egozi *et al.* (1985). These observations suggest that if a correlation exists between muscarinic receptors and cholinesterase levels in glial tumors, it differs from that in the non-malignant mature brain tissue. In addition, the developmental decrease of the cholinesterase:muscarinic receptors ratio indicates that AChE is also involved in functions other than cholinergic transmission in the developing human brain.

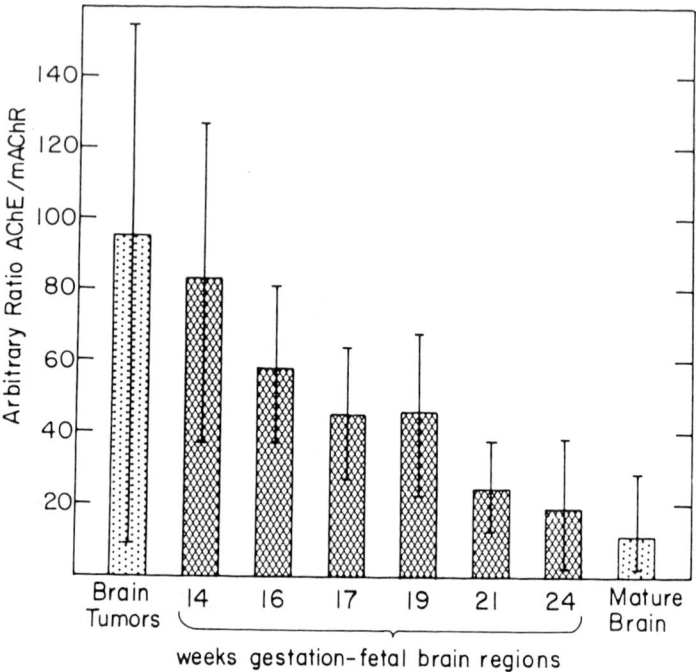

Fig. 11.5 Average arbitrary ratios between the specific activity of cholinesterases and the density of muscarinic receptors in various brain tissues. Cholinesterase activities were assayed on (^{3}H)-acetylcholine, and the density of muscarinic receptors was measured by binding of (^{3}H)-4NMPB, as detailed by Egozi *et al.* (1985). The columns represent average values calculated for collections of brain tumor tissues (Gurwitz *et al.*, 1984), of discrete brain regions from different gestational ages (Zakut *et al.*, 1985), or from mature post-mortem brain tissue samples (Razon *et al.*, 1984). Standard deviation is noted by bars for each value.

11.5 Acetylcholinesterase as a Putative Marker for Alzheimer's Disease

Many clinical and basic research studies have been performed in recent years in an attempt to find out whether cholinesterases could serve as markers for senile dementia of the Alzheimer type (SDAT). SDAT has been shown to be accompanied by loss of neurons in the magnocellular basal nucleus, which is composed of cholinergic cortical-projection cell groups in the basal forebrain (Whitehouse *et al.*, 1982; Perry *et al.*, 1984; Saper and Chelimsky, 1984). Also, clinical evidence has been accumulated for dysfunction in the midtemporal cortex areas innervated by these neurons (Perry *et al.*, 1978). Various cholinesterase measurements were therefore tested as indicators of altered cholinergic function in the Alzheimer brain. However, the observations reached by determination of total cholinesterase activities were rather inconsistent, with no significant pattern.

Thus, recent measurements of total AChE or ψChE activity in plasma, erythrocytes and cerebrosipinal fluid of patients with SDAT did not provide a useful index of alterations in central cholinergic function in SDAT patients (Marquis et al., 1985), in contradiction to earlier reports (Soininen et al., 1981). A different, more significant, picture was obtained when the composition of AChE molecular forms was examined in particular brain areas. A selective loss of AChE tetramers (the 10S form) was reported to take place in the neocortex of Alzheimer patients (Atack et al., 1983; Fishman et al., 1985), as examined by sucrose gradient centrifugation of brain extracts. It is interesting to note that the same tetrameric form of AChE is also the one which is secreted by neural tube cells early in human embryonic development (Bonham and Atack, 1983). There is, therefore, good reason to believe that this is a functionally important form of the enzyme in human brain neurons and that a significant indicator for SDAT could be provided by measurements of the fraction of AChE activity represented by the tetrameric form. This should be done by a simple, rapid technique which is appropriate for adaptation into a widely used clinical method (such as a specific radioimmunoassay). If, indeed, the subunits composing various forms of human brain AChE are produced from distinct polypeptides, as suggested by our in vitro and in ovo mRNA translation experiments (see previous sections for details), it is probable that there are also differences in the amino acid sequences of particular domains in these subunits. Antibodies elicited against such form-specific domains should, in principle, be highly selective for the specific forms of AChE which include these domains. To find these putative form-specific domains, it is necessary to reveal the detailed amino acid sequence of the various subunits composing the different molecular forms of AChE in the human brain. DNA sequencing is today relatively simple, as compared with protein sequencing, particularly when a scarce protein such as AChE is pursued. The sequence determination should hence be done by isolation and characterisation of cDNA clones encoding for the various forms of human brain AChE. Using this approach, we hope that the basic research work described in the first part of this chapter will eventually lead to the development of a simple and rapid method for the clinical diagnosis of senile dementia of the Alzheimer type.

Acknowledgements

We are grateful to Drs M. Sokolovsky, D. Zevin-Sonkin, E. Schejter, R. Achiron, N. Saunders and K. Djiegielewska for their contributions to this work, and to Ms R. Zisling for her excellent technical assistance. The research was supported by the US Army Medical Research and Development Command (Contract 17-85-C-5025, to H.S) and by the Edith Wolfson Hospital Research Fund (H.Z.).

References

Aldridge, W. L., and Reiner, E. (1972). *Enzyme Inhibitors as Substrates.* North-Holland, Amsterdam.

Atack, J. R., Perry, E. K., Bonham, J. R., Perry, R. H., Tomlinson, B. E., Blessed, G., and Fairbairn, A. (1983). Molecular forms of acetylcholinesterase in senile dementia of Alzheimer type: Selective loss of the intermediate (10S) form. *Neurosci. Lett.,* **40,** 199–204.

Austin, L., and Berry, W. K. (1953). Two selective inhibitors of cholinesterase. *Biochem. J.,* **54,** 695–700.

Bonham, J. R., and Atack, J. R. (1983). A neural tube defect specific form of acetylcholinesterase in amniotic fluid. *Clin. Chem. Acta.,* **135,** 233–7.

Brock, D. J. H., and Beder, P. (1983). The use of commercial antisera in resolving the cholinesterase bands of human amniotic fluids. *Clin. Chem. Acta.,* **127,** 419–22.

Djiegielewska, K. M. D., Saunders, N. R., and Soreq, H. (1985). Messenger ribonucleic acid from developing rat cerebellum directs *in vitro* biosynthesis of plasma proteins. *Dev. Brain Res.* (in press).

Djiegielewska, K. M. D., Saunders, N. R., Schejter, E. J., Zakut, H., Zevin-Sonkin, D., Zisling, R., and Soreq, H. (1986). Synthesis of plasma proteins in foetal, adult and neoplastic human brain tissues. *Dev. Biol.* (in press).

Egozi, Y., Sokolovsky, M., Matzkel, A., Schejter, E., Blatt, I., Zakut, H., and Soreq, H. (1985). Divergent regulation of muscarinic binding sites and acetylcholinesterase in discrete regions of the developing human foetal brain. *Cell. Molec. Neurobiol.* (in press).

Ellman, G. L., Cortney, D. K., Anders, V., and Featherstone, R. M. (1961). A new and rapid colorimetric determination of acetylcholinesterase activity. *Biochem. Pharmacol.,* **7,** 88–95.

Fambrough, D. M., Engel, A. G., and Rosenberry, T. L. (1982). Acetylcholinesterase of human erythrocytes and neuromuscular junctions: Homologies revealed by monoclonal antibodies. *Proc. Natl Acad. Sci. USA,* **79,** 1078–82.

Fishman, E. B., Siek, G. C., MacCallum, R. D., Bird, E. D., Volicer, L., and Marquis, J. K. (1985). Distribution of the molecular forms of acetylcholinesterase in human brain: Alterations in dementia of the Alzheimer type. *Annals of Neurol.* (in press).

Gennari, K., and Brodbeck, U. (1985). Molecular forms of acetylcholinesterase from human caudate nucleus: Comparison of salt-soluble and detergent-soluble tetrameric enzyme species. *J. Neurochem.,* **44,** 697–704.

Giveon, D., and Soreq, H. (1984). *In vitro* translation of mRNA and analysis of translation products. In Soreq, H. (ed.), *Molecular Biology Approach to the Neurosciences,* IBRO Handbook Series: Methods in the Neurosciences, Vol. 7. John Wiley & Sons, Chichester, New York, pp. 187–94.

Gurdon, J. B., Lane, C. D., Woodland, H. R., and Marbaix, G. (1971). Use of frog eggs and oocytes for the study of messenger RNA and its translation in living cells. *Nature,* **233,** 177–82.

Gurwitz, D., Razon, N., Sokolovsky, M., and Soreq, H. (1984). Expression of muscarinic receptors in primary brain tumors. *Dev. Brain Res.,* **14,** 61–70.

Hodgkin, W. E., Giblett, E. R., Levine, H., Baner, W., and Motulsky, A. G. (1965). Complete pseudocholinesterase deficiency: Genetic and immunologic characterization. *J. Clin. Invest.,* **44,** 486–97.

Johnson, C. D., and Russell, R. L. (1975). A rapid, simple radiometric assay for cholinesterase, suitable for multiple determinations. *Anal. Biochem.,* **64,** 229–38.

Klose, R., and Gustensohn, G. (1976). Treatment of alkyl phosphate poisoning with purified serum cholinesterase. *Prakl. Anasth.,* **11,** 1–7.

Libermann, T. A., Razon, N., Bartal, A. D., Yarden, Y., Schlessinger, J., and Soreq, H. (1984). Expression of epidermal growth factor receptors in human brain tumors. *Cancer Res.,* **44,** 753–60.

Lund, P. K., Goodman, R. H., and Habener, J. F. (1981). Pancreatic preproglucagons are encoded by two separate mRNAs. *J. Biol. Chem.,* **256,** 6515–18.

Marquis, J. K., Volicer, L., Mark, K. A., Direnfeld, L. K., and Freedman, M. (1985). Cholinesterase activity in plasma, erythrocytes and cerebrospinal fluid of patients with dementia of the Alzheimer type. *Biol. Psych.*, **20**, 605–10.

Massoulié, J., and Bon, S. (1982). The molecular forms of cholinesterase and acetylcholinesterase in vertebrates. *Ann. Rev. Neurosci.*, **55**, 57–106.

Meflah, K., Bernard, S., and Massoulie, J. (1984). Interactions with lectins indicate differences in the carbohydrate composition of the membrane-bound enzymes acetylcholinesterase and 5-nucleotidase in different cell types. *Biochimie.*, **66**, 59–69.

Nawa, H., Kitamura, N., Hirose, T., Asai, M., Inayama, S., and Natanishi, S. (1983). Primary structure of bovine liver low molecular weight kininogen precursors and their two mRNAs. *Proc. Natl Acad. Sci. USA*, **80**, 90–4.

Pelham, H. R. B., and Jackson, R. J. (1976). An efficient mRNA-dependent translation system from reticulocyte lysates. *Eur. J. Biochem.*, **67**, 247–56.

Perry, E. K., Tomlinson, B. E., Blessed, G., Bergman, K., P. H., and Perry, R. H. (1978). Correlation of cholinergic abnormalities with senile plaques and mental test scores in senile dementia. *Br. Med. J.*, **2**, 1457–9.

Perry, E. K., Atack, J. R., Perry, R. H., Hardy, J. A., Dodd, P. R., Edwardson, J. A., Blessed, G., Tomlinson, B. E., and Fairbairn, A. F. (1984). Intralaminar neurochemical distributions in human midtemporal cortex: Comparison between Alzheimer's disease and the normal. *J. Neurochem.*, **42**, 1402–10.

Razon, N., Soreq, H., Roth, E., Bartal, A., and Silman, I. (1984). Characterisation of levels and forms of cholinesterases in human primary brain tumors. *Exp. Neurol.*, **84**, 681–95.

Rosenberry, T. L., and Scoggin, D. M. (1984). Human erythrocyte acetylcholinesterase is an amphipathic protein whose short membrane-binding domain is removed by papain digestion. *J. Biol. Chem.*, **250**, 5643–52.

Saper, C. B., and Chelimsky, T. C. (1984). A cytoarchitectonic and histochemical study of nucleus basalis and associated cell groups in the normal human brain. *Neuroscience*, **13**, 1023–29.

Silver, A. (1974). *The Biology of Cholinesterases.* North-Holland, Amsterdam.

Soininen, H., Halonen, T., and Reikkinen, P. J. (1981). Acetylcholinesterase activities in cerebrospinal fluid of patients with senile dementia of Alzheimer type. *Acta Neurol. Scand.*, **64**, 17–224.

Soreq, H. (1984). Bioassays of oocyte-produced brain enzymes. In Soreq, H. (ed.), *Molecular Biology Approach to the Neurosciences*, IBRO Handbook Series: Methods in the Neurosciences, Vol. 7. John Wiley & Sons, Chichester, New York, pp. 187–94.

Soreq, H. (1985). The biosynthesis of biologically active proteins in mRNA-injected *Xenopus* oocytes. *CRC Critical Reviews in Biochemistry*, **18**, 199–238.

Soreq, H., Parvari, R., and Silman, I. (1982). Biosynthesis and secretion of active acetylcholinesterase in *Xenopus* oocytes microinjected with mRNA from rat brain and from *Torpedo* electric organ. *Proc. Natl Acad. Sci. USA*, **79**, 830–4.

Soreq, H., Zevin-Sonkin, D., and Razon, R. (1984). Expression of cholinesterase gene(s) in human brain tissues: translational evidence for multiple mRNA species. *The EMBO Journal*, **3**, 1371–5.

Soreq, H., Djiegielewska, K. M. D., Zevin-Sonkin, D., and Zakut, H. (1986). Expression of cholinesterase gene(s) in foetal human tissues: evidence for post-translational processing of different polypeptide products. (Submitted).

Soreq, H., Zevin-Sonkin, D., Goldberg, O., and Prody, C. (1986). Molecular biology approach to the expression and properties of mammalian cholinesterases. In Heinemann, S., and Patrick, J. (eds.), *Current Topics in Neurobiology: Molecular Neurobiology*. Plenum Publishing (in press).

Soreq, H., Zevin-Sonkin, D., Avni, A., Hall, L. M. C., and Spierer, P. (1985). A human acetylcholinesterase gene identified by homology to the *Drosophila* gene. *Proc. Natl Acad. Sci. USA*, **82**, 1827–31.

Weitz, M., Bjerrum, O. J., and Brodbeck, J. (1984). Characterization of an active hydrophilic erythrocyte membrane acetylcholinesterase obtained by limited proteolysis of the purified enzyme. *Biochem. Biophys. Acta*, **776**, 65–74.

Whitehouse, P. J., Price, D. L., Struble, R. G., Clark, A. W., Coyle, J. T., and DeLong, M. R. (1982). Alzheimer's disease and senile dementias: loss of neurons in the basal forebrain. *Science*, **215**, 1237-9.

Zakut, H., Matzkel, A., Schejter, E., Avni, A., and Soreq, H. (1985). Polymorphism of acetylcholinesterase in discrete regions of the developing human fetal brain. *J. Neurochem.*, **45**, 382-9.

Zevin-Sonkin, D., Avni, A., Zisling, R., Koch, R., and Soreq, H. (1985). Expression of acetylcholinesterase gene(s) in the human brain: molecular cloning evidence for cross-homologous sequences. *J. Physiol. (Paris)*, **80**, 221-8.

12

An Immunohistochemical Study Comparing Selected Features of the Anatomy of Cholinergic Innervation in the Cerebral Cortex of Six Mammalian Species

F. Eckenstein

12.1 Introduction

Many different investigators have contributed over the last five decades to establishing acetylcholine (ACh) as a neurotransmitter in cerebral cortex. Besides ACh itself, all biochemical correlates of cholinergic function, such as the ACh synthesising and degrading enzymes, choline acetyltransferase (ChAT) and acetylcholinesterase (AChE), respectively, as well as ACh receptors and the high affinity uptake mechanism have all been shown to be present in cortex. In addition, cortical neurons have been found to be sensitive to extracellular application of ACh (for reviews see Emson and Lindvall, 1979; Parnavelas and McDonald, 1983; Eckenstein and Baughman, 1986).

In spite of this wealth of biochemical and physiological data on cholinergic mechanisms in cerebral cortex, little information on anatomical features of cholinergic cortical innervation has been available. Progress has recently been made, however, due to the introduction of specific and sensitive immunohistochemical methods for the localisation of a specific marker, ChAT, for cholinergic neurons (Eckenstein and Thoenen, 1982; Houser et al., 1983; Levey et al., 1983). ChAT-immunohistochemistry, often combined with retrograde tracing techniques, has now clearly demonstrated that basal forebrain nuclei innervate the entire cortical mantle in a topographically organised way (Mesulam *et al.*, 1983a,b; Woolf *et al.*, 1983; Saper 1984), and that a minor cholinergic projection originating in the midbrain tegmentum innervates medial frontal cortex (Mesulam *et al.*, 1983b; Vincent *et al.*, 1983). In addition, in rat cerebral cortex interneurons of bipolar shape have been found to stain for both ChAT and vasoactive intestinal polypeptide (VIP; Eckenstein and Baughman, 1984).

Patients suffering from Alzheimer's disease show marked reductions in cholinergic parameters in cortex, including hippocampus, and in the basal forebrain, due to degeneration of the cholinergic basalo-cortical projection (Davies, 1979; Coyle *et al.*, 1983). It is now important to determine which animal species can serve as a good model system for studying the effects of experimental manipulation of this cholinergic projection. One of the obvious questions is whether ChAT-positive cortical interneurons are found in the rat only, or are present in other species also.

We have studied this question by means of immunohistochemical localisation of both ChAT and VIP in the rat, mouse, guinea pig, rabbit, cat, and monkey. Of all these species, ChAT-positive cortical neurons were found in rat and mouse only. VIP-positive cells, however, were found in the cortex of all species analysed. The organisation of the basal forebrain cholinergic nuclei was remarkably similar in all species studied. Taken together, these findings suggest that the guinea pig might be the preferred small, rodent animal model system for analysing the effects of experimental manipulation on cortical cholinergic parameters, as the cortical cholinergic innervation of this species is more similar to that of the primate, than is that of the rat or mouse.

12.2 Materials and Methods

Long-Evans rats, CD-mice, Hartley guinea pigs, New Zealand rabbits, cats, and macaque monkeys (at least two animals per species) were used for this study. Animals were deeply anaesthetised and perfused through the heart with 4 % paraformaldehyde in 100 mM sodium phosphate, pH 7.2, containing 15 % (sat.) picric acid. Brains were dissected immediately and postfixed for 30 to 60 min in the same fixative. Brains or blocks of appropriate size were washed overnight at 4 °C in 100 mM sodium phosphate, pH 8.2, and sunk first in 15 %, then in 30 % sucrose in the same buffer. 50 μm thick sections were cut on a freezing microtome.

12.3 Immunohistochemistry

Sections were incubated overnight in either a mouse or rat antiserum to ChAT or a rabbit antiserum to synthetic porcine VIP, all of established specificity. They were then washed for 3 × 5 min, and incubated for 60 min in secondary antibody, washed as above, incubated for 90 min in PAP, washed, and the secondary antibody and PAP-steps were then repeated. After the final wash, sections were reacted for 10 min with 1 mg diaminobenzidine in 100 mM sodium phosphate, pH 8.2, containing 0.01 % hydrogen peroxide, and then washed and mounted on slides. Antiserum dilutions were 1:1000, secondary antibodies and PAP were diluted 1:50. The dilution buffer contained 100 mM Tris, 150 mM sodium chloride, 10 % of an appropriate blocking serum and 2 % bovine serum albumin, pH 7.4. Triton X-100 concentrations were 0.5 % for primary, and 0.2 % for secondary antibodies and PAP-solutions. Controls included substitution of non-immune serum for the primary antiserum and preabsorption of the antiserum with the appropriate antigen. Both types of controls exhibited negligible, faint background staining.

12.4 Results

ChAT-positive structures were observed in the CNS of all species studied. Long–Evans rat, for which species the staining protocol used had been optimised, showed the most intense staining, but well-labelled cell bodies, fibres and terminals were also found in mouse, guinea pig, rabbit, cat and monkey.

VIP-staining was also observed in all species studied. Staining intensity was similar in all species but the monkey, where labelling of cortical structures was more faint. This difference in staining-intensity might reflect differences in actual concentration of VIP, as no marked difference in amino-acid sequence between primate and non-primate VIP has been reported.

In the basal forebrain of all species investigated, large, multipolar neurons stained intensely for ChAT (Fig. 12.1). In no case were these cells VIP-positive. The topological organisation of these cells into distinct nuclei was very similar for all species. Most of the stained cells were found in loosely defined nuclei in the septal area, specifically in the medial septal nucleus, the vertical and horizontal limbs of the diagonal band; and in the general area of the substatia innominata and the globus pallidus, specifically in the nucleus basalis of Meynert (Fig. 12.2).

In all of the species most of the ChAT-positive fibres fanned out diffusely from the basal forebrain nuclei to reach their cortical target, but the stained fibres in a medial pathway originating in the septal area and innervating cingulate cortex, were organised in a well-formed bundle. This bundle was most obvious in saggital sections of rat brain, but could easily be found in all the other species (not shown).

ChAT-positive terminals were found in all cortical areas of all species studied (Fig. 12.3). The quality of staining differed between species, and the laminar distribution of stained terminals could only reliably be analysed in rat. In many cortical areas of this species, ChAT-positive terminals were densest in layer V, followed by layers I-III. Layers IV and VI clearly contained less stained ter-

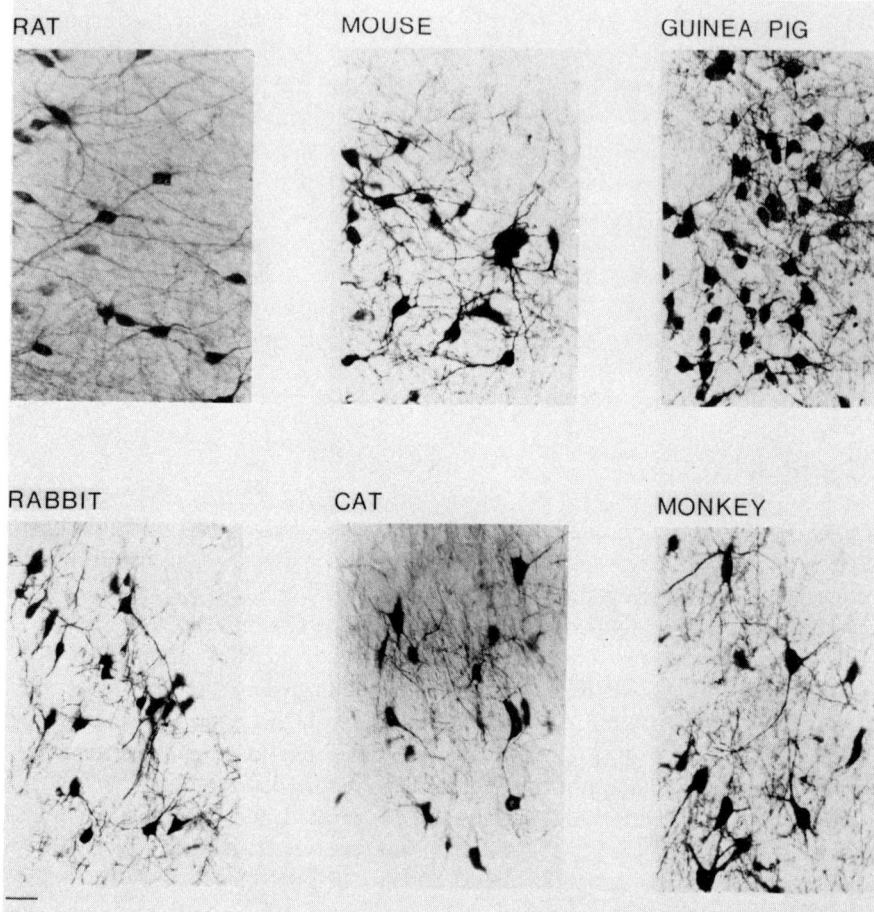

Fig 12.1 Immunohistochemical localisation of ChAT in the horizontal limb of the diagonal band of Broca of six mammalian species. Numerous large (30–40 μm diameter), multipolar neurons are heavily stained. These neurons are arranged in a characteristic pattern formed by the intermingling of stained cholinergic cells with unstained non-cholinergic structures. The morphology of the labelled cells is similar in all species studied. The bar (bottom left) represents 60 μm.

minals (Fig. 12.4). A marked increase in the density of stained terminals was found in entorhinal cortex of all of the species.

The only marked difference between the species observed concerned the presence of ChAT-positive cortical interneurons. These neurons were present in moderate densities in rat cortex, where they were mostly found in layers II, III and IV. The stained cells were of small size (10 μm diameter) and had long, vertical dendrites spanning, in many cases, almost the entire cortical depth (Fig. 12.3). We have earlier shown that the majority of these neurons also

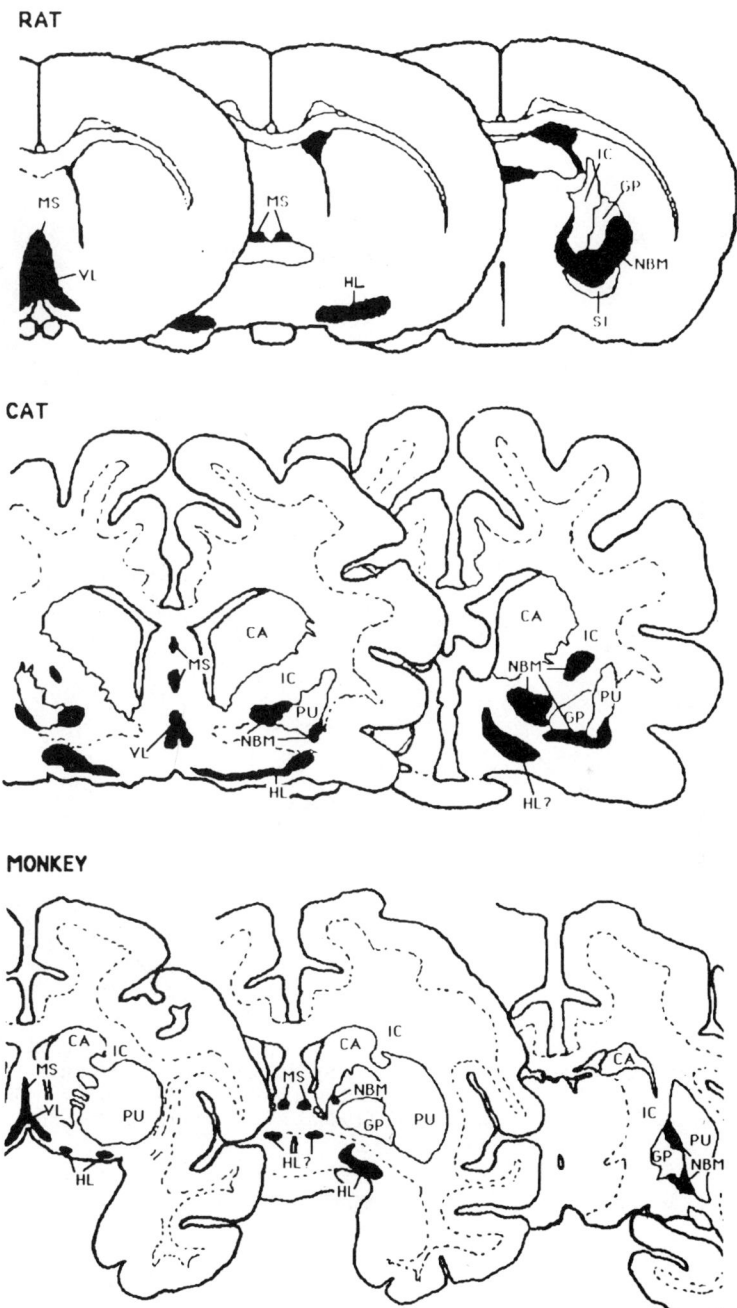

Fig. 12.2 Schematic drawings illustrating the areas (in black) in the basal forebrain where ChAT-positive neurons are found in high density. Note the similar distribution of these areas in rat, cat, and monkey. Abbreviations are: CA, caudate; GP, globus pallidus; HL, horizontal limb of the diagonal band; IC, internal capsule; MS, medial septal nucleus; NBM, nucleus basalis; SI, substantia innominata; and VL, vertical limb of the diagonal band.

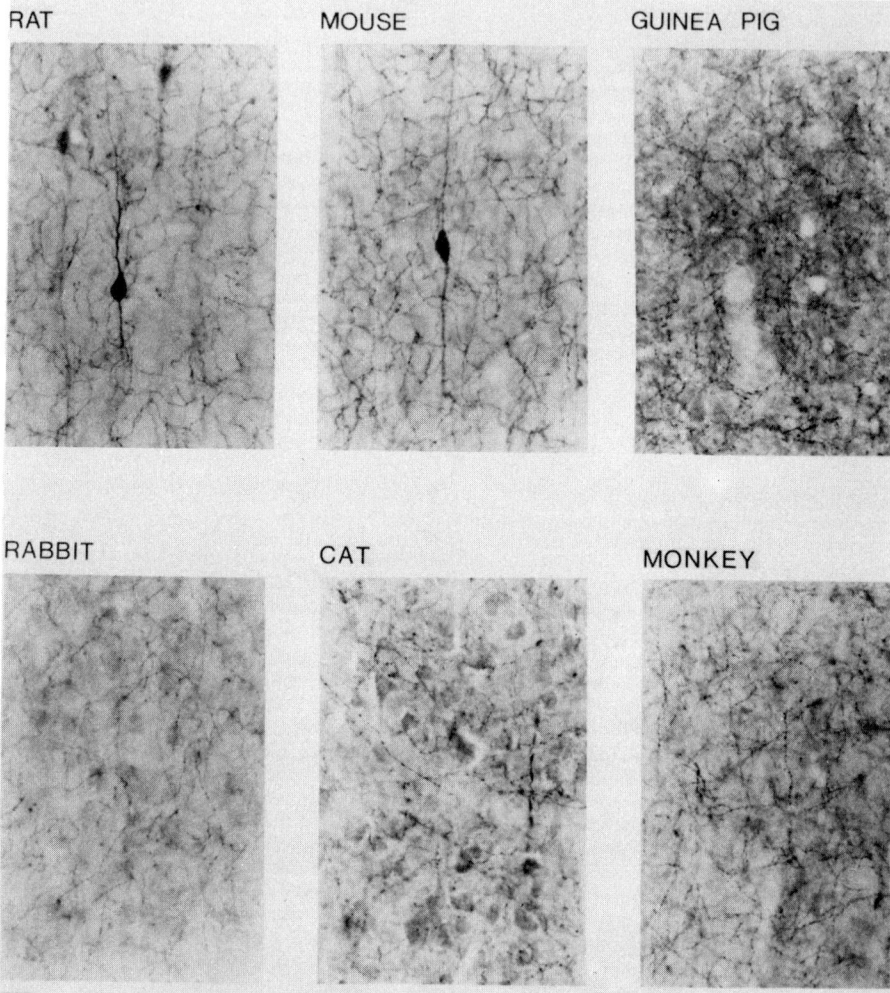

RAT   MOUSE   GUINEA PIG

RABBIT   CAT   MONKEY

Fig. 12.3   Immunohistochemical localisation of ChAT-positive structures in cerebral cortex of six mammalian species. Labelled fibres, many of them containing varicosities which represent likely sites of ACh-release, are present in a moderately high density in all species. Stained cortical neurons of small diameter (10 μm) and of bipolar shape are found in rat and mouse cortex only. The bar represents 15μm.

contain VIP, and it is thus not surprising that a similar number of VIP-positive neurons of similar shape and distribution were found in rat cortex. Small neurons staining for VIP were found in similar numbers in all species studied. In most

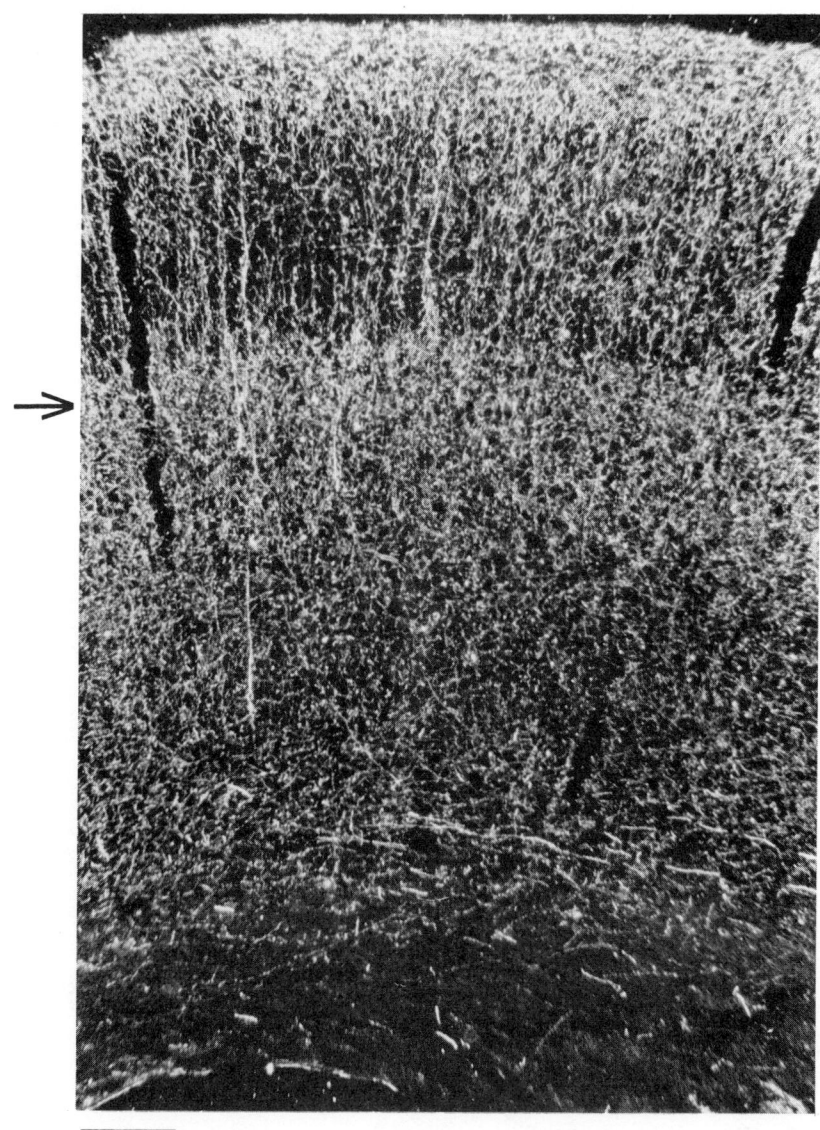

Fig. 12.4   The distribution of ChAT-positive fibres and terminals is shown in this darkfield photomicrograph of rat cerebral cortex. Terminal density is highest in cortical layer V, closely followed by layer I, whereas terminal density is lowest in layers IV and VI. The arrow indicates the border between layer IV and V. The bar represents 200 μm.

RAT   MOUSE   GUINEA PIG

RABBIT   CAT   MONKEY

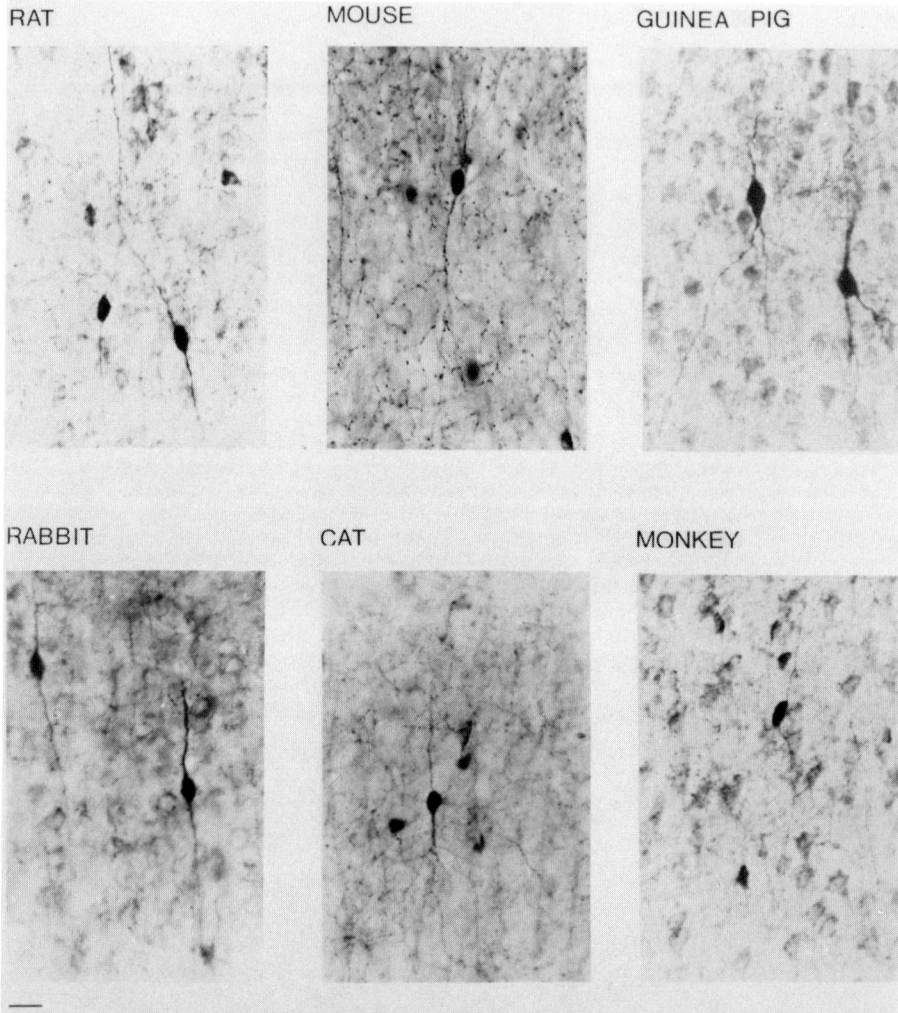

Fig. 12.5 Immunohistochemical localisation of VIP-positive structures in the cerebral cortex of six mammalian species. Small neurons (10 μm in diameter) mostly of bipolar shape, as well as fibres and terminals, are stained. The morphology and distribution of stained elements is similar in all species. Note, however, that the staining intensity in monkey is faint compared to that seen in the other species. The bar (bottom left) represents 15 μm.

of the species the cells were mostly of typical bipolar shape, except in the monkey, where the round cell bodies were stained (Fig. 12.5), ChAT-positive cortical bipolar cells were, however, only found in rat and mouse. Even local cortical injection of colchicine did not reveal neurons staining for ChAT in other species (Fig. 12.3).

12.5 Discussion

The major part of cholinergic cortical innervation is known to be derived from a projection from basal forebrain nuclei (Johnston *et al.*, 1979; Lehmann *et al.*, 1980; Mesulam *et al.*, 1983a,b; Woolf *et al.*, 1983; Saper, 1984), and it has also become clear that a minor cholinergic projection from midbrain tegmentum innervates medial frontal cortex (Mesulam *et al.*, 1983b; Vincent *et al.*, 1983). In addition, ChAT-immunoreactivity containing cortical neurons of mostly bipolar shape have recently been found in rat cerebral cortex (Eckenstein and Thoenen, 1983; Houser *et al.*, 1985). Here, we have analysed the distribution of ChAT-immunoreactivity containing structures in the cerebral cortex and basal forebrain of six different species (rat, mouse, guinea pig, rabbit, cat, and monkey).

In all species studied, large, multipolar neurons staining intensely for ChAT were found mainly in the medial septal nucleus, the diagonal band nuclei and in the nucleus basalis of Meynert. A considerable number of stained neurons of similar morphology were, however, present in the areas between these nuclei, making the exact definition of borders of the cholinergic nuclei difficult in some cases. These results are in good agreement with previous data originating from analysis of single species (for reviews see Fibiger, 1982; Eckenstein and Baughman, 1986). It has been suggested that the anatomical organisation of the basalocortical projection is more refined in more complex brains, such as the monkey's. For example, the NBM of the monkey has earlier been found to be composed of at least five anatomically different substructures. This has been taken as an indication that the topographic organisation of the cholinergic basal-forebrain projection to cortex is more precise in more highly evolved mammalian species (Mesulam *et al.*, 1983a). This argument remains, however, to be evaluated carefully, as it has become clear that the cortical areas innervated by the five subgroups of the NBM overlap considerably in the monkey (Mesulam *et al.*, 1983a), which is not dissimilar to the loosely defined topographical organisation observed in the rat. In addition, we have recently found that in rat the boundaries between cortical areas receiving input from different basal-forebrain nuclei can be very precise (Eckenstein *et al.*, in preparation). We therefore favour the view that the apparent higher complexity of the cholinergic nuclei in the basal forebrain of primates does not *a priori* demonstrate a more precise topographical organisation of the projection to cortex. With closer inspection, it appears that the NBM of the rat, for example, also might contain different subgroups analogous to those observed in the monkey, but that they are harder to notice, due to the lesser differentiation of fibre patterns in the rat forebrain.

The basal-forebrain fibres follow different pathways to reach their cortical target. In rat, fibres originating from the NBM were found to fan out laterally and to form a diffuse system innervating the majority of cortical areas. Fibres from the septal area (mainly innervating cingulate cortex) were, however, observed to form a precise bundle. To our surprise, these different pathways were highly conserved among all species studied. Again, in all species studied, most cortical areas showed a similar density of cholinergic terminals, with the exception of entorhinal cortex where a significant increase of stained terminals was observed.

The observation that both the anatomical organisation of the cholinergic basal-forebrain nuclei and the pathways by which they reach their cortical target area are highly conserved during mammalian evolution might indicate the physiological importance of this system.

Bipolar ChAT-positive cells were only found in rat and mouse cortex. The absence of these cells in other species, even after local application of colchicine, appears not to be due to methodological problems, as well-stained ChAT-positive terminals were observed in cerebral cortex of all species studied. We had earlier shown that at least 80 % of the ChAT-positive cortical cells in rat also contain VIP-immunoreactivity (Eckenstein and Baughman, 1984). In good agreement with earlier observations (Loren *et al.*, 1979), VIP-positive cortical neurons of similar distribution were found in all species here studied, showing only small differences among species in staining intensity and morphology (with the exception of monkey, where VIP-positive cortical structures were stained only faintly, possibly indicating a lower concentration of VIP-immunoreactive material in primate cortex). Interestingly, it has recently been suggested that these neurons innervate, besides neuronal targets, cortical blood vessels (Eckenstein and Baughman, 1984), and that they influence local cortical metabolic processes (Magistretti *et al.*, 1981). It is puzzling why these cortical neurons express a cholinergic phenotype in only some species, especially when we assume that their function is similar in different mammalian species.

Degeneration of the cholinergic basalo-cortical projection is prominent among the pathological changes observed in Alzheimer's disease (Davies, 1979; Coyle *et al.*, 1983). In the present study we have shown that the cholinergic innervation of rat and mouse cerebral cortex differs from that of primates by the presence of cholinergic neurons in cortex. Analogous neurons are present in the primate; they contain, however, VIP only. These neurons appear not to be affected by Alzheimer's disease (Rossor *et al.*, 1980).

One of the interests in research on Alzheimer's disease is to characterise the effects of experimental manipulation on cortical cholinergic parameters. The cholinergic cortical innervation of the guinea pig resembles more closely that of the primate than does that of either rat or mouse, and this species might therefore represent a valuable animal system to which to address such questions.

12.6 Acknowledgements

I would like to thank Dr R. W. Baughman for support and advice, and J. Quinn for expert technical assistance. Supported by ADRDA (FSA 85-011).

References

Coyle, J. T., Price, D. L., and DeLong, M. R. (1983). Alzheimer's disease: a disorder of cortical cholinergic innervation. *Science*, 219, 1184–90.

Davies, P. (1979). Neurotransmitter-related enzymes in senile dementia of the Alzheimer type. *Brain Res.*, 171, 319–27.

Eckenstein, F., and Baughman, R. W. (1984). Two types of cholinergic innervation in cerebral cortex, one co-localised with vasoactive intestinal polypeptide. *Nature*, 309, 152–5.

Eckenstein, F., and Baughman, R. W. (1986). Cholinergic cortical innervation. In Peters and Jones, (eds.), *The Cerebral Cortex*. Pergamon (in press).

Eckenstein, F., and Thoenen, H. (1982). Production of specific antisera and monoclonal antibodies to choline acetyltransferase: characterisation and use for identification of cholinergic neurons. *EMBO J.*, 1, 363–8.

Eckenstein, F., and Thoenen, H. (1983). Cholinergic neurons in the rat cerebral cortex demonstrated by immunohistochemical localization of choline acetyltransferase. *Neurosci. Lett.*, 36, 211–15.

Emson, P. C., and Lindvall, O. (1979). Distribution of putative neurotransmitters in cortex. *Neurosci.*, 4, 1–30.

Fibiger, H. C. (1982). The organization and some projections of cholinergic neurons of the mammalian forebrain. *Brain Res. Rev.*, 4, 327–88.

Houser, C. R., Crawford, G. D., Salvaterra, P. M., and Vaughn, J. E. (1985). Immunocytochemical localization of choline acetyltransferase in rat cerebral cortex: a study of cholinergic neurons and synapses. *J. Comp. Neurol.*,

Houser, C. R., Crawford, G. D., Barber, R. P., Salvaterra, P. M., and Vaughn, J. E. (1983). Organization and morphological characteristics of cholinergic neurons: an immunocytochemical study with a monoclonal antibody to choline acetyltransferase. *Brain Res.*, 266, 97–119.

Johnston, M. V., McKinney, M., and Coyle, J. T. (1979). Evidence for a cholinergic projection to neocortex from neurons in the basal forebrain. *Proc. Natl Acad. Sci. USA*, 76, 5392–6.

Lehmann, J. H, Nagy, S., Atmadja, S., and Fibiger, H. C. (1980). The nucleus basalis magnocellularis: the origin of a cholinergic projection to the neocortex of the rat. *Neurosci.*, 5, 1161–1174.

Levey, A. I., Armstrong, D. M., Atweh, S. F., Terry, R. D., and Wainer, B. H. (1983). Monoclonal antibodies to choline acetyltransferase: production, specificity and immunohistochemistry. *J. Neurosci.*, 3, 1–9.

Loren, I., Emson, P. C., Fahrenkrug, J., Bjorklund, A., Alumets, J., Hakanson, R., and Sundler, F. (1979). Distribution of vasoactive intestinal polypeptide in the rat and mouse brain. *Neurosci.*, 4, 1953–76.

Magistretti, P. J., Morrison, J. H., Shoemaker, W. J., Sapin, V., and Bloom, F. E. (1981). Vasoactive intestinal polypeptide induces glycogenolysis in mouse cortical slices: a possible regulatory mechanism for the local control of energy metabolism. *Proc. Natl Acad. Sci. USA*, 78, 6535–9.

Mesulam, M. M., Mufson, E. J., Levey, A. I., and Wainer, B. H. (1983a). Cholinergic innervation by the basal forebrain: cytochemistry and cortical connections of the septal area, diagonal band nuclei, nucleus basalis (substantia innominata), and hypothalamus in the rhesus monkey. *J. Comp. Neurol.*, 214, 170–97.

Mesulam, M. M., Mufson, E. J., Wainer, B. H., and Levey, A. I. (1983b). Central cholinergic pathways in the rat: an overview based on an alternative nomenclature (Ch. 1–Ch. 6) *Neurosci.*, 10, 1185–201.

Parnavelas, J. G., and McDonald, J. K. (1983). The cerebral cortex. In Emson, P. C. (ed.), *Chemical Neuroanatomy*. Raven Press, New York, pp. 505–49.

Rossor, M. N., Fahrenkrug, J., Emson, P. C., Mountjoy, C., Iversen, L. L., and Roth, M. (1980). Reduced cortical choline acetyltransferase activity in senile dementia of Alzheimer's type is not accompanied by changes in vasoactive intestinal polypeptide. *Brain Res.*, 201, 249–53.

Saper, C. B. (1984). Organization of cerebral cortical afferent systems in the rat. 1: Magno-cellular basal nucleus. *J. Comp. Neurol.*, **222**, 313–42.

Vincent, S. R., Satoh, K., Armstrong, D. M., and Fibiger, H. C. (1983). Substance P in the ascending cholinergic reticular system. *Nature*, **306**, 688–91.

Woolf, N. J., Eckenstein, F., and Butcher, L. L. (1983). Cholinergic projections from the basal forebrain to the frontal cortex: a combined fluorescent tracer and immunohisto-chemical analysis in the rat. *Neurosci. Lett.*, **40**, 93–8.

13

Cell Biology of the Forebrain Cholinergic Neurons: Effects of NGF, Triiodothyronine and Gangliosides

F. Hefti

13.1 Introduction

Alzheimer's disease is associated with a selective loss of cholinergic neurons located in the basal forebrain. Even though other neuronal systems are also partly affected, the loss of cholinergic neurons is regarded by most investigators as being the principal factor responsible for the memory loss that is characteristic of Alzheimer's disease (Bartus *et al.*, 1982; Coyle *et al.*, 1983; Davies, 1985). In attempting to find the cause of and treatment for the disease, I decided to study the cell biology of cholinergic neurons of the forebrain and to characterise their requirements for survival and maintenance of function. A culture system was developed in which cholinergic neurons from rat brains are grown and studied under controlled conditions and are easily accessible for observation. Using these cultures, the effects of other cell types, growth factors, hormones and drugs on survival, growth and differentiation of cholinergic cells are investigated. These studies will lead to a characterisation of the conditions required by cholinergic neurons to survive and maintain their function *in vitro*. Conditions and compounds found to affect cholinergic neurons *in vitro* will later be assessed in living animals with specific lesions of the cholinergic systems. The *in vitro* studies first focussed on the effects of NGF and thyroxine, which were both reported to influence cholinergic neurons, and on gangliosides, which were claimed to promote neuronal survival and regeneration.

13.2 Cultures

Cholinergic neurons giving rise to the ascending cholinergic projections of the
basal mammalian forebrain (Mesulam *et al.*, 1983; Wainer *et al.*, 1984) were
studied in cultures of dissociated cells from the septal area of foetal rat brains.
Culture conditions were optimised to give maximal yield and differentiation of
cholinergic neurons. The septal area was dissected either from foetal rats of
embryonic age E16–E17 or from neonatal rats taken at the day of birth. Tissue
pieces were minced and cells were dissociated using mechanical and enzymatic
procedures. Cells were plated in culture dishes coated with polylysine and were
grown in a modified L-15 medium. The preparation of the cultures and the
medium were described in detail in Hefti *et al.* (1985a).

In the studies with NGF and gangliosides, cultures were grown in the modified L-15 medium supplemented with 5 % horse serum and 1 % rat serum. To
study the effects of thyroxine and its analogues, a serum-free medium was used.
For these experiments, the modified L-15 medium was supplemented with
0.5 mg/l insulin, 10 mg/l transferrin, 1.6 mg/l putrescine, 0.63 µg/l progesterone,
0.52 µg/l sodium selenite, 400 mg/l bovine serum albumin, and 25 ml/l of a
soybean lipid mixture (Gibco).

Cholinergic neurons were identified using immunocytochemical visualisation
of choline acetyltransferase (ChAT) and cytochemical demonstration of acetylcholinesterase (AChE; see Fig. 13.1). For visualisation of ChAT, cultures were
treated with a monoclonal antibody to ChAT and then with a biotinylated second
antibody and an avidin–biotin conjugate of horseradish peroxidase (Vectastain).
The peroxidase was visualised by incubating the cultures with diaminobenzidine
and hydrogen peroxide. AChE cytochemistry was performed as described in
Hefti *et al.* (1985a) using acetylthiocholine as substrate. AChE is a reliable
marker for cholinergic neurons in cultures of septal cells, since 96 % of all
AChE-positive cells were found to be co-stained for ChAT (Hefti *et al.*, 1985a).
Astrocytes growing in the cultures were identified by immunocytochemical
visualisation of glial fibrillary acid protein (GFAP). For biochemical measurements of ChAT activity, cultures were homogenised and aliquots of the homo-
genate were taken for the determination of ChAT activity according to Fonnum
(1975) and protein content according to Bradford (1976).

13.3 Nerve Growth Factor (NGF)

Findings obtained in recent years by several investigators suggest that forebrain
cholinergic neurons are influenced by nerve growth factor (NGF). These findings
are surprising, since NGF is believed normally to be a selective neurotrophic
factor for peripheral sympathetic and sensory neurons (Greene and Shooter,
1980; Thoenen and Barde, 1980). The following evidence for a role of NGF in
the function of cholinergic neurons was obtained. First, NGF as well as the

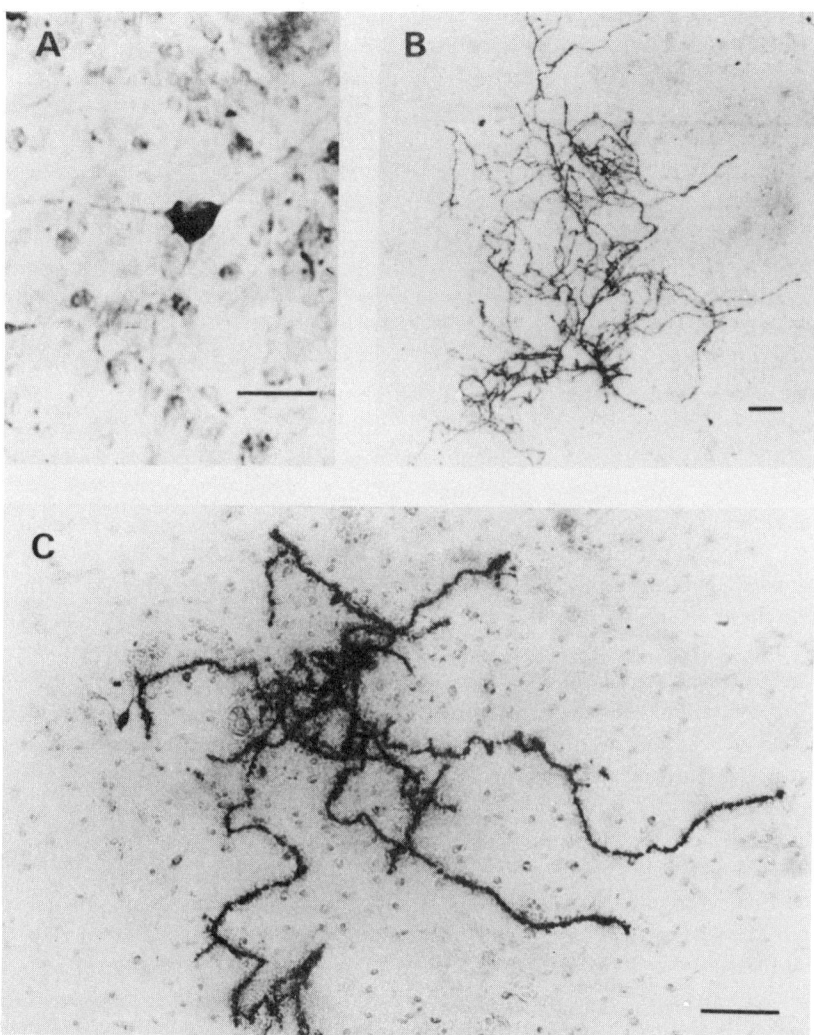

Fig. 13.1 Cholinergic neurons in cultures of dissociated cells from the septal area. (A) immunocytochemical visualisation of ChAT using a monoclonal antibody followed by a biotinylated second antibody and a biotin–avidin conjugate of horseradish peroxidase (bar = 40 μm); (B), (C) cytochemical visualisation of AChE (bars = 100 μm).

mRNA coding for NGF are present in the rat brain and their levels seem to be highest in the hippocampus, i.e. in a target area of forebrain cholinergic neurons (Crutcher and Collins, 1982; Shelton and Reichardt, 1984). Second, NGF injected into target areas of forebrain cholinergic neurons (i.e. hippocampus and

cortex) is taken up by nerve terminals and is transported in a retrograde fashion
to the cholinergic cell bodies located in the basal forebrain (Schwab *et al.*, 1979;
Seiler and Schwab, 1984). Since NGF uptake is mediated by specific receptors,
these findings suggest the existence of NGF receptors on cholinergic neurons.
Third, stimulation of NGF receptors on cholinergic neurons results in an elevation of the activity of choline acetyltransferase (ChAT), the key enzyme in the
synthesis of acetylcholine, in aggregate cultures containing cholinergic neurons
of the foetal rat forebrain (Honegger and Lenoir, 1980a), in the brain of new-
born rats (Gnahn *et al.*, 1983), in the brain of adult rats with partial lesions of a
cholinergic pathway (Hefti *et al.*, 1984), and in adult rats receiving transplants
of foetal septal tissue (Toniolo *et al.*, 1985). Fourth, the notion that NGF acts
as a neurotrophic factor for forebrain cholinergic neurons is supported by results
from lesion studies. Destruction of the cholinergic input to the hippocampus
results in an ingrowth of peripheral sympathetic fibres which matches the
previous distribution of cholinergic terminals in the hippocampus (Loy and
Moore, 1977; Stenevi and Bjorklund, 1978; Crutcher *et al.*, 1979). Since peripheral sympathetic neurons react to NGF, it has been postulated that the hippocampal signal attracting sympathetic fibres is identical to NGF and that, in intact
brains, NGF acts upon and is taken up by the cholinergic terminals in this area
(Crutcher and Davies, 1981).

Part of the studies I have carried out in recent years has focussed on the
effects of NGF on cholinergic neurons in cultures of dissociated cells. In initial
experiments, cultures were prepared from foetal rat brains. Addition of NGF to
the culture medium did not affect the number of cholinergic neurons surviving
in these cultures. Furthermore, NGF failed to influence the general morphological appearance and the number of processes of cholinergic neurons. However, NGF elevated the biochemically measured activity of ChAT two to three
fold (*see* Fig. 13.2 and Table 13.3). The NGF-mediated increase in ChAT was
dose dependent, with an ED_{50} of 4×10^{-10} M. The increase was highly specific
for NGF, since it was blocked by antibodies to NGF and since epidermal growth
factor, insulin and other control proteins failed to exert a similar effect. NGF
had to be present for at least three days in the culture medium in order to raise
ChAT activity, suggesting that the increase was due to an elevated ChAT synthesis
rather than to an activation of the enzyme. These findings have been reported in
detail in Hefti *et al.* (1985a).

Recently, evidence has been obtained which indicates that NGF affects
survival of central cholinergic neurons after axonal transsections *in vivo*. NGF
was given intraventricularly to rats with lesions of the septo-hippocampal pathway. Such lesions reduced the number of cholinergic cell bodies in the septum.
Chronic application of NGF over several weeks was found to prevent this lesion-
induced degeneration of cholinergic neurons (F. Hefti, unpublished results).
Given these findings, it was hypothesised that NGF promotes survival of cholinergic neurons after axonal injury. In order to test this hypothesis *in vitro*,
cholinergic neurons were dissociated from the septal area of postnatal animals,

i.e. at a developmental stage when the septal cholinergic neurons had already started to invade hippocampal tissue (Nadler *et al.*, 1974; Crutcher, 1982; Milner *et al.*, 1983). Neurons taken for culture from such animals lost their processes during the dissociation procedure and they were therefore comparable to neurons submitted to axonal transsection *in vivo*. NGF significantly elevated the number of cholinergic neurons surviving in these cultures (Table 13.1). The stimulatory effect of NGF was prevented by the addition of an antiserum to NGF, indicating that the effect was specific for NGF. Cultures grown in the presence of both NGF and anti-NGF, or in the presence of anti-NGF alone, contained significantly fewer cholinergic cells than control cultures. These findings suggest that NGF is formed by neurons or glial cells growing in the cultures in sufficient quantities to support the survival of an intermediate number of cholinergic cells. The ED_{50} of NGF's effect on survival of cholinergic neurons was found to be approximately 4×10^{-10} M. This concentration is in the range of concentrations necessary to stimulate NGF receptors on sympathetic and sensory neurons (Greene and Shooter, 1980; Thoenen and Barde, 1980).

The findings obtained in culture provide further evidence for an important role of NGF in the function of forebrain cholinergic neurons. The studies show that NGF can stimulate the expression of ChAT activity or promote survival of cholinergic neurons, dependent upon the conditions under which these cells are studied. I have earlier hypothesised that the selective loss of cholinergic neurons in Alzheimer's disease might be caused by a lack of availability of NGF to these neurons and drew attention to the possibility that NGF, or drugs mimicking NGF's actions, might be useful in the treatment of Alzheimer's disease (Hefti,

Table 13.1   Effect of NGF and anti-NGF on survival of cholinergic neurons in cultures of septal cells dissociated from newborn rats

	cholinergic neurons per dish
controls	21.0 ± 0.9
NGF 3 ng/ml	26.7 ± 4.4
10 ng/ml	33.3 ± 4.2*
30 ng/ml	32.5 ± 3.2*
100 ng/ml	37.1 ± 2.8*
1000 ng/ml	38.5 ± 3.4*
NGF 100 ng/ml + anti-NGF[1]	8.6 ± 4.2*
anti-NGF[1]	9.2 ± 1.3*

means $\pm$ S.E. M.; n = 5–12
*different from controls, $p < 0.05$ (analysis of variance)
[1] 2 μl/ml of a sheep anti-mouse NGF serum (Suda *et al.*, 1978)
Cultures were grown over 10 days. Additions were present during the entire culture period. Cholinergic neurons were visualised using AChE-cytochemistry.

1983). The new findings which indicate that NGF is able to promote survival of cholinergic neurons strongly support this notion.

13.4 Triiodothyronine (T3)

The presence of the thyroid hormones thyroxine and triiodothyronine (T3) is essential for the normal development of the brain (Grave, 1977), and these hormones have been reported to influence axonal regeneration in adult animals (Kiernan, 1979). Several findings indicate that thyroid hormones affect central cholinergic neurons. First, thyroid deficiency is associated with a reduction of ChAT activity in various brain areas of experimental animals (Valcana, 1971; Kojima *et al.*, 1981; Kalaria and Prince, 1985). Second, T3 has been found to increase ChAT activity in aggregating cultures of rat brain cells (Honegger and Lenoir, 1980b). These findings prompted me to investigate the effects of thyroid hormones on the survival and differentiation of forebrain cholinergic neurons in culture.

Cultures prepared from foetal rat brains were grown in serum-free medium, since serum contains variable amounts of thyroid hormones as well as their carrier proteins. Cholinergic neurons survived and differentiated in these cultures in the absence of thyroid hormones. The addition of T3 to the culture medium did not result in a higher number of surviving cholinergic neurons (data not shown). However, the presence of T3 elevated the biochemically determined ChAT activity. The ED_{50} of this action of T3 was 3×10^{-9} M (Fig. 13.2). NGF potentiated the T3-induced increase in ChAT activity (Fig. 13.2). The effects of T3 and NGF at concentrations producing maximal increases of ChAT activity alone were additive, suggesting that the two treatments stimulate the expression of ChAT activity of cholinergic neuron cultures by acting through different mechanisms.

Since thyroid hormones affect developing cholinergic neurons and seem to promote axonal regeneration in adult animals, I hypothesised that these hormones might be useful in preventing the degeneration of cholinergic neurons as it occurs in Alzheimer's disease. However, application of thyroid hormones to patients with normal thyroid function would result in a multitude of undesired effects given the fact that these hormones influence the function of most organs. This problem might be circumvented if thyroxine analogues selectively stimulating central cholinergic neurons became available. To test the feasibility of this approach, an attempt was made to characterise the structural requirements of the receptor mediating the effects of thyroid hormones on central cholinergic neurons. Several analogues of T3 were tested for their ability to elevate ChAT activity of cholinergic neurons in culture. Their relative potency in elevating ChAT activity was then compared with their known antigoiter activity determined *in vivo* and the binding affinity to the hepatic nuclear receptor measured *in vitro* (Cheung, 1985; Jorgensen, 1978).

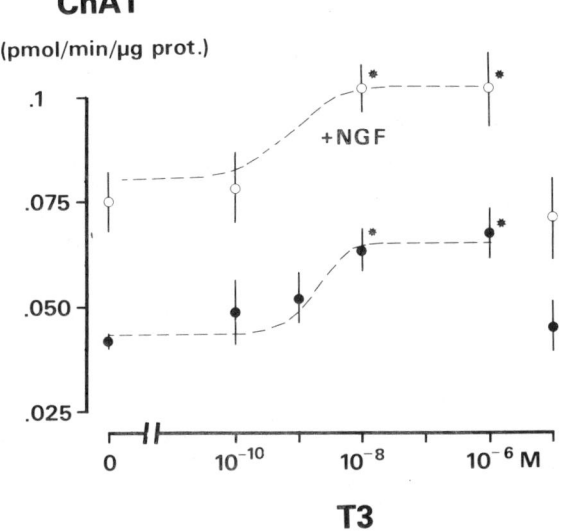

ChAT

(pmol/min/µg prot.)

Fig. 13.2 Effect of triiodothyronine (T3) and NGF on ChAT activity in cultures of dissociated septal cells from foetal rat brains. Cultures were grown for seven days in a serum-free medium. Additions were present during the entire culture time. Bars represent S.E.M.; $n = 5-12$; asterisks indicate values significantly different from corresponding control values measured in absence of T3 ($p < 0.05$, analysis of variance); all values of the groups treated with NGF were significantly different from the corresponding values for the groups not treated with NGF ($p < 0.05$).

The L-form of T3 was slightly more potent than the D-isomer in elevating CAT activity of cholinergic neurons in culture (Table 13.2). Removal of the iodine from the outer ring of T3 (resulting in 3,5-diiodothyronine, T2), removal of the 4' hydroxylic group from the outer ring, and replacement of the amino acid side chain by a carboxylic acid side chain reduced the activity of T3 to a large extent. Substitution of the iodine in the outer ring by an isopropyl group (resulting in 3'-isopropyl-T2) produced the most potent analogue. Reverse substituted analogues, i.e. compounds with one halogen or isopropyl side chain in the inner ring and two such substituents in the outer ring, were virtually inactive. Iodine alone was ineffective. These findings indicate that the structural requirements of the receptor mediating the effects of T3 on cholinergic neurons are identical to those of the hepatic nuclear receptor and of the receptors mediating the antigoiter activity *in vivo* (Jorgensen, 1978; Cheung, 1985). It therefore appears unlikely that analogues of T3 can be developed which selectively affect central cholinergic neurons without exhibiting the other characteristic properties of thyroid hormones.

Table 13.2   Relative potency of thyroxine analogues in stimulating ChAT activity of cholinergic neurons in culture

	relative potency
3,5-diiodo-3'-isopropyl-L-thyronine	1.6
3,5,3'-triiodo-L-thyronine (T3)	1
3,5,3'-triiodo-D-thyronine	0.76
3,5,3'-triiodo-thyropropionic acid	0.098
3,5,3'-triiodo-4'-hydrogen-DL-thyronine	0.031
3,3'-diisopropyl-5'-bromo-DL-thyronine	0.009
3,3'-dibromo-5'-isopropyl-L-thyronine	0.003
3,5-diiodo-L-thyronine	0.001
3-bromo-3',5'-diisopropyl-L-thyronine	<0.001
3-isopropyl-3',5'-dibromo-DL-thyronine	<0.001
3,3',5'-trimethyl-DL-thyronine	<0.001
sodium iodide	<0.001

ED_{50} values were obtained for all analogues. Relative potencies are based on the ED_{50} value determined for T3 (3.2 nM). Values shown are derived from two or three experiments per compound.

13.5 Gangliosides

Gangliosides are glycosphingolipids which are highly abundant in the CNS. The fact that they are differentially regulated during development is suggestive of an important role in CNS development and function (Ando, 1983). Several recent reports indicate that exogenously administered gangliosides might accelerate regeneration and sprouting of neuronal fibres in animals with experimentally induced lesions (Ceccarelli et al., 1976; Gorio et al., 1983; Toffano et al., 1983). Furthermore, exogenously administered gangliosides have been shown to accelerate the functional recovery of animals with lesions which produce behavioural deficits (Ceccarelli et al., 1976; Agnati et al., 1983; Karpiak, 1983). In support of these findings which were obtained in vivo, gangliosides have been reported to stimulate fibre formation of neuroblastoma cells in vitro (Morgan and Seifert, 1979; Byrne et al., 1983; Rybak et al., 1983). Given these findings, I decided to assess the effects of gangliosides on growth and morphology of forebrain cholinergic neurons in vitro. Furthermore, since it has been hypothesized that gangliosides potentiate the action of growth factor (Gorio et al., 1983), the influence of gangliosides on the NGF-mediated increase in ChAT activity was analysed.

Purified ganglioside mixtures were added to the culture medium and were present during the entire culture time. The gangliosides failed to affect survival of cholinergic neurons in these cultures, since cultures grown in the presence of gangliosides contained the same number of cholinergic neurons as control cultures (data not shown). Furthermore, the morphological appearance of cholinergic neurons grown in the presence of gangliosides did not differ from that of neurons grown in control dishes. However, cultures grown in the presence of gangliosides exhibited a higher activity of ChAT (measured biochemically) as compared to controls (Table 13.3). This effect became manifest after ten days in culture. The elevations mediated by NGF and gangliosides were not additive, suggesting that the level reached by NGF-treatment represents a maximal value or, alternatively, that the two treatments act at least in part through a common mechanism.

While gangliosides failed to affect the morphology of cholinergic neurons, these compounds produced prominent changes in the general morphological appearance of the cultures. In contrast to control cultures, which contained many process-bearing cells and a confluent layer of flat, non-neuronal cells, there were no flat cells in cultures grown in the presence of gangliosides (0.2–0.8 mg/ml medium). Using immunocytochemical visualisation of the astro-cytic marker glial fibrillary acid protein (GFAP), it was shown that all astrocytes in cultures grown in the presence of gangliosides exhibited the morphology of process-bearing cells, whereas in control cultures astrocytes represented the majority of the flat cells. Furthermore, gangliosides strongly reduced the pro-liferation of astrocytes. The lower number of astrocytes was reflected by a decrease in protein content of the cultures (Table 13.3). Astrocytic growth and morphology were affected by ganglioside mixtures of various sources and com-position and also by the pure gangliosides GM_1 and GD_{1a}, whereas lipid and carbohydrate components of gangliosides were ineffective. The findings obtained with gangliosides have been described in detail by Hefti et al. (1985b).

The findings indicate that gangliosides differentially affect glial and neuronal cells in cultures of dissociated septal cells. The transformation of flat astrocytes

Table 13.3 Effects of NGF and of gangliosides on ChAT activity in cultures of septal cells prepared from foetal rats

	Proteins (μg/dish)	ChAT Activity	
		(pmol/min/dish)	(pmol/min/μg prot.)
Controls	238 ± 6	4.7 ± 0.3	0.020 ± 0.001
Gangliosides	194 ± 10[1]	7.8 ± 0.6*	0.040 ± 0.001*
NGF	236 ± 9	11.5 ± 0.9*	0.049 ± 0.003*
NGF + gangliosides	213 ± 5[1]	10.9 ± 0.4*	0.051 ± 0.001*

m ± S.E.M.; n = 12
[1] The presence of gangliosides resulted in a slight but significant ($p < 0.01$) reduction in protein content of the cultures, reflecting the inhibitory effect of gangliosides on prolifer-ation of astrocytes.
*Significantly different from controls, $p < 0.01$ (analysis of variance).
Dissociated cells were grown in culture for ten days. NGF (0.5 μg 2.5S NGF/ml, purified from mouse salivary glands) and gangliosides (0.5 mg/ml of a ganglioside mixture containing 27 % GM_1, 40 % GD_{1a}, 16 % GD_{1b}, 17 % GT_{1b}, Fidia) were added to the medium and were present during the entire culture time.

into process-bearing cells was the most prominent change caused by the ganglio-sides, and the simulation of ChAT activity might be secondary to this effect on astrocytes. ChAT activity in septal cultures rises with increasing cell density (Hefti *et al.*, 1985a), suggesting a stimulatory effect of cell–cell interaction on the expression of this enzyme. The reduction of astrocyte number in ganglio-side-treated cultures favours neuron–neuron interactions, which could result in elevated ChAT activity.

13.6 Conclusions

Cultures of dissociated septal cells represent a suitable system for assessing the effects of various compounds and treatments on the survival and maintenance of function of central cholinergic neurons. Findings obtained so far indicate that the cholinergic neurons giving rise to the ascending cholinergic neurons of the basal forebrain are affected by NGF, thyroid hormones and gangliosides. NGF was found to elevate the expression of ChAT activity of cholinergic neurons in cultures prepared from foetal rat brains. In cultures prepared from newborn rats, NGF had a promoting effect on the survival of cholinergic neurons. Both these effects were specific for NGF and were not shared by other growth factors or control proteins. Thyroid hormones stimulated the expression of ChAT activity by cholinergic neurons by a mechanism apparently independent of that of NGF. The receptor mediating the effects of thyroid hormones on central cholinergic neurons seems to have the same structural requirements as the nuclear receptor for these hormones in hepatic cells and the receptors mediating their antigoiter activity. Addition of gangliosides to the culture medium resulted in a stimula-tion of ChAT activity by cholinergic neurons. This effect, however, might be secondary to a pronounced inhibitory effect of gangliosides on the proliferation of astrocytes in these cultures.

Acknowledgement

These studies were supported by the National Parkinson Foundation, Miami FL, USA.

References

Agnati, L. F., Fuxe, K., Calza, L., Benefanti, F., Cavicchioli, L., Toffano, G., and Goldstein, M. (1983). Gangliosides increase the survival of lesioned nigral dopamine neurons and favour the recovery of dopaminergic synaptic function in striatum of rats by collateral sprouting. *Acta Physiol Scand.*, 119, 347–63.
Ando, S. (1983). Gangliosides in the nervous system. *Neurochem. Int.*, 5, 507–37.
Bartus, R. T., Dean, R. L., Beer, B., and Lippa, A. S. (1982). The cholinergic hypothesis of geriatric memory dysfunction. *Science*, 217, 408–17.

Bradford, M. M. (1976). A rapid and sensitive method for the quantitation of microgram quantities of protein utilizing the principle of protein-dye binding. *Anal. Biochem.*, 72, 248–54.

Byrne, M. C., Ledeen, F. J., Roisen, F. J., York, G., and Scalafani, J. R. (1983). Ganglioside-induced neuritogenesis: verification that gangliosides are the active agents, and comparison of molecular species. *J. Neurochem.*, 41, 1214–22.

Ceccarelli, B., Aporti, F., and Finesso, M. (1976). Effects of brain gangliosides on functional recovery in experimental regeneration and reinnervation. *Adv. Exp. Med. Biol.*, 71, 275–93.

Cheung, E. N. (1985). Thyroid hormone action: determination of hormone-receptor interaction using structural analogs and molecular modeling. *Trends Pharmacol. Sci.*, Jan. 1985, 31–4.

Coyle, J. T., Price, D. L., and DeLong, M. R. (1983). Alzheimer's disease: a disease of cortical cholinergic innervation. *Science*, 219, 1184–9.

Crutcher, K. A. (1982). Development of the rat septohippocampal projection: a retrograde fluorescent tracer study. *Dev. Brain Res.*, 3, 145–50.

Crutcher, K. A., and Collins, F. (1982). *In vitro* evidence for two distinct hippocampal growth factors: basis of neuronal plasticity? *Science*, 217, 67–70.

Crutcher, K. A., and Davis, J. N. (1981). Sympathetic noradrenergic sprouting in response to central cholinergic denervations. *Trends Neurosci.*, 4, 70–2.

Crutcher, K. A., Brothers, L., and Davis, J. N. (1979). Sprouting of sympathetic nerves in the absence of afferent input. *Exp. Neurol.*, 66, 778–83.

Davies, P. (1985). Is it possible to design rational treatment for the symptoms of Alzheimer's disease? *Drug Develop Res.*, 5, 69–75.

Fonnum, F. (1975). A rapid radiochemical method for the determination of choline acetyltransferase. *J. Neurochem.*, 24, 407–9.

Gnahn, H., Hefti, F., Heumann, R., Schwab, M., and Thoenen, H. (1983). NGF-mediated increase of choline acetyltransferase (ChAT) in the neonatal forebrain; evidence for a physiological role of NGF in the brain? *Dev. Brain Res.*, 9, 45–52.

Gorio, A., Marini, P., and Zanoni, R. (1983). Muscle reinnervation. III. Motoneuron sprouting capacity, enhancement by exogenous gangliosides. *Neuroscience*, 8, 417–29.

Grave, G. D. (1977). *Thyroid Hormones and Brain Development*, Raven Press, New York.

Greene, L. A., and Shooter, E. M. (1980). The nerve growth factor: biochemistry, synthesis and mechanism of action. *Ann. Rev. Neurosci.*, 3, 353–402.

Hefti, F. (1983). Alzheimer's disease caused by a lack of nerve growth factor? *Ann. Neurol.*, 13, 109–10.

Hefti, F. Dravid, A., and Hartikka, J. (1984). Chronic intraventricular injections of nerve growth factor elevate hippocampal choline acetyltransferase activity in adult rats with partial septo-hippocampal lesions. *Brain Res.*, 293, 305–9.

Hefti, F., Hartikka, J., and Frick, W. (1985b). Gangliosides alter morphology and growth of astrocytes and increase the activity of choline acetyltransferase in cultures of dissociated septal neurons. *J. Neurosci.*, 5, 2086–94.

Hefti, F., Hartikka, J., Eckenstein, F., Gnahn, H., Heumann, R., and Schwab, M. (1985a). Nerve growth factor (NGF) increases choline acetyltransferase but not survival or fiber growth of cultured septal cholinergic neurons. *Neuroscience*, 14, 55–68.

Honegger, P. and Lenoir, D. (1980a). Nerve growth factor (NGF) stimulation of cholinergic telencephalic neurons in aggregating cell cultures. *Dev. Brain. Res.*, 3, 229–38.

Honegger, P., and Lenoir, D. (1980b). Triiodothyronine enhancement of neuronal differentiation in aggregating fetal rat brain cells cultured in a chemically defined medium. *Brain Res.*, 199, 425–34.

Jorgensen, E. C. (1978). In Li, C. H. (ed.), *Hormonal Proteins and Peptides*, Vol. 6. Academic Press, New York, pp. 108–204.

Kalaria, R. N., and Prince, A. K. (1985). The effects of neonatal thyroid deficiency on acetylcholine synthesis and glucose oxidation in rat corpus striatum. *Dev. Brain Res.*, 20, 271–9.

Karpiak, S. E. (1983). Ganglioside treatment improves recovery of alteration behavior after unilateral entorhinal cortex lesion. *Exp. Neurol.*, 81, 330–9.

Kiernan, J. A. (1979). Hypotheses concerned with axonal regeneration in the mammalian nervous system. *Biol. Rev.*, 54, 155–97.

Kojima, M., Kim, J. S., Uchimurea, H., Hirano, M., Nakahara, T., and Matsumoto, T. (1981). Effect of thyroidectomy on choline acetyltransferase in rat hypothalamic nuclei. *Brain Res.*, **209**, 227–30.

Loy, R., and Moore, R. Y. (1977). Anomalous innervation of the hippocampal formation by peripheral sympathetic axons following mechanical injury. *Exp. Neurol.*, **57**, 645–50.

Mesulam, M. M., Mufson, E. J., Wainer, B. H., and Levey, A. I. (1983). Central cholinergic pathways in the rat: an overview based on an alternative nomenclature (Ch. 1–Ch. 6). *Neuroscience*, **10**, 1185–201.

Milner, T. A., Loy, R., and Amaral, D. G. (1983). An anatomical study of the development of the septo-hippocampal projection in the rat. *Dev. Brain Res.*, **8**, 343–71.

Morgan, J. I., and Seifert, W. (1979). Growth factors and gangliosides: a possible new perspective in neuronal growth control. *J. Supramolec. Struc.*, **10**, 111–24.

Nadler, J. V., Mattews, D. A., Cotman, C. W., and Lynch, G. S. (1974). Development of cholinergic innervation in the hippocampal formation of the rat. *Dev. Biol.*, **36**, 142–54.

Rybak, S., Ginzburg, I., and Yavin, E. (1983). Gangliosides stimulate neurite outgrowth and induce tubulin mRNA accumulation in neural cells. *Biochem. Biophys. Res. Commun.*, **116**, 974–80.

Schwab, M., Otten, U., Agid, Y., and Thoenen, H. (1979). Nerve growth factor (NGF) in the rat CNS: absence of specific retrograde axonal transport and tyrosine hydroxylase induction in locus coeruleus and substantia nigra. *Brain Res.*, **168**, 473–83.

Seiler, M., and Schwab, M. E. (1984). Specific retrograde transport of nerve growth factor (NGF) from neocortex to nucleus basalis in the rat. *Brain Res.*, **300**, 33–6.

Shelton, D. L., and Reichardt, L. F. (1984). Expression of the nerve growth factor gene correlates with the density of sympathetic innervation in effector organs. *Proc. Natl Acad. Sci. USA*, **81**, 7951–5.

Stenevi, U., and Bjorklund, A. (1978). Growth of vascular sympathetic axons into the hippocampus after lesions of the septo-hippocampal pathway; a pitfall in brain lesion studies. *Neurosci. Lett.*, **7**, 219–24.

Suda, K., Barde, Y. A., and Thoenen, H. (1978). Nerve growth factor in mouse and rat serum: correlation between bioassay and radioimmunoassay determinations. *Proc. Natl Acad. Sci. USA*, **75**, 4042–6.

Thoenen, H., and Barde, Y. A. (1980). Physiology of nerve growth factor. *Physiol. Rev.*, **60**, 1284–335.

Toffano, G., Savoini, G., Moroni, G., Lombardi, G., Calza, L., and Agnati, L. F. (1983). GM_1 ganglioside treatment reduces dopamine cell body degeneration in the substantia nigra after unilateral hemitranssection in rat. *Brain Res.*, **296**, 233–9.

Toniolo, G., Dunnett, S. B., Hefti, F., and Will, B. (1985). Acetylcholine-rich transplants in the hippocampus: influence of intrinsic growth factors and application of NGF on choline acetyltransferase activity. *Brain Res.*, **345**, 141–6.

Valcana, T. (1971). Effect of neonatal hypothyroidism on the development of acetylcholinesterase and choline acetyl transferase activity in rat brain. In Ford, D. H. (ed.), *Influence of Hormones on the Nervous System.* S. Karger, Basel, pp. 174–84.

Wainer, B. H., Levey, A. I., Mufson, E. F., and Mesulam, M. M. (1984). Cholinergic systems in mammalian brain identified with antibodies against choline acetyltransferase. *Neurosci. Int.*, **6**, 163–82.

14

Dissociated Monolayer Cultures of Human Spinal Cord

A. C. Kato, L. Erkman and G. Touzeau

14.1 Introduction

Recently, we began an investigation on the aetiology of amyotrophic lateral sclerosis (ALS) using neuronal cultures as a tool. Our initial study was done on 'motoneuron-like' cells, the ciliary ganglion neurons from the chick embryo (Touzeau and Kato, 1983). Since ALS is a human disease principally affecting spinal motoneurons, it seemed appropriate to develop a culture system for human spinal cord neurons. This paper reports some of the morphological, biochemical and electrophysiological characteristics of these cultures.

The culture of neurons from human brain and peripheral nervous tissue has been described by several groups using either explants (Murray and Stout, 1947; Crain et al., 1980; Baron-Van Evercooren et al., 1982) or dissociated cell cultures (Kim et al., 1979; Kennedy et al., 1980; Baron-Van Evercooren et al., 1982; Zeevalk et al., 1982; Louis et al., 1983; Dickson et al., 1984). As far as human spinal cord is concerned, other workers have not been successful in culturing neurons from dissociated spinal cord using embryonic tissue from the 15th to the 21st week (Kennedy et al., 1980). Their cultures contained astrocytes, oligodendrocytes, fibroblasts and macrophages, but none of the cells were positive for tetanus toxin binding (a marker for neurons). The authors state that the central nervous system neurons are probably extremely sensitive to anoxia and consequently do not survive. We believe that the age of the embryos is critical, since few neurons from foetuses older than 9 weeks survived in culture; after 11 weeks of age, we could not identify any neuronal cells. Therefore, the majority of our experiments were done using spinal cords from 8- to 9-week-old embryos; foetuses younger than 8 weeks were difficult to stage and the small quantity of tissue was limiting for a biochemical study.

Using cell-type specific markers, it was possible to identify both neurons and glial cells in the culture; tetanus toxin binding and antibodies to neurofilament protein were used to label the neurons, whereas antibodies to glial fibrillary acidic protein (GFAP) were used to identify astrocytes.

Since we intend to use these cultures as a model system for the study of ALS, it was important to show that cholinergic neurons survive and develop under these culture conditions (Kato *et al.*, 1985). We have examined the effect of serum from ALS patients on these cultures (Touzeau and Kato, 1986) and we have begun to purify motoneurons on Percoll gradients.

14.2 Results and Discussion

14.2.1 General Characteristics of the Culture

Figure 14.1 (A) shows a photograph of human spinal cord cells 13 days in culture as viewed with Nomarski optics. Processes are seen to extend from the neuronal cell bodies and appear to grow on top of the non-neuronal cells. In the presence alone of collagen as a substrate, rather than collagen plus polyornithine, the cells form small aggregates with networks of neurites between the cell masses.

Figure 14.1 (B) shows a similar culture but in this case the cells were labelled with a monoclonal antibody for neurofilament protein. This antiserum labelled all cells that would have been classified as neurons by phase-contrast optics.

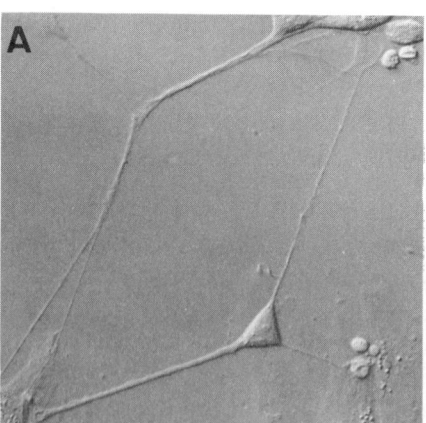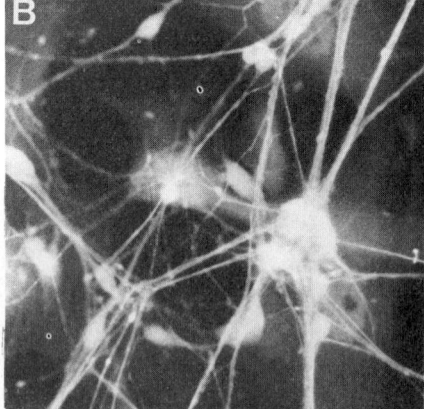

Fig. 14.1 (A) Photograph of human spinal cord cells in culture for 13 days taken with Nomarski optics. (B) Immunofluorescence staining of neurofilament protein in cells cultured for 21 days.

None of the non-neuronal cells were labelled with this antiserum apart from a nuclear binding which is characteristic of this antibody.

In order to test that the cells morphologically identified as neurons had the electrophysiological properties of neurons, recordings were made with patch electrodes using the whole-cell recording method (Hamill *et al.*, 1981; Bader *et al.*, 1983). Figure 14.2 is a current clamp recording showing the effect of

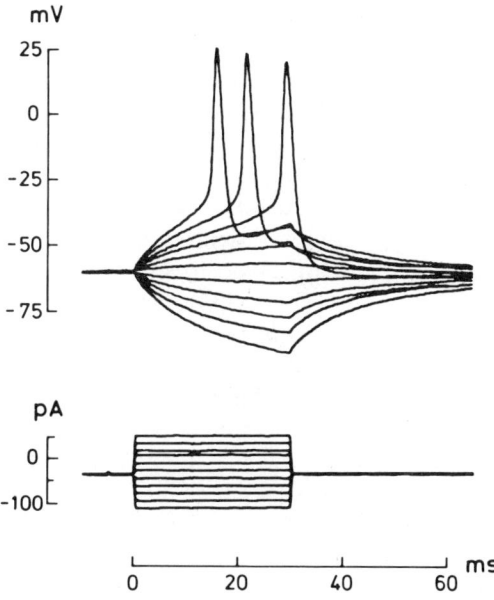

Fig. 14.2 Action potentials in a human spinal cord neuron. The neuron was 20 days in culture. Superfusion was with control medium. The solution in the patch electrode contained (in mM): potassium acetate (130); KCl (20); Hepes (5); glucose (5); and EGTA (5; pH 7.3); the pH was 7.05. The membrane resting potential was −46 mV. The cell was held at −59 mV by injecting a constant hyperpolarising current of 36 pA. Hyperpolarising and depolarising current steps were applied (bottom trace) and the corresponding voltage responses were recorded (upper traces).

constant current injection on the membrane potential of a human spinal cord neuron. The membrane currents in these neurons were studied in voltage clamp experiments. Three types of voltage-dependent currents were observed: a sodium current; a potassium current made up of two components, I_A and I_K; and a calcium current.

14.2.2 Evidence for Cholinergic Neurons

Since our primary interest is to study motor neuron disease (amyotrophic lateral sclerosis), it was important to demonstrate that putative motoneurons existed in the cultures. Since these are cholinergic neurons, we used as markers the enzyme choline acetyltransferase (ChAT) and the synthesis and accumulation of acetylcholine (ACh) using extracellular (^{3}H)choline as a precursor.

The levels of ChAT in spinal cord cells cultured for 7 to 13 days was 65 pmoles of (^{3}H)ACh synthesised per 100,000 cells plated per hour. Bromoacetylcholine, which is a specific inhibitor of ChAT, blocked the enzymatic activity by 82 %. This level of ChAT activity is similar to that found in spinal cord cultures of chick (Berg and Fischbach, 1978) and rat (Smith and Appel, 1983) embryos.

The kinetics of (^{3}H)ACh synthesis, using (^{3}H)choline as a precursor, were analysed in order to determine optimal conditions for the time of incorporation of the precursor and also the concentration of the precursor in the culture medium. As shown in Fig. 14.3(A) and (B), the synthesis and accumulation of (^{3}H)ACh reached a plateau at approximately 100 min and at a choline concentration of 100 to 200 μM. Therefore, in subsequent experiments, an incorporation time of 60 min and a choline concentration of 100 μM were chosen as standard conditions for (^{3}H)ACh synthesis. These results agree favourably with those reported by Berg (1978) for dissociated cultures of chick spinal cord cells.

The number of spinal cord cells plated varied from one experiment to the next. Consequently, we determined whether (^{3}H)ACh synthesis in spinal cord cells was directly proportional to the number of cells initially plated. Figure 14.4 illustrates an experiment using cells cultured at various densities for 19 days. Over the range of 10^5 to 4×10^5 cells plated per 16 mm well, the rate of synthesis increased linearly from 0.4 to 2.5 pmoles of (^{3}H)ACh per dish per hour.

Cultured neurons obtained from embryonic material usually show some degree of development in culture. In particular, spinal cord cells from chick embryos showed an increase in their ability to synthesise and store (^{3}H)ACh (Berg, 1978). We determined whether this cholinergic index would also increase in human spinal cord cells. Figure 14.4(B) shows that the production of (^{3}H)ACh increased 1.4-fold between 3 and 15 days in culture. This development of the cholinergic cells appears to be slower than reported for chick spinal cord cultures (Berg, 1978), where there was, approximately, a 4-fold increase in (^{3}H)ACh synthesis over the same time period.

The synthesis of (^{3}H)ACh was compared in cultures prepared from the anterior and posterior parts of the spinal cord from an eight-week old embryo. After one week in culture, there was already more ACh synthesised in the anterior part; it is possible that the observed increase in ACh synthesis is due to an enrichment of the cholinergic motoneurons which are situated in the anterior part of the cord.

14.2.3 Other Neurotransmitters

It has been well-established that GABAergic neurons exist in the spinal cord of both embryonic and adult tissue. Examination of autoradiographs of (^{3}H)GABA uptake suggests that approximately 60 % of the neurons are labelled by

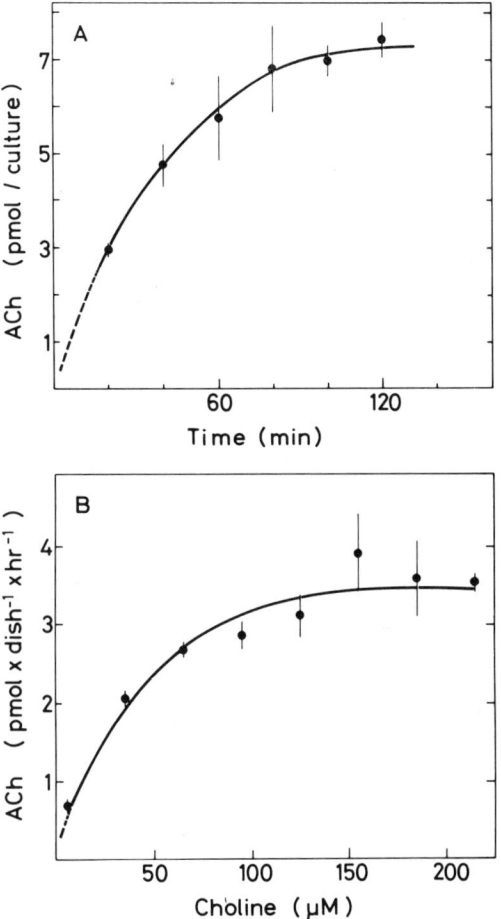

Fig. 14.3 (^{3}H)ACh synthesis as a function of time and choline concentration. (A) Human spinal cord cells were cultured for 12 days and then incubated for various times in the presence of 100 μM (^{3}H)choline (0.33 Ci/mmole) in a medium that contained 5.4 mM KCl. The cell extracts were analysed for (^{3}H)ACh formation, and the specific activity of the (^{3}H)choline was used to calculate the amount of product present. All values for ACh are expressed on a per culture basis. (B) Human spinal cord cells cultured for 14 days were incubated for 1 h in the presence of varying concentrations of (^{3}H)choline in 5.4 mM KCl. The cell extracts were analysed for (^{3}H)ACh formation. Each point represents the mean of three sister cultures, and the bars in the figure indicate the S.E.M.

(^{3}H)GABA. There are no noradrenergic neurons in the cultures, as there was no uptake of (^{3}H)Norepinephrine (NE), nor any synthesis of (^{3}H)NE using (^{3}H)tyrosine as a precursor. Also, neurons with enkephalin and somatostatin have been identified in these cultures by Y. Charnay (Lyon, France).

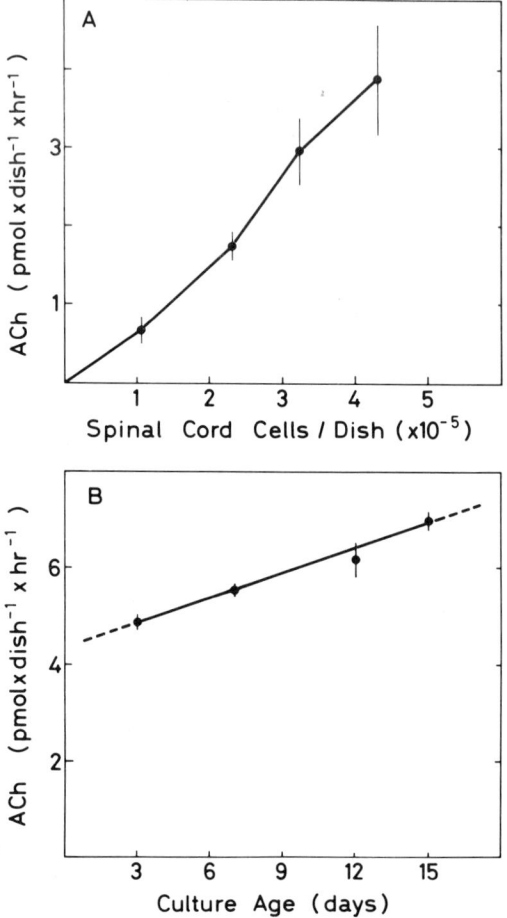

Fig. 14.4 (³H)ACh synthesis as a function (A) of the number of spinal cord neurons plated; and (B) of time in culture.

14.2.4 Effect of Serum from Controls and ALS Individuals

Since the human spinal cord cells grow in the presence of a standard tissue culture medium which contains 13 % decomplemented human serum, we decided to examine the effects of ALS sera on the cultures (Touzeau and Kato, 1986). Biochemical measurements were used to assess the viability of the cells: ChAT activity was used as a measure of health of the cholinergic neurons; GAD as an index of the GABAergic neurons in the culture, and lactate dehydrogenase as a measure of the overall growth of the cultures. All three enzymes could be measured in each culture well.

The cells were grown for 20 to 24 days in the presence of serum from control, ALS and neurological control individuals. At the end of this period, the cells were scraped and analysed for the three enzymatic activities. On the basis of these biochemical measurements, there was no detectable difference between the effects of the three types of sera on the cultures.

14.2.5 Percoll Gradients of Quail Spinal Cord Cells

Since the human spinal cord preparation is composed of a heterogeneous population of cells, there are probably trophic factors secreted by the non-neuronal cells which can affect the neurite-outgrowth and the survival of the neurons. This could be an explanation for the negative findings reported here. Therefore, we have begun a series of experiments to purify and culture the motoneuron population. We have initiated our studies using quail embryonic spinal cord cells.
As shown in Fig. 14.5, the cells separated into two main peaks of LDH activity. Peak I ($d = 1.0335$) contains 65 % of the total ChAT activity, whereas peak II

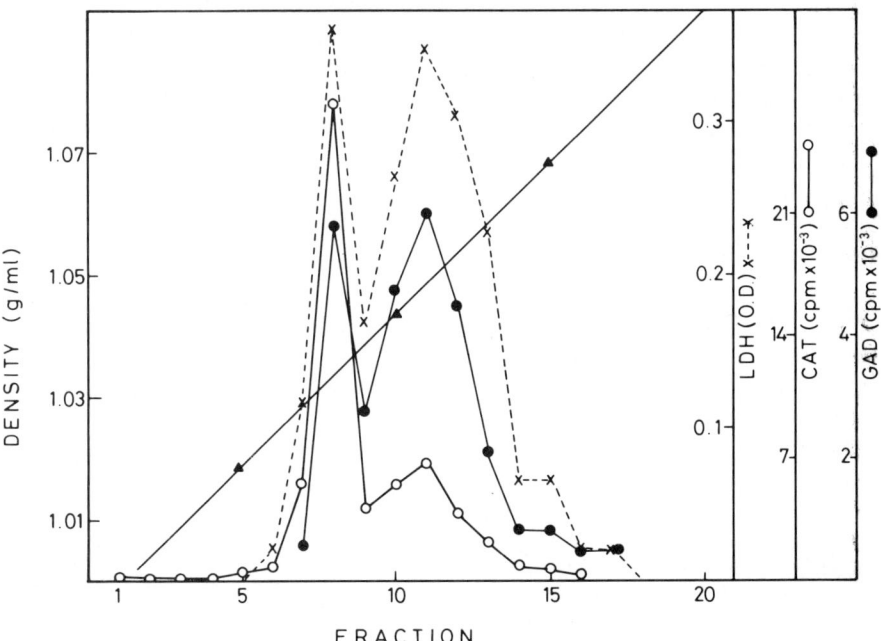

Fig. 14.5 Sedimentation profile of LDH (x - - x), GAD (●—●) and ChAT (○—○) activities from dissociated quail spinal cord cells centrifuged on a 0–60 % Percoll gradient. A cell suspension (500 μl) of dissociated spinal cord cells (3 × 10⁶) from eight-day quail embryos was applied to a 6 ml linear Percoll gradient (0–60 % in MEM). After centrifugation for 15 min at 4000 rev/min (Sorvall HB 4), 20 fractions were collected and analysed for the three enzymatic activities. The straight line shows the density of each fraction in g/ml.

(d = 1.0485) contains only 35 %. In contrast, only 29 % of the total GAD activity was found in peak I and 71 % in peak II. Therefore, peak I is enriched in cholinergic cells, with little contamination by GABAergic neurons. The density of this peak corresponds to that described for chick spinal cord neurons (Schnaar and Schaffner, 1981). Similar experiments are underway using human spinal cord cells.

Conclusion

The study of neurological diseases affecting the human brain and spinal cord is complicated by the inability to do experiments directly on the neural tissue. Therefore, important questions about the possible role of toxic substances or a defect in trophic factors in neurological diseases cannot be addressed in a simple manner. An *in vitro* preparation composed of human tissue may be a useful tool for the characterization of the conditions necessary for neuronal survival, the testing of pathological material, and the study of pharmacological agents.

A suitable system for the achievement these goals is the dissociated monolayer culture of neural tissue. Although the cellular organization in this preparation differs from the *in vivo* situation, it permits the best possible control of the extracellular environment. In this study, we show that dissociated spinal cord cells from 8- to 9-week-old human embryos can survive for up to 7 weeks in monolayer cultures and we are using these cultures as a model system to study Amyotrophic Lateral Sclerosis.

Acknowledgements

We are most grateful to C. R. Bader and D. Bertrand for the electrophysiological experiments. We thank F. Steimer and F. Pillonel for their excellent technical assistance. This work was supported by grants from the Amyotrophic Lateral Sclerosis Society of America (ALSSOA, USA), the NIH (USA: No. NS21652-02), the Fondation de Reuter (Geneva) and the Swiss National Science Foundation (3.582-0.84).

References

Bader, C. R., Bertrand, D., Dupin, E., and Kato, A. C. (1983). Development of electrical membrane properties in cultured avian neural crest. *Nature*, 305, 808–10.
Baron-Van Evercooren, A., Kleinman, H. K., Ohno, S., Marangos, P., Schwartz, J. P., and Dubois-Dalcq, M. E. (1982). Nerve growth in human factor, Laminin and Fibronectin promote neurite growth in human fetal sensory ganglia cultures. *J. Neurosci. Res.*, 8, 179–93.
Berg, D. K. (1978). Acetylcholine synthesis by chick spinal cord neurons in dissociated cell culture. *Dev. Biol.*, 66, 500–12.

Berg, D. K., and Fischbach, G. D. (1978). Enrichment of spinal cord cell cultures with motoneurons. *J. Cell Biol.*, 77, 83–98.

Crain, S. M., Peterson, E. R., Leibman, M., and Schulman, H. (1980). Dependence of nerve growth factor of early human fetal dorsal root ganglion neurons in organotypic cultures. *Exp. Neurol.*, 67, 205–14.

Dickson, J. G., Flanigan, T. P., and Walsh, F. S. (1984). Antigen expression in human neuronal primary cell cultures and human x mouse neuronal cell hybrids. In Rose, F. C. (ed.), *Research Progress in Motor Neurone Disease*. Pitman Press, Bath, pp. 388–404.

Hamill, O. P., Marty, A., Neher, E., Sakmann, B., and Sigworth, F. J. (1981). Improved patch clamp techniques for high resolution current recording from cells and cell-free membrane patches. *Pfluegers Arch.*, 391, 85–100.

Kato, A. C., Touzeau, G., Bertrand, D., and Bader, C. R. (1985). Human spinal cord neurons in dissociated monolayer cultures: Morphological, biochemical and electrophysiological properties. *J. Neurosci.*, 5, 2750–61.

Kennedy, P. G. E., Lisak, R. P., and Raff, M. C. (1980). Cell type-specific markers for human glial and neuronal cells in culture. *Lab. Invest.*, 43, 342–51.

Kim, S. U., Warren, K. G., and Kalia, M. (1979). Tissue culture of adult human neurons. *Neurosci. Lett.*, 11, 137–41.

Louis, J. C., Langley, K., Anglard, P., Wolf, M., and Vincendon, G. (1983). Long-term culture of neurons from human cerebral cortex in serum-free medium. *Neurosci. Lett.*, 41, 313–19.

Murray, M. R., and Stout, A. P. (1947). Adult human sympathetic ganglion cells cultivated in vitro. *Am. J. Anat.*, 80, 225–50.

Schnaar, R. L., and Schaffner, A. E. (1981). Separation of cell types from embryonic chicken and rat spinal cord: Characterization of motoneuron-enriched fractions. *J. Neurosci.*, 1, 204–17.

Smith, R. G., and Appel, S. H. (1983). Extracts of skeletal muscle increase neurite outgrowth and cholinergic activity of fetal rat spinal motor neurons. *Science*, 219, 1079–81.

Touzeau, G., and Kato, A. C. (1983). Effects of amyotrophic lateral sclerosis sera on cultured cholinergic neurons. *Neurol.*, 33, 317–22.

Touzeau, G., and Kato, A. C. (1986). ALS sera have no effect on three enzymatic activities in cultured human spinal cord neurons. *Neurol.*, 36, 573–6

Zeevalk, G. D., Cederqvist, L. L., and Lyser, K. M. (1982). The ultrastructure of human fetal sympathetic ganglion cells in serum free medium. *Dev. Brain Res.*, 4, 248–52.

15

A Glycoprotein from Muscle-conditioned Medium Involved in the Differentiation of Rat Cholinergic Neurons in Culture: Partial Purification and Regulation of Neurotransmitter Metabolism Enzymes in Central-Nervous-System Cultures

M. C. Giess, J. C. Martinou, B. Raynaud, C. Delteil, A. Le Van Thai, S. Vidal and M. Weber

15.1 Introduction

The identification, purification and study of the mode of action of macro-molecular factors responsible for the survival, neurite outgrowth and differentiation of neurons in culture is nowadays a field of intense research (for a review, see Berg, 1985). Cell culture systems can indeed constitute valuable biological assays for the identification of neuronotrophic factors in various biological fluids or tissue homogenates. Except for nerve growth factor (NGF), the role played by these factors during *in vivo* development or ageing is still unknown, but they are good candidates for the mediation of retrograde trophic interactions between defined groups of neurons and their field of innervation. A defect in such retrograde factors may be involved in certain degenerative neurological diseases, such as motor neuron disease or Alzheimer's disease (see Chapters 13, 14 and 16).

We have for several years been studying a glycoprotein which is released in culture by a variety of rat non-neuronal cells, and which is involved in the differentiation of cholinergic neurons in cultures prepared both from the PNS and the CNS of immature rats (Patterson and Chun, 1977a,b; Weber, 1981). In this article, we first briefly review our present knowledge on the action of this factor on cultures of new-born rat sympathetic and sensory ganglia and present recent data on its action on rat embryo CNS cultures.

15.2 Materials and Methods

15.2.1 Sympathetic and Sensory Neuron Cultures

The superior cervical and nodose ganglia from new-born rat were dissociated into single cells by a treatment with Dispase (2 %) at 37 °C and cultured on a collagen film in an L15 medium containing 5 % adult rat serum. The medium used for sympathetic neurons also contained 1 μg/ml 7S-nerve growth factor (Swerts et al., 1983; Mathieu et al., 1984). The cultures were treated between days 0 and 6 with 10 μM cytosine arabinoside to prevent the proliferation of ganglionic non-neuronal cells.

15.2.2 CNS Cultures

The CNS of E14 rat embryos was divided into three parts corresponding to the spinal cord, the hindbrain (minus cerebellum) and the mid- and forebrain. After mechanical dissociation, the cells were cultured in a modified L15 medium containing 5 % each foetal calf serum and horse serum (Giess and Weber, 1984) in plastic trays treated with poly-L-lysine, at an initial cell density of 2×10^5 cells/dish.

The medial septum region, the olfactory lobes and the hippocampus were dissected from E17–E19 rat embryos and cultured as above.

15.2.3 Enzymatic Assays

The cultures were scraped from the culture dish with a rubber policeman and homogenised in 0.1 ml 0.2 M NaCl, 0.2 % Triton X-100. After a brief centrifugation in a top bench centrifuge, the supernatant was used for enzymatic assays. Choline acetyltransferase and acetylcholinesterase activities were measured by the methods of Fonnum (1975) and Ellman et al. (1961), respectively. Dopa decarboxylase activity was measured by the method of Lamprecht and Coyle (1972). Glutamate decarboxylase activity was measured as described by Kato et al. (see Chapter 14). Protein was measured by the method of Lowry et al. (1951), or of Wallace and Partlow (1978) for non-collagen protein.

15.3 Results and Discussion

15.3.1 Characterization and Partial Purification of a Cholinergic Differentiation Factor

Sympathetic neurons from new-born rats acquire many characteristics of mature noradrenergic neurons when cultured in the absence of non-neuronal cells. A marginal, but significant, increase in choline acetyltransferase (ChAT) activity is also observed in such cultures. However, ChAT activity develops at a 20- to 100-fold higher rate in sister cultures grown in the presence of muscle- or heart-conditioned medium (CM). Simultaneously, some noradrenergic characters of the neurons, including the levels of activity of norepinephrine synthesising enzymes, are depressed. On the other hand, CM has no effect on neuronal survival and growth in these cultures (Patterson and Chun, 1977a,b; Landis; 1976, 1980; Swerts *et al.*, 1983, 1984).

The biological activity of the cholinergic differentiation factor from muscle-CM can thus be measured by the stimulation of ChAT activity in sympathetic neuron cultures grown in the presence of the factor between days 2 and 12. Using this, or similar assays, the cholinergic factor has been purified several thousand-fold from heart- or muscle-CM containing 10 % foetal calf serum (Weber, 1981; Weber and Le Van Thai, 1982), as indicated in Table 15.1. Recently, Fukada (1985) has purified the factor from serum-free CM to homogeneity by using four steps from Table 15.1 followed by SDS-gel electrophoresis. We have determined its sedimentation coefficient (2.1 S) and partial specific volume ($\bar{v} = 0.68$ ml/g) on sucrose gradients made in H_2O and D_2O according to Martin and Ames (1961). Its Stockes' radius, determined on molecular sieving columns, is identical to that of ovalbumin (27.6 Å) (Weber, 1981; Weber *et al.*, 1985; Fukada, 1985). Once these three parameters were known, the molecular weight was calculated according to Siegel and Monty (1966). The calculated value is 21.000 daltons (Weber *et al.*, 1985). The discrepancy between the calculated value and the *apparent* molecular weight determined on Sephadex columns (Weber, 1981; Fukada, 1985) results from the slightly elongated shape ($f/f_o = 1.6$) of the molecule (Weber *et al.*, 1985). About half of the mass of the factor is composed of carbohydrates (Fukada, 1985).

15.3.2 Regulation of Neurotransmitter Metabolism Enzymes in Cultured Sympathetic Neurons

Swerts *et al.* (1983, 1984) have carried out an extensive comparison of neurotransmitter metabolism enzymes in sister sympathetic neurons grown with and without CM (or purified cholinergic factor). As expected from earlier data (Patterson and Chun, 1977a), the factor has no influence on neuronal survival and overall growth as measured by cell countings and determinations of lactate dehydrogenase activity. As expected, the factor stimulates ChAT activity in a

Table 15.1   Flow-chart for the partial purification of the cholinergic factor

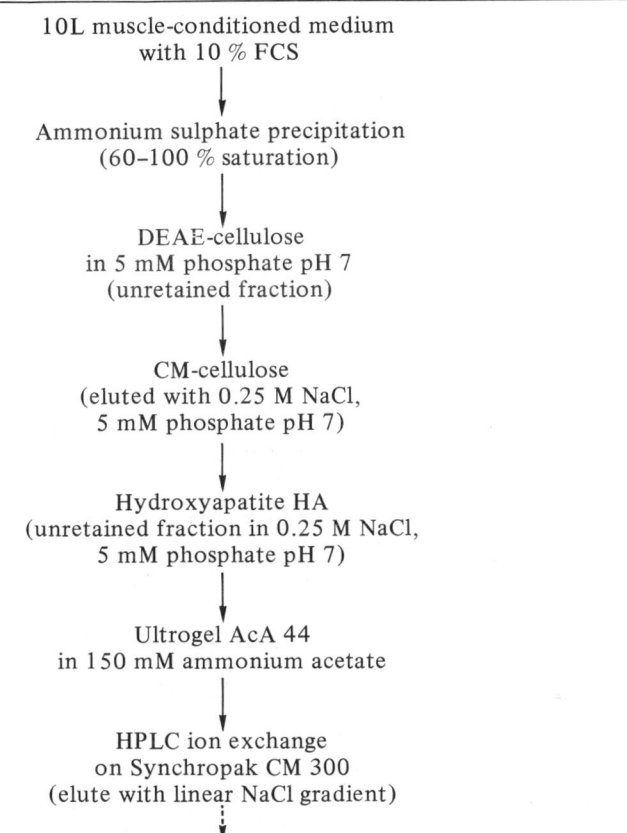

10L muscle-conditioned medium
with 10 % FCS

↓

Ammonium sulphate precipitation
(60–100 % saturation)

↓

DEAE-cellulose
in 5 mM phosphate pH 7
(unretained fraction)

↓

CM-cellulose
(eluted with 0.25 M NaCl,
5 mM phosphate pH 7)

↓

Hydroxyapatite HA
(unretained fraction in 0.25 M NaCl,
5 mM phosphate pH 7)

↓

Ultrogel AcA 44
in 150 mM ammonium acetate

↓

HPLC ion exchange
on Synchropak CM 300
(elute with linear NaCl gradient)

↓

Primary to tertiary cultures from new-born rat skeletal muscle were grown in L15 medium containing 10 % foetal calf serum. Conditioned medium was collected from dense cultures after a 24 h contact.

dose-dependent manner but, surprisingly enough, it decreases AChE levels in sympathetic neuron cultures. In particular, the development of the asymmetric A_{12} form of AChE is blocked in cultures grown with the factor (Swerts *et al.*, 1984). As far as catecholamine metabolism is concerned, the factor impairs the development of three enzymes in the norepinephrine synthesis pathway: tyrosine hydroxylase (TOH), dopa decarboxylase (DDC) and dopamine-β-hydroxylase. The deficit in TOH activity in cultures grown in CM correlates with a decrease in immunotitrable enzyme molecules, whereas the kinetic parameters of the enzyme, including the apparent K_{m}s for tyrosine and for the cofactor tetra-hydrobiopterine, are identical in homogenates from cultures grown with and without CM (Swerts *et al.*, 1983). This suggests that the effect of CM does not involve a covalent modification, e.g. phosphorylation of TOH. Recently, the deficit in TOH activity in cultures grown with the purified factor has been correlated with a deficit in TOH mRNA level, as measured by Northern blot analysis with a rat TOH cDNA clone (Raynaud *et al.*, unpublished data). It is still not known if the factor decreases the rate of synthesis, or processing, of TOH mRNA or increases its rate of degradation. Cultured sympathetic neurons certainly constitute an interesting model system for the study of the regulation of neurotransmitter-related genes.

15.3.3 *Regulation of Neurotransmitter Metabolism Enzymes in Cultured Primary Sensory Neurons*

Primary sensory neurons from the nodose ganglia do not arise from the neural crest, but from epibranchial placodes. A variety of neurotransmitters/neuromodulators have been identified in this ganglia, but there is no clear-cut evidence for the existence of cholinergic neurons. When placed in cultures, these neurons nevertheless form cholinergic synapses among themselves with high frequency (Baccaglini and Cooper, 1982; Cooper, 1984). It was thus of interest to investigate if they were target cells for the cholinergic factor. Mathieu *et al.* (1984) have indeed demonstrated that the purified cholinergic factor increased ChAT activity by 4–5 fold in nodose neuron cultures. As found with cultured sympathetic neurons, this increase in ChAT activity is accompanied by a decrease in AChE activity. On the other hand, the factor has no effect on neuron survival and lactate dehydrogenase activity in the cultures. It is not known if neurotransmitter phenotypic transitions also occur in these neurons, but it is interesting to note that a small percentage of nodose neurons *in vivo* express immunoreactive TOH, both in embryonic and adult rats (Katz *et al.*, 1983).

15.3.4 *Effects of Muscle-conditioned Medium on Cultures from E14 Rat Embryo CNS*

Early studies of Giller *et al.* (1973, 1977) demonstrated that co-cultured muscle cells increased ChAT activity in mouse embryo spinal cord cultures. This stimulation was reproduced by muscle-CM, suggesting that the effect of muscle CM was mediated by diffusible factor(s). On the other hand, chick muscle-CM has no effect on ChAT activity in chick embryo spinal cord cultures (Berg, 1978). We thus wondered if: (a) such muscle–nerve interaction took place in the case of rat embryo cultures; and (b) if the cholinergic factor we had purified on the basis of its activity on rat sympathetic neurons could also stimulate ChAT activity in rat spinal cord cultures.

As shown in Fig. 15.1, muscle-CM stimulated ChAT activity in cultures prepared from E14 rat embryo spinal cord and hindbrain (minus cerebellum). In cultures from fore- and midbrain, a highly significant stimulation was also

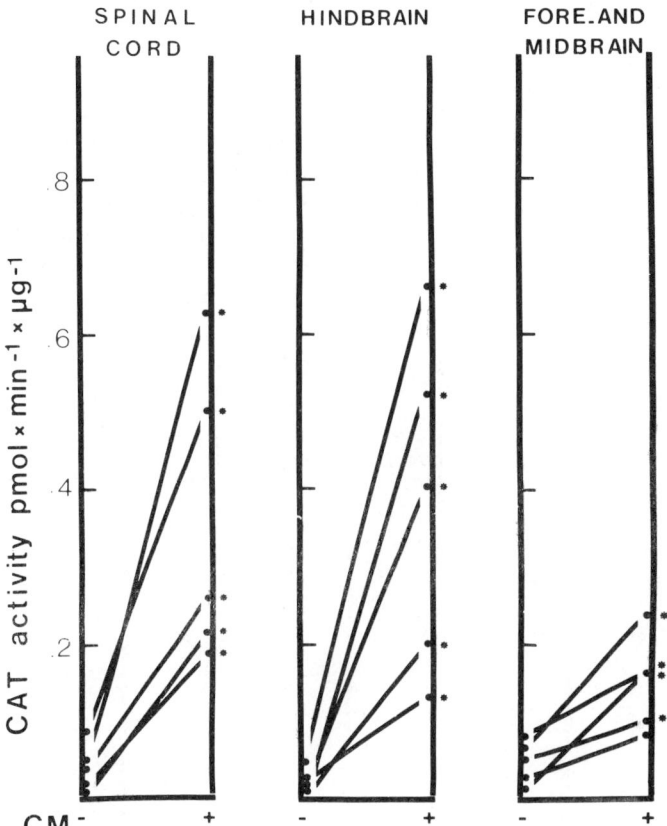

Fig. 15.1 Regulation of ChAT activity in rat embryo CNS cultures. Cultures prepared from E_{14} rat embryo were maintained for 14 days in the absence (−) or presence (+) of 50 % muscle-CM. The activity of ChAT was determined in triplicate in a pool of 2–3 identical cultures. Oblique bars join the means of the values obtained from sister cultures. Asterisks indicate a significant effect of CM ($p < 0.05$ or $p < 0.01$).

observed, but it was distinctly smaller than in the two other types of culture. A decrease in the sensitivity to muscle-CM along the caudo-rostral axis of the CNS has also been reported for mouse embryo (Godfrey *et al.*, 1980).

Several lines of experiments suggested that the ChAT stimulating factors for sympathetic and spinal cord neurons are identical (Giess and Weber, 1984).

(a) The two activities co-purified during at least the first four steps in Table 15.1, leading to an approximately 1500-fold purification.

(b) CM prepared from various types of rat non-neuronal cells displayed the same order of activity on both types of cultures.

(c) As demonstrated for sympathetic neurons (Patterson and Chun, 1977a), mouse heart cell CM was strikingly less active than its rat counterpart on rat spinal cord cultures, suggesting a degree of species specificity for the cholinergic factor.

Figure 15.2 shows that muscle-CM also increased AChE activity in spinal cord and hindbrain cultures. A similar phenomenon may also take place in fore- and midbrain cultures. Giess and Weber (1984) have suggested that the same factor in CM is responsible for the regulation of ChAT and AChE, and the same result holds for hindbrain cultures (Giess, unpublished data). If further purification work confirms this, it would mean that the same ChAT stimulating factor regu-

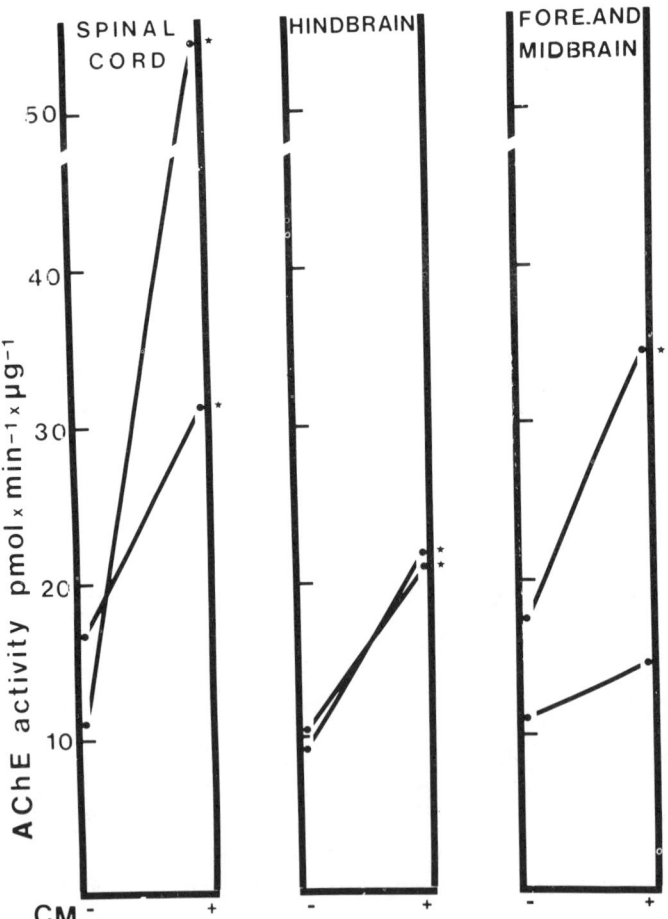

Fig. 15.2 Regulation of AChE activity in rat embryo CNS cultures. The data are presented as indicated in the caption to Fig. 15.1.

lates AChE activity in opposite directions in cultures from sympathetic and nodose ganglia on one hand, and from the CNS on other hand. We speculate that this factor has opposite effects on AChE gene expression in neurons with different embryonic origins.

We then wondered if catecholaminergic/cholinergic transitions (Potter *et al.*, 1980, 1981) might take place in CNS cultures, as in cultured sympathetic neurons. Not surprisingly, neither TOH activity, nor [³H] catecholamine synthesis and accumulation from [³H] tyrosine could be detected in spinal cord cultures (Giess, unpublished data) and these assays remain to be done with the other types of CNS cultures. However, the three types of cultures studied contained detectable levels of dopa decarboxylase (DDC) activity. Figure 15.3 further shows that DDC activity was significantly decreased in CNS cultures

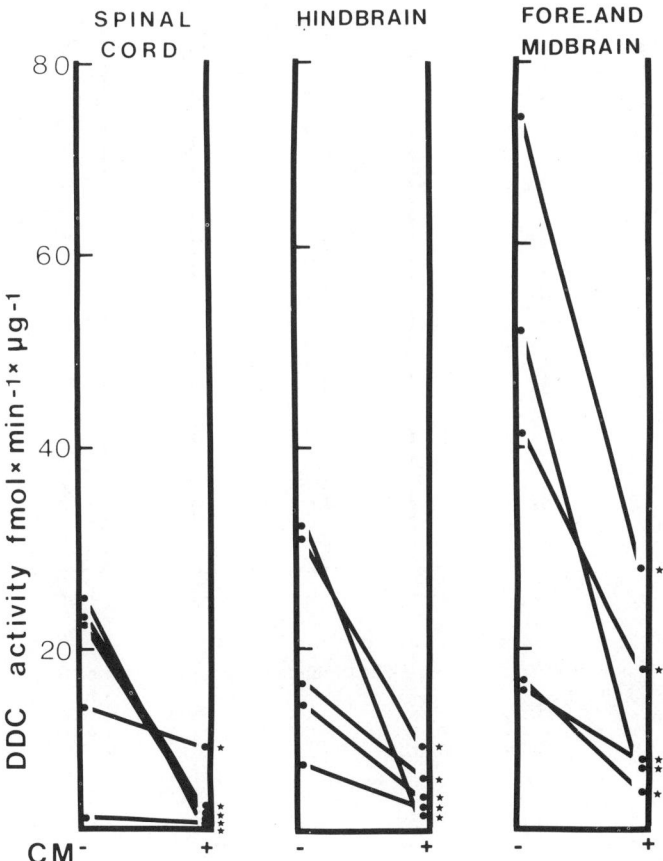

Fig. 15.3 Regulation of DDC activity in rat embryo CNS cultures. Cultures used for ChAT measurements (Fig. 15.1) were also used for DDC determinations.

grown with CM. Preliminary experiments suggest that the purified cholinergic factor reproduces this effect of CM (Giess, unpublished data). On the other hand, CM does not regulate glutamate decarboxylase activity (Fig. 15.4). The

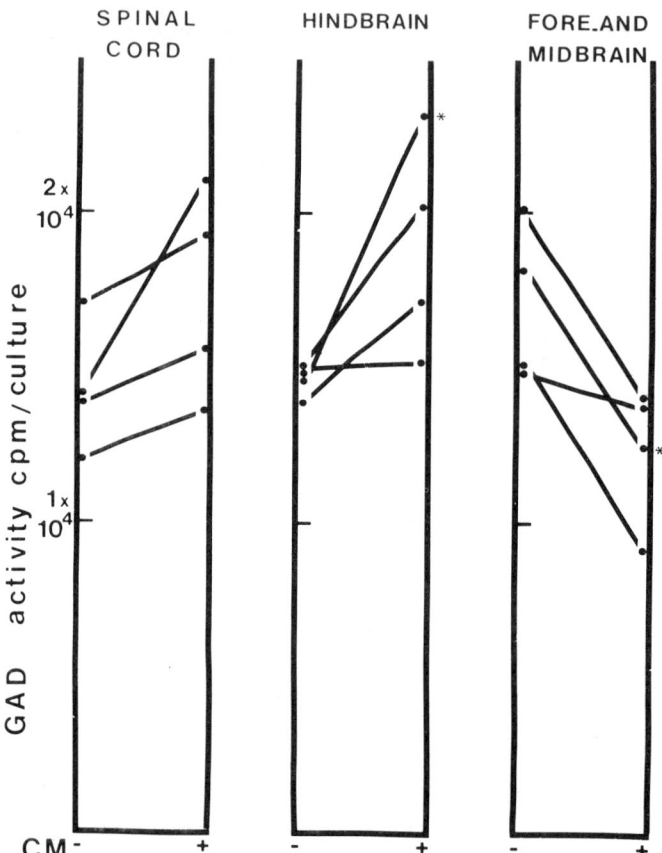

Fig. 15.4 Lack of effects of muscle-CM on glutamate decarboxylase (GAD) activity in rat embryo CNS cultures.

identity of DDC-expressing cells in our CNS cultures is still unknown. If the increase in ChAT activity and the decrease in DDC activity caused by CM occurred in the same neurons, it would suggest that neurotransmitter plasticity, which is well documented among PNS neurons (Patterson, 1978), may also take place in immature CNS neurons.

15.3.5 Regulation of ChAT Activity by Muscle-CM in Cultures from the Medial Septum Region ,

Different batches of muscle-CM were tested in parallel on cultures from E14 spinal cord and E17 medial septum region. The activity of CAT was increased 5-fold in septal cultures grown for 12–15 days with CM. A 5–12-fold increase in ChAT activity was observed in spinal cord cultures with the same CMs (Fig. 15.5).

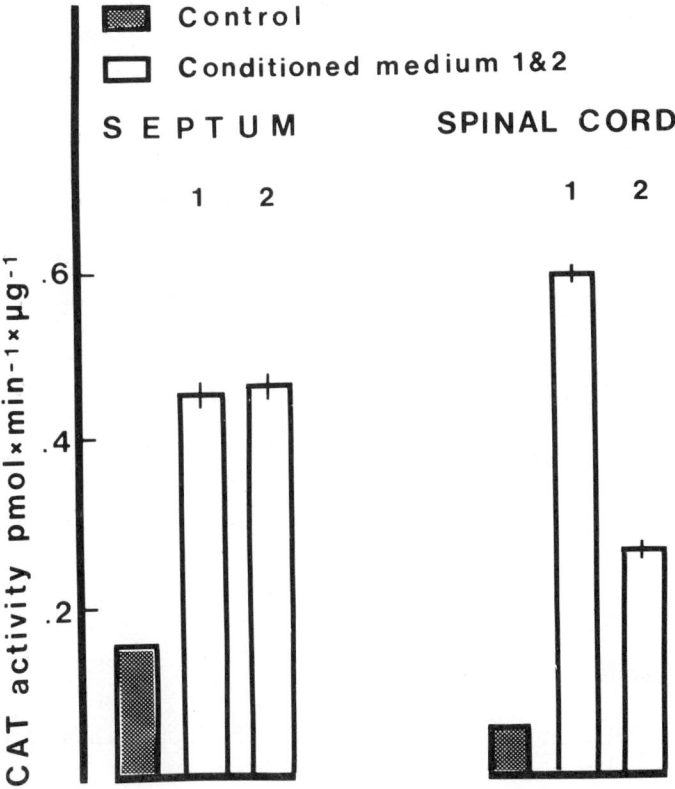

Fig. 15.5   Comparison of the effects of muscle-CM on cultures from the spinal cord and the medial septum region. The spinal cord and the medial septum region were dissected from E14 and E17 rat embryos, respectively. After a mechanical dissociation, the cells were grown in the culture medium described by Giess and Weber (1984) either in the absence (stippled bars) or presence (open bars) of 50 % muscle-CM. CM 1 and 2 are CMs from secondary and tertiary muscle cultures, respectively. For septal and spinal cultures, the stimulations caused by CM are significant at the $p < 0.01$ level.

To further delineate the target cell specificity of these effects, cultures were pre-pared from various regions of E17 embryonic brain. As shown on Table 15.2, no significant ChAT activity was measured in hippocampal cultures grown without CM, and only a marginal one was measured in sister cultures grown with CM. No ChAT activity was present in cultures from the olfactory lobes, neither in the presence or absence of CM. The same batch of CM caused a two-fold increase in ChAT activity in cultures of the septal region from the same rat embryo litter. This is an interesting observation, as ChAT activity in cultures from the septal region is also stimulated by NGF (Honegger and Lenoir, 1982; Gnahn et al., 1983; Hefti et al., 1985 and Ch. 13).

Table 15.2   Effects of muscle-CM on ChAT activity in brain cultures.

	Choline acetyltransferase activity (fmol/min/μg protein)	
	$-$CM	$+$CM
Medial septum region	9.8 ± 0.6	$19.7 \pm 0.3^*$
Hippocampus	<0.5	3.2 ± 0.3
Olfactory lobes	<0.5	<0.5

The medial septum region, the hippocampus and the olfactory lobes were dissected from E17 rat embryos, and dissociated and maintained in cultures, as described for spinal cord cells (Giess and Weber, 1984). Sister cultures were grown for 14 days with (+ CM) or without ($-$ CM) 50 % CM. ChAT activity was measured in tripli-cate on pools of two identical cultures. The data are means ± SEM. (*): $p < 0.001$.

15.4 Conclusion

Our data strongly suggest that a macromolecular factor which has been partially purified by following its stimulation of ChAT development in sympathetic neuron cultures also increases ChAT activity in CNS cultures. In particular, spinal moto-neurons and neurons from the medial septum region are targets for this cholin-ergic factor, as well as unidentified neurons from the hindbrain. However, several questions remain unanswered.

(a) Is the increase in ChAT activity in CNS cultures grown with CM the result of a better survival of cholinergic neurons; or of an increase in ChAT activity in a pool of neurons, the survival of which is not dependent on CM? Cell countings, with appropriate markers for cholinergic neurons (Hefti et al., 1985), are needed in order to answer this question.

(b) What is the identity of cells expressing DDC activity in CNS cultures? Do they also express other catecholamine or serotonin synthesising enzymes? Are the well-identified dopaminergic, noradrenergic or serotoninergic neurons in the CNS target cells for the cholinergic factor? Would this factor induce ChAT activity in these neurons?

(c) What is the role played by the cholinergic factor *in vivo*, during development and/or ageing? The obtention of antibodies against the cholinergic factor would certainly help in understanding which groups of neurons require this factor for their differentiation.

References

Baccaglini, P. L., and Cooper, E. (1982). Electrophysiological studies of new-born rat nodose neurones in cell culture. *J. Physiol. (Lond.)*, **324**, 429–39.

Berg, D. K. (1978). Acetylcholine synthesis by chick spinal cord neurons in dissociated cell culture. *Dev. Biol.*, **66**, 500–12.

Berg, D. K. (1985). New neuronal growth factors. *Ann. Rev. Neurosci.*, **7**, 149–70.

Cooper, E. L. (1984). Synapse formation among developing sensory neurones from rat nodose ganglia grown in tissue culture. *J. Physiol. (Lond.)*, **351**, 263–74.

Ellman, G. L., Courtney, K. D., Andres, V., and Featherstone, R. M. (1961). A new and rapid colorimetric determination of acetylcholinesterase activity. *Biochem. Pharmacol.*, **7**, 88–95.

Fonnum, F. (1975). A rapid radiochemical method for the determination of choline acetyltransferase. *J. Neurochem.*, **24**, 407–9.

Fukada, K. (1985). Purification and partial characterization of a cholinergic neuronal differentiation factor. *Proc. Natl Acad. Sci. USA*, **82**, 8795–9.

Giess, M. C., and Weber, M. J. (1984). Acetylcholine metabolism in rat spinal cord cultures: regulation by a factor involved in the determination of the neurotransmitter phenotype of sympathetic neurons. *J. Neurosci.*, **4**, 1442–52.

Giller, E. L., Schrier, B. K. Shainberg, A., Fisk, H. R., and Nelson, P. G. (1973). Choline acetyltransferase activity is increased in combined cultures of spinal cord and muscle cells from mice. *Science*, **182**, 588–9.

Giller, E. L., Neal, J. H., Bullock, P. N., Schrier, B. K., and Nelson, P. G. (1977). Choline acetyltransferase activity of spinal cord cell cultures increased by co-culture with muscle and by muscle-conditioned medium. *J. Cell Biol.*, **74**, 16–29.

Gnahn, H., Hefti, F., Heumann, R., Schwab, M. E., and Thoenen, H. (1983). NGF-mediated increase of choline acetyltransferase (ChAT) in the neonatal rat forebrain: evidence for a physiological role of NGF in the brain? *Dev. Brain Res.*, **9**, 45–52.

Godfrey, E. W., Schrier, B. K., and Nelson, P. G. (1980). Source and target cell specificities of a conditioned medium factor that increases choline acetyltransferase activity in cultured spinal cord cells. *Dev. Biol.*, **77**, 403–18.

Hefti, F., Hartikka, J., Eckenstein, F., Gnahn, H., Heumann, R., and Schwab, M. (1985). Nerve growth factor (NGF) increases choline acetyltransferase, but not survival of fiber outgrowth of cultured septal cholinergic neurons. *Neuroscience*, **14**, 55–68.

Honegger, P., and Lenoir, D. (1982). Nerve growth factor (NGF) stimulation of cholinergic telencephalic neurons in aggregating cell cultures. *Dev. Brain Res.*, **3**, 229–38.

Katz, D. M., Markey, K. A., Goldstein, M., and Black, I. B. (1983). Expression of catecholaminergic characteristics by primary sensory neurons in the normal adult rat *in vivo*. *Proc. Natl Acad. Sci. USA*, **80**, 3526–30.

Lamprecht, F., and Coyle, J. T. (1972). Dopa decarboxylase in the developing rat brain. *Brain Res.*, **41**, 503–6.

Landis, S. C. (1976). Rat sympathetic neurons and cardiac myocytes developing in microcultures: correlation of the fine structure of endings with neurotransmitter function in single neurons. *Proc. Natl Acad. Sci. USA*, **73**, 4220–4.

Landis, S. C. (1980). Developmental changes in the neurotransmitter properties of disso-ciated sympathetic neurons: a cytochemical study of the effects of medium. *Dev. Biol.*, **77**, 349–61.

Lowry, O. H., Rosebrough, N. J., Farr, A. L., and Randal, R. J. (1951). Protein measure-ment with the Folin phenol reagent. *J. Biol. Chem.*, **193**, 265–75.

Martin, R. G., and Ames, N. A. (1961). A method for determining the sedimentation behavior of enzymes: application to protein mixtures. *J. Biol. Chem.*, **236**, 1372–9.

Mathieu, C., Moisand, A., and Weber, M. J. (1984). Acetylcholine metabolism by cultured neurons from rat nodose ganglia: regulation by a macromolecule from muscle-conditioned medium. *Neuroscience*, **13**, 1373–86.

Patterson, P. H. (1978). Environmental determination of autonomic neurotransmitter func-tions. *Ann. Rev. Neurosci.*, **1**, 1–17.

Patterson, P. H., and Chun, L. L. Y. (1977a). The induction of acetylcholine synthesis in primary cultures of dissociated rat sympathetic neurons. I. Effects of conditioned medium. *Dev. Biol.*, **56**, 263–80.

Patterson, P. H., and Chun, L. L. Y. (1977b). The induction of acetylcholine synthesis in primary cultures of dissociated rat sympathetic neurons. II. Developmental aspects. *Dev. Biol.*, **60**, 473–81.

Potter, D. D., Landis, S. C., and Furshpan, E. J. (1980). Dual function during development of rat sympathetic neurons in culture. *J. exp. Biol.*, **89**, 57–71.

Potter, D. D., Landis, S. C., and Furshpan, E. J. (1981). Adrenergic-cholinergic dual func-tion in cultured sympathetic neurons of the rat. In *Development of the Autonomic Nervous Systems*, Ciba Foundation Symposium 83, pp. 123–38.

Siegel, L. M., and Monty, K. J. (1966). Determination of molecular weight and frictional ratios of proteins in impure systems by use of gel filtration and density gradient centri-fugation. Application to crude preparations of sulfite and hydroxylamine reductases. *Biochim. Biophys. Acta.*, **112**, 346–62.

Swerts, J. P., Le Van Thai, A., and Weber, M. S. (1984). Regulation of enzymes responsible for neurotransmitter synthesis and degradation in cultured rat sympathetic neurons. I: Regulation of 16S acetylcholinesterase by conditioned medium. *Dev. Biol.*, **103**, 230–4.

Swerts, J. P., Le Van Thai, A., Vigny, A., and Weber, M. J. (1983). Regulation of enzymes responsible for neurotransmitter synthesis and degradation in cultured rat sympathetic neurons. I. Effects of muscle conditioned medium. *Dev. Biol.*, **100**, 1–11.

Wallace, L. J., and Partlow, L. M. (1978). A sensitive microassay for protein in cells cultured on collagen. *Anal. Biochem.*, **87**, 1–10.

Weber, M. (1981). A diffusible factor responsible for the determination of cholinergic func-tions in cultured sympathetic neurons. Partial purification and characterization. *J. Biol. Chem.*, **256**, 3447–53.

Weber, M. J., and Le Van Thai, A. (1982). Progress in the purification of a factor involved in the neurotransmitter choice made by cultured sympathetic neurons. In Burger, M. M., and Weber, R. (eds.), *Embryonic Development*. A. R. Liss, New York, **85**B, pp. 473–83.

Weber, M. J., Raynaud, B., and Delteil, C. (1985). Molecular properties of a cholinergic dif-ferentiation factor from muscle-conditioned medium. *J. of Neurochem.*, **45**, 1541–7.

16

Neurite-promoting Factors for Embryonic Spinal Neurons: Studies on Develpoment in the Chick and Possible Importance for the Understanding of Degenerative Disorders of the Nervous System

T. Taguchi and C. E. Henderson

16.1 Introduction

The concept that a given population of neurons might depend for its survival and normal development on the presence of its target tissue is an old one, and remarkably little is yet known of the detailed cellular and molecular interactions that serve to define this trophic relationship. Much attention has been focussed on the possibility that the post-synaptic cells themselves produce retrograde neuronal growth factors to which the innervating neurons respond and for which, possibly, they compete. However, there exists no system in which all the elements of this model have been demonstrated.

The only neuronal growth factor for which a role *in vivo* has been firmly established is the nerve growth factor NGF (Levi-Montalcini and Angeletti, 1968; Thoenen and Barde, 1980). NGF was originally detected by its effects on the survival and differentiation of neurons from sensory and sympathetic ganglia, both *in vivo* and *in vitro*, but it is now clear that it is synthesised and transported in parts of the central nervous system, where its role may be quite different (for a full discussion, see Ch. 13). Proof of the physiological importance of NGF (as opposed to the effects of exogenous NGF) came from experiments with blocking antisera which, administered at appropriate developmental stages, result in massive cell death ('immunosympathectomy') within mammalian sympathetic or sensory ganglia (Levi-Montalcini and Booker, 1960). Recent studies using sensitive two-site enzymeimmunoassays have shown that NGF protein is present at significant levels in sympathetic effector organs and sympathetic ganglia, but not in skeletal muscle or serum (Korsching and Thoenen, 1983a). The NGF found in the ganglia probably derives from the target organ, since specific mRNA for NGF was detected in the effector organs and not the ganglia themselves (Heumann *et al.*, 1984; but see Shelton and Reichardt, 1985) and since endogenous NGF can be shown to be retrogradely transported by sympathetic axons (Korsching and Thoenen, 1983b). Two major unanswered questions concerning NGF are still the exact cellular site of synthesis, and the regulation of NGF levels during the periods of synaptogenesis and cell death in which it supposed to play an important role. Exploitation of currently developing techniques, such as *in situ* hybridisation, should hopefully soon clarify these points.

Many other molecules having an effect on certain parameters of neuronal survival and differentiation *in vitro* are at present under study, and it is not possible to discuss them in detail here (for a review, see Crutcher, 1986). Among those for which the active species have been identified and isolated some, such as the brain-derived neurotrophic factor (Barde *et al.*, 1982) and the ciliary neuronotrophic factor (Barbin *et al.*, 1984), have actions only on certain neuronal populations whereas others, such as laminin (Edgar *et al.*, 1984; Lander *et al.*, 1985), are apparently active in many systems.

The aim of the present article will be to discuss the evidence, not as yet conclusive, that there exist neuronal growth factors for motoneurons of the spinal cord. We will discuss possible roles for such hypothetical factors in the regulation of cell death, synapse formation and regeneration, and consider the evidence that the levels of production of such factors by muscles vary according the state of activity of a given muscle. In conclusion, we will present hypotheses linking possible anomalies in growth factor metabolism to the selective motoneuron death observed in diseases such as amyotrophic lateral sclerosis and the spinal muscular atrophies and, by extension, to the aetiology of other degenerative diseases of the nervous system.

16.2 Evidence for the Existence of Motoneuron Growth Factors

The first evidence that spinal motoneurons depend upon their target muscles for survival came from the classical experiments of Hamburger and colleagues (Hamburger, 1977). Naturally occurring cell death of motoneurons takes place between embryonic days 5 and 9 at lumbar levels in the chick spinal cord, and affects about 50 % of the motoneurons initially generated. Extirpation of a limb bud prior to this period results in an accentuation of the cell death phenomenon: virtually all of the motoneurons corresponding to the operated limb are lost. Implantation of a supernumerary limb, on the other hand, is followed by innervation of the additional muscles and a reduction of cell death in the corresponding motoneuron pool (Hollyday and Hamburger, 1976).

These results (and comparable ones from the cholinergic ciliary ganglion) have been interpreted in terms of a motoneuron growth factor produced by muscle, upon which motoneurons at certain developmental stages depend for their survival. It has frequently been considered that there may be competition at the periphery between motoneurons for a supply of factor which is not sufficient in normal conditions to maintain the whole motoneuron pool. In terms of this hypothesis, it is likely that inactive muscle produces more of the growth factor than does active muscle (*see* Section 16.4), as neuromuscular blockade throughout the cell death period considerably increases numbers of surviving motoneurons (Pittmann and Oppenheim, 1978), while direct stimulation enhances cell death (Oppenheim and Nunez, 1982). However, direct evidence for the existence of peripheral competition of this type is not abundant (Pilar *et al.*, 1980), and some published studies are in apparent conflict with the hypothesis in its simplest form (Lamb, 1979). It is in any case clear that other possibilities, such as central competition and programmed cell death of certain populations, cannot yet be excluded.

Muscle-derived factors may also be of importance in aspects of motoneuron development other than cell death. When the somites of two-day chick embryos were X-irradiated, embryos were generated in which one wing was completely normal whereas the other, although morphologically normal, was devoid of muscle (Lewis *et al.*, 1981). In the irradiated wings, all the main nerve trunks were present and apparently normal, yet specific muscle nerve branches were absent. These results suggest, but do not prove that, although the initial outgrowth of axons from the spinal cord is not apparently muscle-dependent (Oppenheim *et al.*, 1978), later stages of innervation could indeed be regulated over short distances by muscle-derived substances.

The system in which the clearest evidence exists for the action of a muscle-derived factor on motoneuron development *in vivo* is the sprouting observed following partial denervation of adult mammalian skeletal muscles (Brown *et al.*, 1981). Elegant *in vivo* experiments suggest that nerve growth in this situation occurs in response to a 'sprouting signal' released by the denervated muscle fibres and capable of diffusing a limited distance within the muscle. Sprouting, and thus presumably the release of the sprouting signal, is repressed by direct stimulation of partially denervated muscles (Brown and Holland, 1979).

16.3 Neurite-promoting Factors for Spinal Neurons and their Developmental Changes in the Chick

Many different *in vitro* systems have been used in attempts to characterise and study candidates for the role of motoneuron growth factor, and it is not possible to discuss them fully here (for references, see Henderson *et al.*, 1984; Henderson,

1985). In cultures of spinal cord explants, dissociated spinal neurons and identified motoneurons, effects of muscle-derived (and other) substances on such parameters as cell survival, neurite outgrowth and acetylcholine synthesis have been described. We wish in this section to resume our own work on neurite-promoting factors for chicken spinal neurons and to compare the results, where appropriate, with others from the literature. The major problem in doing this is that the *in vitro* systems used differ widely from one laboratory to another and that molecular data are incomplete, thus making comparison unreliable.

Media conditioned over cultures of embryonic chicken myotubes contained neurite-promoting activity (Fig. 16.1) for dissociated embryonic chicken spinal neurons (Henderson *et al.*, 1981). The cultures were performed using neural tubes at an age (4.5 days *in ovo*) at which motoneurons were expected to make up one third to one half of the total neuronal cell population, although we have no direct evidence that the neurite-bearing cells under the conditions of our culture were indeed motoneurons. However, other workers using comparable cultures showed that more than 50 % of the cells were capable of forming functional synapses with myotubes (Berg and Fischbach, 1978) or, using cultures from 7-day embryos, demonstrated retrograde labelling of up to 9 % of total cells by wheatgerm agglutinin–Lucifer Yellow (Calof and Reichardt, 1984).

The active factor(s) in embryonic muscle-conditioned medium was trypsin-sensitive, and associated with species of molecular weight 40,000 and greater. Most other conditioned media which were tested contained only low levels of neurite-promoting activity and, furthermore, the muscle-conditioned medium had little effect on dorsal root ganglia or on PC12 cells, suggesting that the observed activity had at least some selectivity for the interactions of spinal neurons and muscle. It is interesting to compare these results with those of Gundersen and Park (1984), who showed that, of a series of conditioned media tested, only muscle-conditioned media produced a directional growth response in growth cones of neurons in cultures enriched for motoneurons. Calof and Reichardt (1984), too, found that the full effect of muscle-conditioned medium on purified motoneurons could not be reproduced by other media. The apparent discrepancy between our results and those of others (Longo *et al.*, 1982) who demonstrated the presence of laminin-like neurite-promoting factors in virtually all conditioned media, might be explained by the absence in our culture system of a polycationic substratum to which such factors need to bind in order to exert their optimal effects on neurite outgrowth (Collins, 1978).

Comparison of the neurite-promoting activities in embryonic muscle-conditioned media and in high-speed supernatants of homogenates of neonatal chick leg muscle allowed us to study two aspects of their developmental regulation (Henderson *et al.*, 1984). First, the molecules responsible for the neonatal and embryonic activities are apparently different, as revealed by their differential binding affinity for the culture substratum under cell culture conditions. This could mean that, as in other systems (Edgar *et al.*, 1981), different factors regulate different stages of the development of these neurons, although *in vitro*

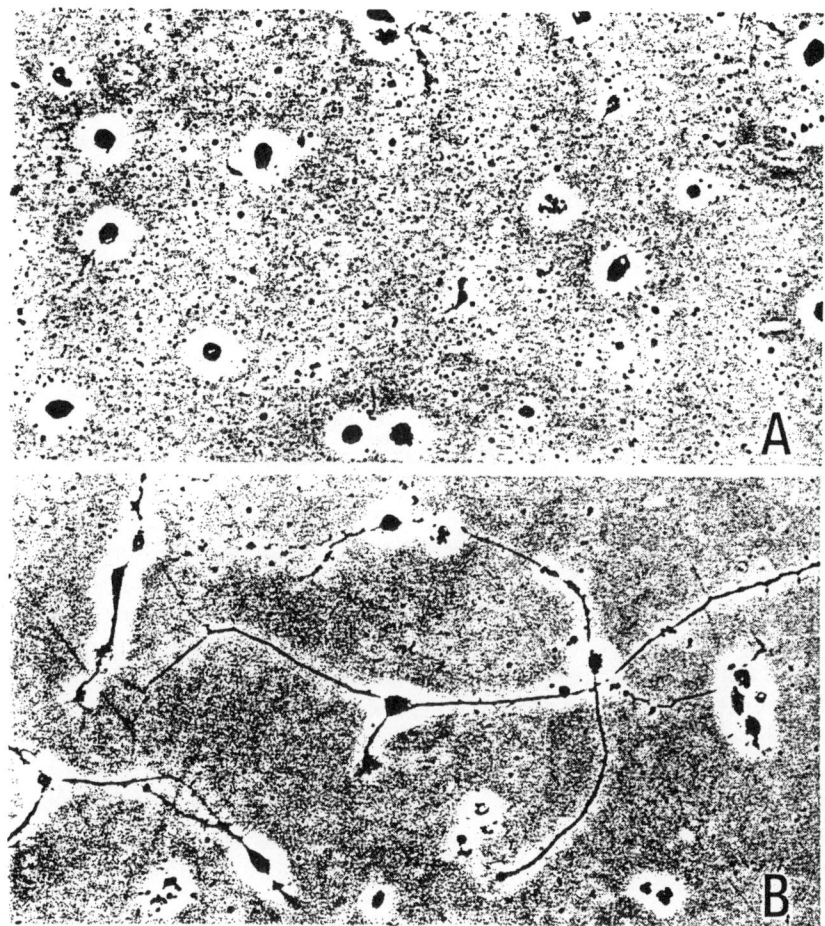

Fig. 16.1 Response of spinal neurons to neurite-promoting activity in extracts of neo-natal chick leg muscle. Dissociated spinal neurons from 4.5-day chicken embryos were cultured as described elsewhere (Henderson *et al.*, 1984). (A) after 20 h of culture in non-conditioned F12 medium; and (B) after 20 h of culture in F12 medium supplemented with neonatal (four days post-hatch) muscle extract at a dilution of 1:2000 (v/v).

data such as these can not prove such a hypothesis. Second, levels of neurite-promoting activity in extracts of leg muscle from post-hatch chicks of different ages increased reproducibly almost ten-fold during the course of the first three or four days of postnatal life, subsequently falling back to basal levels. It is likely that, during this period in the chick, regression of polyneuronal innervation is occurring in the leg, and we have speculated that the peak of activity might be related to the hypothetical factor proposed to stabilise the nerve terminals that will remain in the adult (Gouzé *et al.*, 1983). In order to further test this hypothesis, it will be necessary to establish a quantitative correlation in a single muscle between the evolution of polyneuronal innervation and the levels of this 'neonatal' activity.

No reproducible effect of either 'embryonic' or 'neonatal' activities on the survival of spinal neurons in these conditions has been observed. This does not necessarily mean that the molecules bearing these activities will not turn out to be survival-promoting factors. It is conceivable that the extreme simplicity of the culture conditions we have chosen (no serum, no hormonal supplements, plastic culture substratum), although sufficient for the observation of rapid neurite outgrowth, means that long-term survival is definitively excluded. Indeed, when cultured on extracellular matrix in otherwise similar conditions, many spinal neurons survive up to 15 days in the presence of muscle-conditioned medium, but die rapidly in its absence (C. Pinset and C. E. Henderson, unpublished observations). However, until the active factor(s) has been purified, it will not be possible to determine whether the survival-promoting and neurite-promoting activities are borne by the same molecule.

Purification of the active factor from extracts of denervated muscle (*see* Section 16.4) is currently being undertaken in our laboratory using a combination of conventional and high-pressure chromatography. The most highly purified preparations obtained, after isoelectric precipitation, anion-exchange chromatography, chromatofocussing and gel filtration, are apparently enriched approximately 10^4-fold with respect to total protein, and have specific activities in the neurite outgrowth assay of the order of 10^7 units/mg protein (which are comparable to that, in a different system, of highly purified NGF (10^5–10^6 units/mg protein)). However, as judged by silver staining of SDS gels, these fractions still contain at least 10 polypeptide species, and so complete purification has not been achieved. At this degree of purity, and at low protein concentrations, the activity migrates on gel filtration columns with an apparent molecular weight of 50 000.

16.4 Does Muscle Activity Regulate the Production of Motoneuron Growth Factors?

If one allows the hypothesis that neuronal growth factors are one of the mechanisms by which neuronal connections may be specified, selected or modified, it is tempting to speculate that patterns of expression of growth factors may be modulated by the electrical or mechanical activity of the system. Activity-dependent regulation of this type has been suggested or implied by experimental results and theoretical models concerning a wide variety of neuronal systems, but in no case has it been conclusively demonstrated (Henderson, 1986). This is in contrast with the situation for the acetylcholine receptor, transcription of whose α-subunit gene has been shown to increase in inactive muscle and to decrease in active muscle (Klarsfeld and Changeux, 1985), providing one explanation for the phenomenon of post-denervation hypersensitivity (Lomo and Rosenthal, 1972).

For the neuromuscular junction, three cases have already been described (Sections 16.2 and 16.3) in which activity-dependent regulation of growth factor production has been evoked as a possibility: motoneuron cell death; regression of polyneuronal innervation, and motor nerve sprouting in partially denervated muscles (Changeux and Danchin, 1976). In none of these situations has the active factor been characterised, and thus it was interesting to study the effects of activity on the production of *in vitro* growth-promoting molecules.

We investigated the effects of denervation on the production by muscle of neurite-promoting factors for spinal neurons (Henderson *et al.*, 1983). The sciatic nerve of 6-day post-hatch chicks was sectioned under anaesthesia and muscle extracts were prepared three days later from denervated, contralateral, non-operated and sham-operated leg muscles. All the control extracts gave half-maximal stimulation of neurite outgrowth at about 1.5 μg/ml total protein, whereas only 100 ng/ml of the denervated muscle extract was required to give the same effect (representing an apparent 15-fold increase in specific activity). In other experiments, it was shown that the time course of appearance of this increased activity was consistent with the time that elapses before the first observation of sprouts in paritally denervated mammalian muscles. Similar results have been obtained by other groups working on survival-promoting factors for identified motoneurons *in vitro* (Slack and Pockett, 1982; Nurcombe *et al.*, 1983), and it has recently been claimed that direct stimulation of denervated muscle prevents the observed increase in survival-promoting activity (Hill *et al.*, 1985).

One conclusion which it is possible to draw from these results is that production of neurite-promoting activity is increased in inactive muscle. However, the cellular effects of denervation are extremely complex, and one apposite example of the difficulty in interpreting such results is provided by recent studies on the rat iris. Denervation and explantation of rat irides result in significant increases in the levels of NGF detectable by bioassay (Ebendal *et al.*, 1980). Assay of specific NGF mRNA confirms the increase in messenger levels in explanted (Heumann *et al.*, 1984; Shelton and Reichardt, 1984) but not in denervated irides (Shelton and Reichardt, 1985), suggesting that in the latter case the increase in NGF levels at the level of the target could have arisen as a result of interruption of retrograde transport by sympathetic and sensory axons. A further complication is provided by the observation (Rush, 1984) that in such irides NGF immunoreactivity is associated not with smooth muscle but with Schwann cells in the nerve tracts. The activity-dependent regulation of NGF expression by postsynaptic smooth muscle cells is thus not demonstrated.

In the light of these problems of interpretation, we next measured levels of neurite-promoting activity in two other experimental situations in which the activity of the neuromuscular system should be lowered, but in which the nerve was not experimentally sectioned. The mutant mouse *Paralysé* (Duchen *et al.*,

1983) shows paralysis from four days post-natally and only survives for 12 or 13 days. The muscle weakness and paralysis seem likely to be due to the progressive atrophy of nerve terminals, with eventual denervation of end-plates. The cause of the axonal abnormalities is not yet established. We compared neurite-promoting activities of muscle extracts from mutants and control littermates (Henderson *et al.*, 1986a), and found increases of up to 10-fold in mutant muscles. The effect of the *Paralysé* mutation on neurite-promoting activity tended to increase with age up to death (Fig. 16.2), suggesting that it does not constitute a primary lesion in this mutant.

Tenotomy (section of the distal tendons of the gastrocnemius and soleus muscles) in neonatal rats has been shown to retard the regression of polyneuronal innervation in these muscles (Benoit and Changeux, 1978), as does blockade of nerve activity by local anaesthetic for regenerating neuromuscular junctions (Benoit and Changeux, 1975). In conjunction with results showing that direct stimulation accelerated regression (O'Brien *et al.*, 1978), these experiments were taken to suggest that inactive muscle produced more of a hypothetical nerve

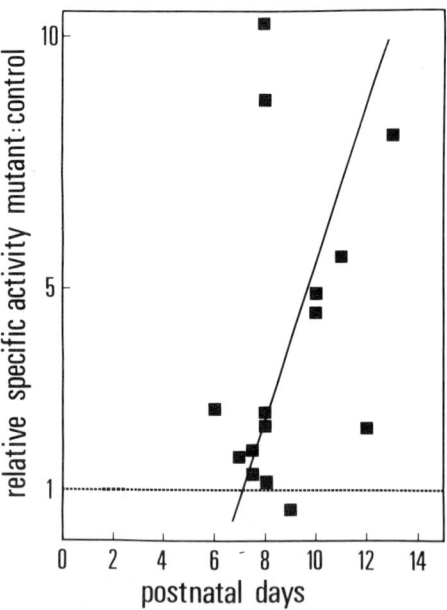

Fig. 16.2 Variation with age of the effect of the *Paralysé* mutation on neurite-promoting activity in muscle extracts. High-speed supernatants of muscle homogenates were prepared in the presence of protease inhibitors as described in Henderson *et al.* (1984). For each point (solid square), dose-response curves were established for a mutant muscle extract and an extract of muscle from a control littermate. Their specific neurite-promoting activities (biological units per mg protein) were expressed as the ratio mutant:control. The experimental line represents the best fit by the linear regression analysis.

terminal stabilisation factor than its active counterpart (Changeux and Danchin, 1976). Using our *in vitro* assay for neurite outgrowth from spinal neurons, we demonstrated that tenotomy caused a reproducible two-fold increase in specific growth-promoting activity, similar to the effects of denervation in this system (Henderson *et al.*, 1986a).

The observation of increases in neurite-promoting activity in muscles whose contractile activity was reduced by three different mechanisms (denervation, tenotomy and the *Paralysé* mutation) suggests, though cannot prove, that there is an activity-dependent regulation of the synthesis of these neurite-promoting factors. The interesting possibility is raised that the corresponding structural genes may be expressed coordinately with other muscle-specific genes, such as those coding for the acetylcholine receptor, during the development of muscle innervation.

16.5 Hypotheses concerning Neuronal Growth Factors and Degenerative Diseases of the Nervous System

The spinal muscular atrophies are inherited disorders of the anterior horn moto-neurons which present clinically as muscle weakness and atrophy. Their cause remains completely unknown. The structural lesion consists of selective degeneration and atrophy of the anterior horn cells of the spinal cord and, more rarely, of the cranial motor nuclei. If human spinal motoneurons at infantile stages do indeed depend upon muscle-derived factors for survival or axonal stabilisation, then the selective motoneuron death might be explained by one of the following mechanisms.

(a) The production by muscles of the growth factor diminishes or stops.

(b) Substances capable of inhibiting growth-factor action appear in the blood, muscle or cerebrospinal fluid.

(c) The motoneurons themselves become incapable of responding to the growth factor.

Recently, we used the spinal neuron neurite outgrowth assay as a first step towards testing the first two of these hypotheses (Henderson *et al.*, 1986b). Many soluble extracts of biopsies from patients with spinal muscular atrophies contained substances capable of inhibiting the action *in vitro* of the chick 'neonatal' neurite-promoting activity but not the 'embryonic'. No comparable inhibition was observed using extracts from biopsies from pathologically or morphologically normal controls. It is possible that these findings might be relevant to the second hypothesis, but extreme care should be taken in interpreting *in vitro* results obtained in a system in which neither the cell types nor the molecules involved are completely defined. In addition, such inhibitory substances could be the secondary result of a quite different primary lesion.

The hypotheses presented can be generalised to the case of any degenerative disorder of the nervous system in which a target-dependance of a specific neuronal population is supposed to exist. Indeed, the first of them has previously been discussed in terms of amyotrophic lateral sclerosis (ALS), Parkinsonism and Alzheimer's disease (Appel, 1981). Gurney and colleagues (Gurney, 1984; Gurney et al., 1984) have reported that sera from some patients with ALS were able to suppress botulinum toxin-induced terminal nerve sprouting from rat muscle and suggested, by immunoblot analysis of sera from three patients, that this blocking activity was mediated by autoantibodies reactive with a protein of 56,000 molecular weight which were present in media conditioned by cultured rat muscle. These results clearly address the second hypothesis. In a recent study (Hauser et al., 1986), however, we failed to confirm the suggestion that anti-56K reactivity is characteristic of ALS.

16.6 Conclusions

Although no growth factor for spinal motoneurons has been characterised thus far, there exists much evidence from both in vivo and in vitro studies that such molecules do exist. Certain molecules detected by their growth-promoting activity in vitro are found in muscles at levels which vary with the developmental stage and state of innervation of the muscle, suggesting that they might play a role in regulating the formation and stabilisation of the neuromuscular junction in vivo.

It has been hypothesised that anomalies in growth factor metabolism could lie at the origin of degenerative disorders such as the spinal muscular atrophies or amyotrophic lateral sclerosis. If central cholinergic neurons depend upon these or (more probably) other growth factors for their survival, then at least some of the characteristic lesions in Alzheimer's disease might result from a selective lack of, or interference with, trophic support.

Acknowledgements

The work described in this article was the collaborative effort of P. Benoît, P. A. Cazenave, J.-P. Changeux, M. Fardeau, S. Hauser, F. Hentati and M. Huchet, to whom we express our gratitude. T. T. was a Boursier of the Japan Society for promoting Science.

References

Appel, S. H. (1981). A unifying hypothesis for the cause of amyotrophic lateral sclerosis, Parkinsonism and Alzheimer Disease. *Ann. Neurol.*, **10**, 499–505.
Barbin, G., Manthorpe, M., and Varon, S. (1984). Purification of the chick eye ciliary neuronotrophic factor. *J. Neurochem.*, **43**, 1468–78.

Barde, Y.-A., Edgar, D., and Thoenen, H. (1982). Purification of a new neurotrophic factor from mammalian brain. *EMBO J.*, 1, 549–53.

Benoît, P., and Changeux, J.-P. (1975). Consequences of tenotomy on the evolution of multiinnervation in developing rat soleus muscle. *Brain Res.*, 99, 354–8.

Benoît, P., and Changeux, J.-P. (1978). Consequences of blocking the nerve with a local anaesthetic on the evolution of multiinnervation at the regenerating neuromuscular junction of the rat. *Brain Res.*, 149, 89–96.

Berg, D. K., and Fischbach, G. D. (1978). Enrichment of spinal cord cell cultures with motoneurons. *J. Cell Biol.*, 77, 83–98.

Brown, M. C., and Holland, R. L. (1979). A central role for denervated tissues in causing nerve sprouting. *Nature*, 282, 724–6.

Brown, M. C., Holland, R. L., and Hopkins, W. G. (1981). Motor nerve sprouting. *Ann. Rev. Neurosci.*, 4, 17–42.

Calof, A. L., and Reichardt, L. F. (1984). Motoneurons purified by cell sorting respond to two distinct activities in myotube-conditioned medium. *Develop. Biol.*, 106, 194–210.

Changeux, J. P., and Danchin, A. (1976). Selective stabilisation of developing synapses as a mechanism for the specification of neuronal networks. *Nature*, 264, 705–12.

Collins, F. (1978). Induction of neurite outgrowth by a conditioned-medium factor bound to the culture substratum. *Proc. Natl Acad. Sci. USA*, 75, 5210–13.

Crutcher, K. A. (1986). The role of growth factors in neuronal development and plasticity. *Crit. Rev. Clinic. Neurobiol.* (in press).

Duchen, L. W., Gomez, S., Guénet, J. L., and Love, S. (1983). *Paralysé*: a new neurological mutant mouse with progressive atrophy and loss of motor nerve terminals. *J. Physiol.*, 345, 166P.

Ebendal, T., Olson, L., Seiger, A., and Hedlund, K. O. (1980) Nerve growth factors in the rat iris. *Nature*, 286, 25–8.

Edgar, D., Barde, Y.-A., and Thoenen, H. (1981). Subpopulations of cultured chick sympathetic neurones differ in their requirements for survival factors. *Nature*, 289, 294–5.

Edgar, D., Timpl, R., and Thoenen, H. (1984). The heparin-binding domain of laminin is responsible for its effects on neurite outgrowth and neuronal survival. *EMBO J.*, 3, 1463–8.

Gouzé, J.-L., Lasry, J.-M., and Changeux, J.-P. (1983). Selective stabilization of muscle innervation during development: a mathematical model. *Biol. Cybern.*, 46, 207–15.

Gundersen, R. W., and Park, K. H. C. (1984). The effects of conditioned media on spinal neurites: substrate-associated changes in neurite direction and adherence. *Develop. Biol.*, 104, 18–27.

Gurney, M. E. (1984). Suppression of terminal sprouting at the neuromuscular junction by immune sera. *Nature*, 307, 546–8.

Gurney, M. E., Belton, A. C., Cashman, N., and Antel, J. P. (1984). Inhibition of terminal axonal sprouting by serum from patients with amyotrophic lateral sclerosis. *New Eng. J. Med.*, 311, 933–9.

Hamburger, V. (1977). The developmental history of the motor neuron. *Neurosci. Res. Progr. Bull.*, 155, 1–37.

Hauser, S. L., Cazenave, P.-A., Lyon-Caen, O., Taguchi, T., Barbier, E., Huchet, M., Nuret, H., Changeux, J.-P., and Henderson, C. E. (1986). Immunoblot analysis of circulating antibodies against muscle proteins in amyotrophic lateral sclerosis and other neurological diseases. *Neurology* (in press).

Henderson, C. E. (1985). Neurite-promoting factors for spinal neurons. In Althaus, H. H., and Seifert, W. (eds.), NATO Advanced Research Workshop: *Glial–neuronal communication in development and regeneration*, Plenum (in press).

Henderson, C. E. (1986). Activity and the regulation of neuronal growth factor metabolism. In Changeux, J. P. and Konishi, M. (eds.), Dahlem Workshop Report: *Neural and Molecular Bases of Learning*, Springer-Verlag (in press).

Henderson, C. E., Huchet, M., and Changeux, J.-P. (1981). Neurite outgrowth from embryonic chicken spinal neurons is promoted by media conditioned by muscle cells. *Proc. Natl Acad. Sci. USA*, 78, 2625–9.

Henderson, C. E., Huchet, M., and Changeux, J.-P. (1983). Denervation increases a neurite-promoting activity in extracts of skeletal muscle. *Nature*, 302, 609–11.

Henderson, C. E., Huchet, M., and Changeux, J.-P. (1984). Neurite-promoting activities for embryonic spinal neurons and their developmental changes in the chick. *Develop. Biol.*, 104. 336–47.

Henderson, C. E., Benoît, P., Huchet, M., Guénet, J. L., and Changeux, J.-P. (1986a). Increase of neurite-promoting activity for spinal neurons in muscles of "paralysé" mice and tenotomised rats. *Dev. Brain Res.*, 25, 65–70.

Henderson, C. E., Hauser, S., Huchet, M., Dessi, F., Taguchi, T., Changeux, J.-P., Hentati, F., and Fardeau, M. (1986b). Spinal muscular atrophies: extracts of muscle biopsies inhibit neurite outgrowth from spinal neurons *in vitro* (submitted).

Heumann, R., Korsching, S., Scott, J., and Thoenen, H. (1984). Relationship between levels of NGF and its messenger RNA in sympathetic ganglia and peripheral target tissues. *EMBO J.*, 3, 3183–90.

Hill, M. A., Dangain, J., and Bennett, M. R. (1985). Motoneurone growth factor activity in muscle regulated by impulse traffic. *Neurosci. Lett. Suppl.*, 19, S71.

Hollyday, M., and Hamburger, V. (1976). Reduction of the naturally occurring motor neuron loss by enlargement of the periphery. *J. Comp. Neurol.*, 170, 311–20.

Klarsfeld, A., and Changeux, J.-P. (1985). Activity regulates the levels of acetylcholine receptor α-subunit mRNA in cultured chicken myotubes. *Proc. Natl Acad. Sci. USA*, 82, 4558–62.

Korsching, S., and Thoenen, H. (1983a). Nerve growth factor in sympathetic ganglia and corresponding target organs of the rat: correlation with the density of sympathetic innervation. *Proc. Natl Acad. Sci. USA*, 80, 3513–16.

Korsching, S., and Thoenen, H. (1983b). Quantitative demonstration of the retrograde axonal transport of endogenous nerve growth factor. *Neurosci. Lett.*, 39, 1–4.

Lamb, A. H. (1979). Evidence that some limb motoneurons die for reasons other than peripheral competition. *Develop. Biol.*, 71, 8–21.

Lander, A. D., Fujii, D. K., and Reichardt, L. F. (1985). Laminin is associated with the 'neurite outgrowth-promoting factors' found in conditioned media. *Proc. Natl Acad. Sci. USA*, 82, 2183–7

Levi-Montalcini, R., and Angeletti, P. (1968). Nerve growth factor. *Physiol. Rev.*, 48, 534–69.

Levi-Montalcini, R., and Booker, B. (1960) Destruction of the sympathetic ganglia in mammals by an antiserum to the nerve growth-promoting factor. *Proc. Natl Acad. Sci. USA*, 42, 384–91.

Lewis, J., Chevallier, A., Kiény, M., and Wolpert, L. (1981). Muscle nerve branches do not develop in chick wings devoid of muscle. *J. Embryol. Exp. Morphol.*, 64, 211–32.

Lomo, T., and Rosenthal, J. (1972). Control of ACh sensitivity by muscle activity in the rat. *J. Physiol.*, 221, 493–513.

Longo, F. M., Manthorpe, M., and Varon, S. (1982). Spinal cord neuronotrophic factors. I. Bioassay of schwannoma and other conditioned media. *Develop. Brain Res.*, 3, 277–94.

Nurcombe, V., Hill, M. A., Eagleson, K., and Bennett, M. R. (1983). Motoneurone survival and neurite extension from spinal cord explants induced by factors released from denervated muscle. *Brain Res.*, 291, 19–28.

O'Brien, R. A. D., Ostberg, A. J. C., and Vrbova, G. (1978). Observations on the elimination of polyneuronal innervation in developing mammalian skeletal muscle. *J. Physiol.*, 282, 571–82.

Oppenheim, R. W., and Nùnez, R. (1982). Electrical stimulation of hindlimb increases neuronal cell death in chick embryo. *Nature*, 295, 57–9.

Oppenheim, R. W., Chu-Wang, I.-W., and Maderdrut, J.-L. (1978). Cell death of motoneurons in the chick embryo spinal cord. The differentiation of motoneurons prior to their induced degeneration following limb-bud removal. *J. Comp. Neurol.*, 177, 87–112.

Pilar, G., Landmesser, L., and Burstein, L. (1980). Competition for survival among developing ciliary ganglion cells. *J. Neurophysiol.*, 43, 233–54.

Pittman, R., and Oppenheim, R. W. (1978). Neuromuscular blockade ꞏ ₋₋ₐses motoneurone survival during normal cell death in the chick embryo. *Natur*, 271, 364–6.

Rush, R. A. (1984). Immunohistochemical localization of endogenous nerve growth factor. *Nature*, 312, 364–6.

Shelton, D. L., and Reichardt, L. F. (1984). Expression of the β-NGF gene correlates with the density of sympathetic innervation in effector organs. *Proc. Natl Acad. Sci. USA*, 81, 7951–5.
Shelton, D. L., and Reichardt, L. F. (1985). Denervation of the rat iris does not increase the level of mRNA encoding Beta Nerve Growth Factor. *Soc. Neurosci. Abstr.*, 11, 939
Slack, J. R., and Pockett, S. (1982). Motor neurotrophic factor in denervated adult skeletal muscle. *Brain Res.*, 247, 138–40.
Thoenen, H., and Barde, Y.-A. (1980). Physiology of nerve growth factor. *Physiol. Rev.*, 60, 1284–335.

17

Molecular Biology as a Possible Approach to Human Inherited Disorders

I. Oberlé

17.1 Introduction

The last ten years have witnessed remarkable progress in the understanding of the structure and function of eukaryotic genes and in the elucidation of the molecular basis of genetic diseases. Whilst some areas, notably haematology, cancer and immunology, have already benefitted from the application of new molecular genetic concepts and techniques, neuroscientists are only now taking advantage of this new approach to old problems.

The human genome is about 3×10^9 pairs long and might contain 2–10×10^4 genes. According to our current knowledge, less than 10 % of the total genome are necessary to code and regulate this number of genes, and the function of most part of the DNA sequences is still unknown. From the study of the complexity of mRNAs in rodent brains, it has been proposed that at least half of the structural gene loci are involved in central nervous system function (Chandhari and Hahn, 1983), which could explain why so many genetic diseases affect the nervous system (about a third of the 1,637 Mendelian genetic diseases so far established (McKusick, 1983)). Up to now, most of these inherited disorders have eluded the characterisation of their primary defect (70 % of the recessive disorders, for instance) or even their mapping on the human genome (only 900 human genes have been assigned to a specific chromosome (McAlpine et al., 1985)).

In this survey, we will try to present an overall view of the possible strategies for the investigation of neurogenetic disorders at the level of the abnormal gene itself. It is not our purpose to explain the technical 'tricks' of all the methodologies used in recombinant DNA, since they are reported elsewhere (Williamson,

1981-3; Maniatis *et al.*, 1982; Watson *et al.*, 1983; Silhavy *et al.*, 1984; Steel, 1984). Two cases will be distinguished. Genes corresponding to some diseases have already been identified and cloned, and we will discuss some of the results obtained from the study of their mutations. In numerous cases, however, the gene involved in a disease has not yet been precisely identified, and we will focus on the strategies which can be used to search for such genes.

17.2 Direct Analysis of Genetic Diseases: The Gene is Cloned

Some inherited disorders were first characterised by the structural and functional study of abnormal protein or by using assays for immunologically cross-reacting materials (CRMs). As soon as recombinant DNA techniques were available, geneticists attempted to isolate and analyse the mutated genes. The main problem in cloning sequences corresponding to a given gene is to devise a strategy for the screening of libraries which contain up to 10^6 different cloned DNA fragments. The logic of these cloning strategies has been reviewed (see, for example, Watson *et al.*, 1983; Heilig and Mandel, 1986). Briefly, one or several of the following are needed: partial aminoacid sequence; specific antibodies; identification of cells with high or inducible levels of mRNA; etc. Genes corresponding to mRNA species present at high level in readily available tissues were the first to be isolated (i.e. globins, albumin, insulin, etc.), since it was relatively easy in such cases to prepare probes for the screening of clones which were well represented in the appropriate library. As illustrated in Table 17.1, the number of cloned genes is increasing at a substantial rate. Therefore, compilations of cloned genes need to be steadily updated (Schmidtke and Cooper, 1985; Willard *et al.*, 1985).

17.2.1 *Methods of Mutation Detection*

The identification of the nucleotide sequence change which is responsible for a given phenotype is a major goal. In the first place, we could think to sequence and compare DNA of a 'normal' gene and of its mutated counterpart. This is a rather blind approach (is the mutation located within coding, intervening or

Table 17.1 Number of human DNA clones mapped to chromosomes which were reported at the last three workshops on human gene mapping*

	Year		
	1981	1983	1985
Cloned genes (with RFLPs)	16(6)	104(35)	249(88)
Anonymous probes (with RFLPs)	35(18)	215(95)	559(245)

*Willard *et al.* (1985).

regulating sequences?) which may make necessary major efforts with very large genes (up to 186 kilobases for the coagulation factor VIII gene) and which usually requires cloning of mutated genes in addition to the normal one. Two other technical approaches are therefore preferentially used: restriction mapping and southern blotting (for detailed description of these procedures and their logic see Southern, 1980; Little, 1981; Antonarakis *et al.*, 1982; Housman *et al.*, 1982; Lewin, 1985). In classical genetics, studying the gene organisation on the chromosome meant establishing a genetic map. As Lewin (1985) pointed out:

> A genetic map identifies a series of sites at which mutations occur. The existence of the sites depends on the fact that changes in base sequence have altered the phenotype. The distance between the sites is determined by recombination frequencies.

Molecular geneticists used to represent the genetic material as a restriction map which

> identifies a linear series of sites in DNA, separated from one another by actual distance along the nucleic acid. A restriction map can be obtained for any sequence of DNA, irrespective of whether mutations have been identified in it or, indeed, whether we have any knowledge of its function.

This physical map is obtained by breaking the DNA molecule at defined points whose distance apart can be accurately determined. These defined cuts are generated by digestion of the DNA with restriction endonucleases. These enzymes recognise a short, specific sequence of bases. For instance, the enzyme EcoRI recognises the sequence 5'-GAATTC-3' and cuts at all such sequences. There are more than 100 different restriction endonucleases. The human genome is cleaved by a given enzyme in 10^6–10^7 distinct restriction fragments which can be separated and sized by electrophoresis. Southern blotting allows the determination of the number and localisation of restriction sites within and around any cloned DNA or RNA sequence (the 'probe'), starting from total genomic DNA (extracted from peripheral blood leukocytes or other cell types).

Restriction mapping can reveal differences between normal and mutated DNA sequences. For example, a deletion or an insertion in a gene will change the size of the restriction fragments in which it lies, provided the changes are big enough to be technically detectable (more than 50 base pairs).

In rare cases some minor changes, as in point mutations, can also be revealed by restriction mapping if this mutation affects a base in the recognition site for a restriction enzyme. Indeed, when 5'-GAATTC-3' becomes 5'-GAGTTC-3', the enzyme EcoRI will not cut DNA, and a probe encompassing this particular restriction site sequence will hybridise to two restriction fragments in normal DNA, whereas in mutated DNA it will recognise a unique fragment whose size accounts for the disappearance of an internal site (*see* Fig. 17.1). Reciprocally, a point mutation can create a new restriction site.

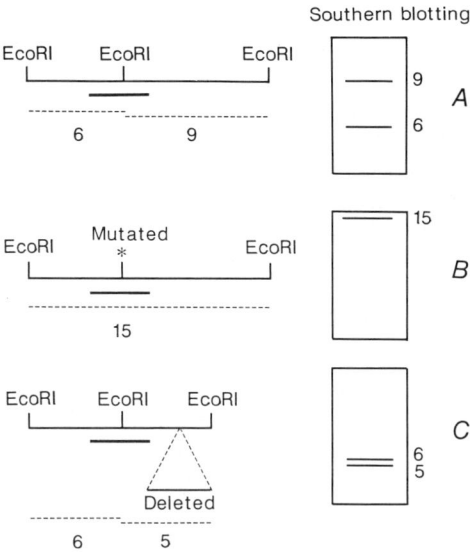

Fig. 17.1 Examples of changes in DNA detectable by Southern blotting. The bold rule indicates the probe (anonymous DNA, cDNA, or cloned gene). The numbers indicate the size of the restriction fragments. (*A*) the probe hybridises to two EcoRI restriction fragments in normal DNA. (*B*) A mutation in one EcoRI site generates a single EcoRI fragment hybridising to the probe. (*C*) A deletion occurs of 4 kb DNA.

When such an approach is inconclusive, one has to clone and sequence the gene and its regulatory sequences from healthy and affected individuals. The problem will be to distinguish the deleterious mutation from changes in DNA sequence which do not have phenotypic consequences (the healthy phenotype may itself be polymorphic, *see below*). For this purpose, functional analysis of the gene and its mutations may orientate the research.

If the tissue which expresses the gene is available, one can analyse the corresponding RNAs (mature messenger or precursors) with respect to levels, structure and function. Tools for the analysis of RNA are the dot blot (which will mainly measure the mRNA level) or Northern blot (which measures in addition the RNA sizes and can distinugish between the primary transcript, the processing intermediates, and the mature mRNA). Finer analysis of the RNA structure can be performed by nuclease S1 mapping or by cDNA synthesis with a specific primer. The mRNA can be assayed in an *in vitro* translation system which will detect nonsense mutations. Discrepancy between the production of a normal-sized protein in the *in vitro* system and its absence *in vivo* might indicate a mutation affecting stability or processing of the protein.

If there is evidence that a large part of a gene is made up of introns and that in an affected individual its mRNA or protein is of normal size and abundance, one can first limit the sequencing efforts to protein coding exons. But if the defect seems to result from a pretranslational block, it will probably be necessary to sequence part of the introns (near the splicing site) and/or 5' flanking sequences. Several processes are emerging which might spare one the cloning of all mutated genes before their sequencing; direct RNA (Kaartinen *et al.*, 1983) and genomic DNA (Church and Gilbert, 1984) sequencing. A more general method of detection of point mutations which reveals 30 % of the single base mismatches between two DNA sequences has been proposed by Myers *et al.* (1985), but this method can explore only a relatively small region and is not yet standard.

17.2.2 Types of Mutation Detected by these Methods

The first hereditary disorder diagnosed by gene analysis was α-thalassaemia and, more generally, haemoglobinopathies were so thoroughly studied that we will consider them as the paradigm of a genetic disease whose gene was cloned.

There are two classes of haemoglobin defects: the structural variants (altered polypeptide chains caused by amino acid substitutions) and the thalassaemias (caused by reduced or absent synthesis of α or β globin chains). All types of lesion have been discovered (Little, 1981; Antonarakis *et al.*, 1982; Orkin and Kazazian, 1984; Antonarakis *et al.*, 1985a): frame-shift or missense mutations, as well as premature termination or protein prolongation. Splicing variants have also been detected, resulting from mutations in the vicinity of a splicing site or from the creation of a new splicing site in an intron or in an exon. Modifications of the polyadenylation signal were shown to impair the maturation of the RNA transcript.

Deletions of one or both α-globin genes within the α-globin locus are the major cause of α-thalassaemias, but deletions are very rare in simple β-thalassaemias (except in India where a partial deletion accounts for 30 % of the thalassaemic genes). Complex β-thalassaemias, such as Hb Lepore δβ or γδβ thalassaemias with or without hereditary persistence of foetal haemoglobin HPFH, are often very large deletions (Antonarakis *et al.*, 1985a). Other diseases have been studied less thoroughly, but deletions do appear to be infrequent (less than 10–20 % of cases). They have been characterised in haemophilias A (Gitschier *et al.*, 1985a) and B (Giannelli *et al.*, 1983), ornithine transcarbamylase deficiency (Rozen *et al.*, 1985), Lesch Nyhan disease (HPRT deficiency) (Yang *et al.*, 1984), type A familial growth hormone deficiency (Phillips *et al.*, 1981), antithrombin III deficiency (Prochownik *et al.*, 1983), and in osteogenesis imperfecta (Barsh *et al.*, 1985; Cheah, 1985). In general, deletions will not allow expression of a protein recognisable by antibodies specific for the normal protein and will thus be CRM^- mutations. However, in the case of collagen genes (types I, II and III), where exons are in phase with the repetitive unit characteristic of the triple helical domain of the protein, deletion of one or two exons in this region will result in the synthesis of a collagen chain of shorter size (Cheah, 1985).

Insertions are much rarer than deletions; however, a 6.5 kilobases DNA insertion was demonstrated in the apolipoprotein A-I gene of patients with premature atherosclerosis (Karathanasis *et al.*, 1983).

17.2.3 Functional Analysis of Mutations

As already mentioned, a functional analysis of the mutation is sometimes desirable before one starts to perform a structural characterisation, but is also useful to understand the phenotype resulting from the detected mutation. In some genes, mutations in non-coding sequences (introns 5′ or 3′ unstranslated) might also affect important regulatory sequences (such as transcription enhancers) or the secondary structure and stability of premessenger or messenger RNAs. A mutation at a degenerate codon position in a protein coding sequence which does not change the protein structure might create an alternate splice site as, for example, the translationally silent change T-A in codon 24 of the β-globin gene. A very good example of a mutation with a dual effect is the β^E mutation which creates an amino acid change and modifies the electrophoretic mobility of haemoglobin Hb E. The mutation had been characterised already at the protein sequence level, but a puzzling feature was that the β^E gene was expressed at relatively low levels and was hence comparable to a mild β^+ thalassaemia gene. It was thus originally thought that an additional thalassaemia mutation was present in the gene. However, DNA sequencing showed that the β^E mutation was located within a sequence resembling a donor splice site. Functional analysis showed that the mutation activated this cryptic splice site and, in fact, was responsible for the decreased expression, since part of the primary RNA transcript was processed incorrectly.

If appropriate patient tissue is not available, it is possible to analyse function using the cloned gene sequences. *In vitro* transcription systems can be used to analyse some of the promoter elements (e.g. the TATA box). More efficiently, it is possible to clone the gene in an appropriate eukaryotic expression vector and introduce it in cultured cells, allowing the analysis of the transcription and maturation of the RNA product. This has been very fruitful, for instance in the analysis of β-thalassaemia mutations which create new splice sites within introns or exons (Treisman *et al.*, 1982). However, it is important to realise that in many expression systems some regulatory sequences are not necessary which are nonetheless important within the organism. For instance, in a $\gamma\delta\beta$ thalassaemia with deletion of the γ and δ gene, the remaining β gene appeared normal as tested by nucleotide sequencing and expression of the cloned gene in cells. In contrast, this gene was not detectably expressed in the erythroid cells of the patient and was present in an inactive chromatin conformation, as shown by nuclease sensitivity studies and analysis of DNA methylation.

17.2.4 Application of Recombinant DNA Techniques to Diagnosis

17.2.4.1 Advantages of DNA Analysis

DNA analysis has transformed the perspective of diagnosis, including carrier and prenatal diagnosis, and this domain is rapidly progressing.

Direct diagnosis of inherited diseases usually involved biochemical, enzymatic or immunological studies of the gene product in tissues or cells, and at the given developmental stage at which the gene responsible for the disease is expressed. For example, diagnosis of haemoglobinopathies required foetal blood sampling and the study of globin chain synthesis (Alter, 1981). DNA analysis allows the identification of the specific genetic defect after amniocentesis (16–18 weeks of pregnancy) or, better, after chorionic villus biopsy (8–10 weeks of pregnancy).

DNA analysis can thus be performed with any type of nucleated cells. An identical basic methodology will serve for different diseases (only probes vary) and, although this technology is still quite costly and labour intensive, it is being adopted by an increasing number of laboratories. Furthermore, simplifications can be expected: non-radioactive stable probes (Leary *et al.*, 1983; Tchen *et al.*, 1984) might replace the ^{32}P-probe; and some automation could be anticipated if liquid-phase hybridisation substitutes for blotting experiments. In contrast, biochemical diagnosis involves specific techniques for each disease and, in some cases, only very few laboratories in the world are able to carry out accurately a particular diagnosis. The most important advantage of diagnosis at the DNA level, however, is its applicability to diseases for which the primary defect and biochemical mechanisms are unknown. It can also be applied to presymptomatic diagnosis of diseases with late onset (*see below*).

17.2.4.2 Direct Detection of the Deleterious Mutation

As already stated, the characterisation of point mutations represents a major effort for most genetic diseases since, in general, many different lesions can cause the same disease: sickle-cell anaemia (β^s) or α-antitrypsin deficiency are exceptional examples of diseases caused by a single (β^s) or predominant (α-antitrypsin phenotype PI Z (Kurachi *et al.*, 1981)) point mutation. In contrast, more than 35 different mutations have so far been identified in β-thalassaemias (Antonarakis *et al.*, 1985a). In fact, a β-thalassaemia 'homozygote' is often a compound heterozygote with two distinct mutations on its two chromosomes. In several other diseases, one can already predict that a different mutation will exist in each family. Indeed, in X-linked severe diseases (Duchenne muscular dystrophy, haemophilias, etc.), or in dominant diseases which affect reproductive fitness (neurofibromatosis, Marfan syndrome or dominant forms of osteogenesis imperfecta), an important proportion of cases are due to new mutations which are lost after a few generations (Vogel and Motulsky, 1979). In contrast, it is thought that a small number of independent mutations are at the origin of the Huntington's chorea (Conneally, 1984). The main limitation of a direct mutation detection as a diagnostic approach is therefore due to the heterogeneity of mutations in a given disease.

In those conditions where extensive genetic material is deleted from the genome, as for the major variety of α-thalassaemias in South-East Asia, direct diagnosis by restriction mapping is straightforward. But when more subtle genetic defects are involved, specific assays must be designed. Sickle-cell anaemia provides a particularly illustrative example. The glutamic acid to valine substitution, in the sixth codon of the β^S chain results from an A-T nucleotide change in the DNA. This change alters the sequence of a region normally recognised and cleaved by three different restriction enzymes (MnlI, DdeI and MstII). Southern-blot analysis of normal and sickle-cell DNAs will yield restriction fragments of different sizes provided the appropriate DNA probe is used. Unfortunately, most forms of β-thalassaemia are not directly detectable by restriction analysis (Antonarakis et al., 1985a).

When the sequence change of a particular form of β-thalassaemia has been identified in a family or a population at risk, short oligonucleotide probes are synthesised. These oligomers are homologous either to the 'healthy' sequence or the 'mutated' one. Under carefully controlled hybridisation conditions, such pairs of probes will identify their complementary counterpart in restriction digest of human DNA (cf. Fig. 1 from Orkin, 1984; and Conner et al., 1983; Piratsu et al., 1983). Prenatal diagnosis of ZZ status in α-antitrypsin deficiency has also been performed using a synthetic probe (Kidd et al., 1984). As specific globin mutations are concentrated in particular ethnic groups, judicious probe panels may be devised by the diagnostic laboratories depending on the population to be examined. In order to identify those mutations present in a population, efficient use can be made of the presence of polymorphic restriction sites within or near the genes, as shown in the example of haemoglobinopathies.

17.2.5 Polymorphic Restriction Sites and Haplotypes

The coexistence in the population of more than one variant for a given locus is called genetic polymorphism. We have shown that restriction maps of the 'wild-type' and 'mutated' alleles may sometimes be differentiated. We have already mentioned that the 'wild-type' may itself by polymorphic in the sense that different sequence variants can be distinguished by Southern-blotting experiments which are not detected as phenotypic variants: these fortuitous variations in DNA sequence, pre-existing in the population at large, result in restriction fragment length polymorphisms (RFLPs). Because the restriction map is largely independent of gene function, these RFLPs can be detected irrespective of whether the sequence change affects the phenotype and, due to the great proportion of non-coding or non-regulating DNA sequences in human genome, only a minority of RFLPs actually affect the phenotype. Therefore, differences in restriction map between individuals are remarkable genetic markers.

The main advantages of the above are the following. RFLPs are numerous (estimates of DNA variation are in the range 1 nucleotide per 100–500 (Jeffreys, 1979; Murray *et al.*, 1983; Cooper *et al.*, 1985; Oberlé *et al.*, 1986b), and they therefore allow the extension of classical linkage analysis which was impaired by the low number of phenotypically polymorphic markers like red blood cell antigens, electrophoretic protein variants or phenotypic traits such as Daltonism. They are co-dominant genetic markers, i.e. one allele does not conceal another, so both alleles can be scored in heterozygous individuals (we can directly assess the genotype of an individual). They also keep the advantages noticed above for DNA analysis: a small amount of biological material is needed and DNA can be extracted from any nucleated cells. Restriction mapping can be carried out with 5 μg of DNA. Now, about 50 μg of DNA is routinely extracted per ml of blood, and chorionic villus biopsy or amniocyte cultures yield 10 to 50 μg of DNA.

In 1979, Kan and Dozy reported that many negroes suffering from sickle-cell anaemia lacked a HpaI site at the 3' flanking region of their β-globin gene. The linkage disequilibrium (i.e. non-random association) between this RFLP and the sickle-cell mutation in this ethnic group has led to a more extensive study of DNA polymorphisms in the β-globin cluster. Not less than 17 polymorphic restriction sites have been detected. It is probably relevant to note that only one such RFLP lies within the coding portion of the β-globin gene (Orkin and Kazazian, 1984). Although this could in theory give $2^{17} \simeq 130,000$ different combinations (haplo-types), only a relatively small number have been observed in human populations (due to the existence of linkage disequilibrium between the different sites). Why was it interesting to 'haplotype' the β-globin cluster? By analyzing many polymorphic sites within and around genes we increase the likelihood of distinguishing 'wild-type' and mutated chromosomes without cloning and sequencing them or even using a large panel of oligonucleotide probes. Orkin *et al.* hypothesised that, since β-thalassaemias are restricted to some ethnic groups, they should have occurred relatively recently, and might thus be found predominantly associated with particular haplotypes (Orkin *et al.*, 1982). In a preliminary study of β-thalassaemia in Mediterraneans, nine mutant globin genes present on nine different haplotypes were isolated and sequenced, revealing eight different mutations. In a subsequent study, Kazazian *et al.* (1984) used synthetic oligonucleotide probes specific for ten different β-thalassaemia mutations known to be present in Mediterraneans to detect directly by analysis of genomic DNA the type of mutation present in each of 162 Mediterranean β-thalassaemia genes, and determined in parallel the restriction site haplotypes. 156 of the 162 β genes contained one of the ten mutations. On average, about 85 % of cases with a given mutation corresponded to a single haplotype and, conversely 85 % of the mutations within a given haplotype were of a single type (Antonarakis *et al.*, 1985a). This systematic strategy was extended to other ethnic groups by cloning and sequencing one or two globin genes from each different haplotype. Twenty-three new uncharacterised mutations were found (out of 30 genes analysed), showing the great power of this approach. In fact, when a mutation is present in two haplotypes, this can in general be explained by a single recombination event occurring in a region, 5' to the β-globin gene, which is thought to be a 'hot spot' for crossing over. A similar analysis on the β^s mutation showed that it can be found associated with three major haplotypes which cannot derive from each other by a few recombination events. These 3 β^s-bearing chromosomes are in fact concentrated in different geographic regions of Africa, which strongly suggests three independent origins for β^s mutation in Africa. Moreover, it was recently demonstrated, by such haplotype studies, that a single, relatively recent, mutational event probably originated the Z allele of α-antitrypsin in Caucasians (Cox *et al.*, 1985).

17.2.6 Polymorphic Restriction Sites and Diagnosis

RFLPs detected by Southern-blotting experiments using a gene-specific probe provide a powerful diagnostic tool, especially in diseases where great mutational heterogeneity is expected. Since the RFLPs are usually not the result of the mutation, it is necessary in each family at risk to perform a minimal segregation analysis in order to identify the allele associated with the mutated gene. The two main limitations of this method are related to the informativeness of the family material and the informativeness of the RFLPs.

This will be illustrated with an example of prenatal diagnosis for the X-linked disease haemophilia B. The defective gene responsible for haemophilia B is coding for the coagulation factor IX, and the cDNA of this gene was shown to detect a two-allele RFLP in DNAs digested with the TagI restriction enzyme (Camerino *et al.*, 1984). The two allelic restriction fragments are 1.8 and 1.3 kilobases (kb) long, and 40 % of the population (here, 40 % of the women) are heterozygous at the locus. This latter figure can be considered, in first approximation, as the 'informativeness' of the probe. In the family examined by Tønnesen *et al.* (Fig. 17.2 is from Tønnesen *et al.*, 1984), haemophilia B was associated with the allele of 1.8 kb, since the affected individual III6 has this allelic pattern. Unfortunately, in the obligate carrier women II1 and II4, it was impossible to differentiate the two X chromosomes since they are homozygous. In other terms, they are 'uninformative' and the carrier status of their daughters could not be established by DNA analysis. Nevertheless, DNA analysis allowed a first-trimester prenatal diagnosis in this particular example, since the pregnant woman (III3) was heterozygous for the TaqI RFLP. Indeed, her male foetus (IV1) was shown to have received the 1.3 kb allele from his healthy grandfather. Other successful carrier diagnoses have been reported using this TaqI RFLP (Grunebaum *et al.*, 1984), but the need for improved informativeness of the factor IX probe has led to a search for other polymorphic restriction sites within the factor IX gene. It can be estimated that the combined use of XmnI, HinfI or DdeI (Winship *et al.*, 1984) and MspI (Camerino *et al.*, 1985) RFLPs will enable prenatal and carrier diagnosis in 65–70 % of haemophilia-B families.

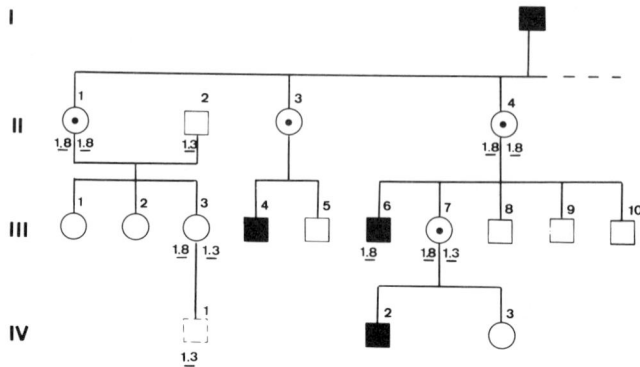

Fig 17.2 Exclusion of haemophilia B in the male foetus by analysis of a DNA polymorphism within the coagulation factor IX gene. In the illustrated partial pedigree of the family studied, the open squares denote normal males, the closed squares affected males and the dotted circles obligate female carriers. The daughter (III 3) of an obligate carrier (II 1) consulted in the eighth week of pregnancy. Coagulation assays to identify her carrier status were inconclusive. After chorionic villus biopsy (ninth week), her male foetus (IV 1) was shown to have received the 1.3 kb allele from his healthy maternal grandfather (II 2).

In some cases, such diagnosis will not be possible if the only affected sib or one or both parents are dead or unavailable. Useful information, however, can be gained from an unaffected sib (especially in X-linked diseases), from grandparents (who are often essential for the obtention of the coupling phase between the polymorphic marker and the defective gene in X-linked or autosomal dominant diseases), or from other family members. Thus, genetic counsellors and physicians should be aware of the importance of establishing complete pedigrees and of keeping blood samples from affected or aged individuals in families likely to ask for prenatal diagnosis in the future. This latter recommendation extends to diseases for which no diagnosis is available at present.

17.3 Indirect Analysis of Genetic Disease: The Deficit is Unknown

A most important problem that geneticists still face concerns the diseases for which we have no knowledge about the corresponding gene or protein (cystic fibrosis, Huntington's chorea, Duchenne muscular dystrophy, etc.). Considerable efforts have been devoted to seeking out the molecular defect in these inherited diseases, but recombinant DNA techniques provide a new expedient for approaching it by reviving the mapping of human genome; we can already forecast that isolation of the causative gene in many hereditary disorders will stem from their mapping in the genome.

17.3.1 Physical Mapping of Human Genome

17.3.1.1 Hybrid Panels

Panels of human–rodent somatic cell hybrids can be successfully used for the chromosomal or subchromosomal mapping of cloned probes (Ruddle, 1981). If DNAs from the various cell lines are blotted on a re-usable support (such as DBM paper or nylon membranes), a localisation can be obtained in a few days. Contrary to the use of enzymatic markers, mapping with cloned probes is independent of the expression of the gene in cultured cells, and it is always possible to find a restriction enzyme that will differentiate between the pattern of the rodent and human sequence. Subchromosomal mapping is possible if one uses hybrid cell lines which contain various portions of a given chromosome derived from translocations (Oberlé *et al.*, 1986b), X irradiation (Goss and Harris, 1975), or chromosome transfer (Miller and Ruddle, 1978; Klobutcher and Ruddle, 1981). Such lines are, however, rare for chromosomes which lack a selectable marker, such as the HPRT gene (for the X chromosome) or the thymidine kinase gene (for chromosome 17). Selectable markers might be introduced by transformation with cloned DNA (corresponding antibiotic resistance genes, the bacterial XGPT gene, etc) (Athwal *et al.*, 1985). Combined with the technique of microcell mediated chromosome transfer this could allow the construction of hybrids containing a single human chromosome (or portion of chromosome) in a rodent background (Saxon *et al.*, 1985). Such hybrids might in turn be very useful for obtaining DNA sequences mapping in a particular chromosome region.

17.3.1.2 In situ Hybridisation

In recent years, *in situ* hybridisation with tritium-labelled probes (Gerhard *et al.*, 1981) has become an extremely efficient way of mapping genes with an increasing resolution (which may be improved in the future by the use of non-radioactive probes). *In situ* hybridisation is also possible with abnormal chromosomes, allowing the mapping of a cloned gene with respect to a translocation breakpoint or a fragile site (Lindgren *et al.*, 1984; Mattei *et al.*, 1985a, 1985b).

17.3.1.3 Gene Dosage

The Southern-blotting technique can be used in gene dosage experiments with DNAs from patients having unbalanced translocations or interstitial deletions (De Martinville *et al.*, 1985). There, too, it might be useful to constitute panels of appropriate cell lines for each chromosome. Many such lines are now available through the Human Cell Repository in Camden (NJ). It should be pointed out that when a large number of probes is available for a given chromsome, the information gained can be extremely useful for the ordering of translocation breakpoints with respect to each other, for characterising the extent of interstitial deletions, and for defining the minimal extent of a deletion or a partial trisomy associated with a specific clinical sympatomatology (deletions associated with retinoblastoma (Benedict *et al.*, 1983), Wilms tumor (Francke *et al.*, 1979, 1985), Prader Willi syndrome (Ledbetter *et al.*, 1982), etc.).

17.3.2 Linkage Mapping of Human Genome

Human gene mapping by linkage analysis combines traditional methods of Mendelian genetics, with RFLPs as genetic markers provided by modern molecular biology. As illustrated in Fig. 17.3, segregation analysis will consider the inheritance of traits such as hair colour or sequence variations in genomic DNA segments. If the locus defining, say, the hair colour and the locus detecting the RFLP are 'linked enough' (*see below*) they will tend to be inherited together through meiosis. As physical mapping of any cloned DNA probe is easy, we can also infer the physical mapping of the phenotypic trait we examine (here the hair colour).

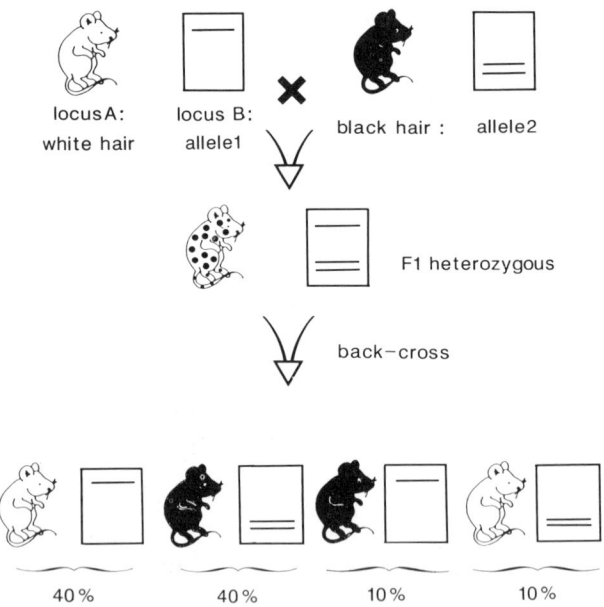

Fig. 17.3 Use of restriction polymorphisms as genetic markers to measure recombination frequencies from phenotypic markers. Homozygous individuals (for the restriction marker and for the phenotypic trait) are crossed. Their progeny (F1 generation) are heterozygous. After a back-cross (genetic cross between the F1 individuals and their homozygous parents), one observes 80 % of mice with the parental type and 20 % recombinants; the restriction marker, then, is 10 map units from the locus responsible for hair color.

17.3.2.1 RFLPs as Genetic Markers

Botstein *et al.* (1980) proposed a general strategy for mapping the human genome using such markers, both by constructing a marker-to-marker linkage map and by testing for linkage of these markers with genetic diseases. Although it was initially estimated that 200 polymorphic probes located 20 centimorgans apart would be sufficient to cover the whole genome, a much larger number will be necessary since the markers are not evenly spaced, and because a single marker is often not informative enough to detect linkage efficiently.

The number of DNA probes which detect RFLPs is increasing at a very rapid pace (*see* Table 17.1). These can correspond to cloned gene sequences (cDNA or genomic probes) with known function, or to random DNA segments ('anonymous' probes). The latter can be obtained from total genomic libraries (Maniatis *et al.*, 1978), but a very efficient way of obtaining many markers for a given chromosome is to use libraries of genomic DNA highly enriched in sequences of this chromosome. Such libraries can be prepared using DNA from mitotic chromosomes purified on a cell sorter (Carrano *et al.*, 1979), or from hybrid cells containing a single human chromosome (or chromosome fragment) (Olsen *et al.*, 1980). Chromsome-specific libraries of either type have been prepared for many chromosomes (Davies *et al.*, 1981; Krumlauf *et al.*, 1982; Cavanee *et al.*, 1984). It is now possible to prepare libraries of overlapping DNA fragments from sorted chromosomes (Kunkel *et al.*, 1985b), and this should facilitate genome walking by decreasing the size of the libraries which have to be screened. A project is underway at the Lawrence Livermore Laboratory in Los Alamos (USA) to prepare chromosome-specific libraries for each of the human chromosomes which will be made available to the scientific community.

About one base position in 100 to 500 will show variation in the human population, so that it is in general possible to find RFLPs with any unique sequence probe if enough different restriction enzymes are used (20 or more). Some regions, however, appear particularly devoid of polymorphisms (e.g. thyroglobulin (Baas *et al.*, 1984) and coagulation factor VIII (Gitschier *et al.*, 1985b)).

Most RFLPs studied are two allele polymorphisms which have a limited informativeness in linkage analysis, since at most 50 % of the individuals will be homozygous for such a marker. Therefore, in a typical nuclear family (two parents and the affected proband), these two-allele markers will be useful for diagnosis in 50 % of the cases for an X-linked disease, and in 43.7 % and 31.2 % of the cases for recessive or dominant autosomal diseases, respectively. Higher figures will be obtained if the recessive disease occurs in a consanguineous family, or if more family members can be studied. As already stated, it is possible to extend the informativeness of a probe by searching for additional RFLPs with additional enzymes and/or by using contiguous DNA segments (as was done for the β-globin cluster and its 17 different RFLPs). However, this approach is cumbersome as different probes and restriction enzyme digests must be used for a single locus and the existence of linkage disequilibrium between closely located polymorphic sites restricts the informativeness of the additional RFLPs.

Much more interesting for linkage analysis are probes that reveal multiple alleles with a single restriction enzyme digest. Such a probe was initially described by Wyman and White (1980), but similar loci initially proved rare; other examples were found near the insulin gene, the Ha-ras-1 gene, the α-related globin gene, and in the q28 region of the X chromosome (Bell et al., 1982; Capon et al., 1983; Goodbourn et al., 1983; Oberlé et al., 1985a). For the four latter cases sequence analysis revealed that the polymorphism was due to the presence of a satellite-like sequence (i.e. tandem repeats of a short sequence element) with variation in the number of repeat units in different alleles. Recently, a more systematic search for such sequences using as a starting probe a minisatellite sequence found within the human myoglobin gene allowed Jeffreys et al. to isolate probes which can detect several unlinked hypervariable loci (Jeffreys et al., 1985a). It has been calculated that the probability of observing an identical pattern in two individuals with one of the probes is less than 10^{-10} (Jeffreys et al., 1985b). Such markers have the additional advantage that the genotype of deceased family ancestors can often be deduced. These hypervariable loci should be extremely valuable for linkage analysis. See, for example, the use of the St14 probe for mapping diseases in the Xq28 region (Boué et al., 1985; Oberlé et al., 1985b, 1986a), and the startling very recent discovery of close linkage between the polycystic kidney disease locus and the minisatellite sequence close to the α-globin locus (Reeders et al., 1985).

17.3.2.2 Linkage Analysis and Genetic Distances

As already stated, traditional Mendelian genetics determines distance between loci of a genetic map as recombination frequencies, which implies the introduction of statistical evaluation of the experimental data. This requirement results from the experimental procedure used in linkage analysis.

Linkage analysis involves tracing the inheritance of genetic markers in families and correlating the data with the inheritance of the disease gene. One tries to identify, by trial and error, the genetic markers passed on to progeny which are most frequently associated with the disease. Occasionally, a recombination event between the two loci will reassert the linked alleles (hence the experimental estimate of recombination fraction). Therefore, very large families are studied preferentially, in order to obtain statistically significant scores of coinheritance for the marker and the disease. Another prerequisite is the careful clinical analysis of the tested families, in order to ascertain the exact status of the largest number of individuals (normal, affected, carrier, etc.).

Usually, data concerning linkage between two loci are reported as their lod score. The probability of observing one allele of the RFLP and the disease in a family, given no linkage, is calculated (recombination fraction = 0.5). This is compared with the probability of observing the same combination of traits over a selective range of recombination fractions, assuming linkage. The logarithm of the ratio of these likelihoods is referred as the lod score. Lod scores from different families can be added and, the statistical significance improved by further analysis. A lod score of +3 indicates 1,000 to 1 odds in favour of linkage at a particular value of recombination, whereas a lod score of -2 means that independent segregation of both loci is 100 times more likely at that recombination value than linkage.

An example of such linkage analysis is shown in Fig. 17.4 (from Oberlé *et al.*, 1985b). In this family, haemophilia A and allele 4 of the TaqI RFLP, as detected by the anonymous probe St14, always segregate together through three generations. This close linkage between St14 and haemophilia A was also observed in eleven other families; this is unlikely to happen by chance and yields odds in favour of linkage of 4.4×10^9 to 1 (lod score = 9.65). The 95 % confidence interval for the recombination frequency between these two loci is 0 to 6.5 percent. Further linkage analysis increased the lod score to 28.65 and narrowed the 95 % confidence interval (Gitschier *et al.*, 1985b).

17.3.3 Successful Mapping of some Neurogenetic Disorders

17.3.3.1 Huntington's Disease (or Chorea)

Huntington's chorea (HD) highlights the potentialities of linkage analysis to RFLPs for mapping a neurogenetic disorder whose underlying deficit and chromosomal location were unknown. This autosomal dominant disease is characterised by a late age of onset (usually 30–50 years), which poses tremendous problems in genetic counselling. Gusella *et al.* (1983) reported linkage between G8, a random probe, and HD. The G8 probe was then localised, by hybridisation to DNAs from a hybrid panel, to the short arm of chromosome 4.

Two polymorphic restriction sites were initially detected by the enzyme HindIII (Gusella *et al.*, 1983), one more is detected by PstI, and two others by EcoRI (cited in Folstein *et al.*, 1985). Approximately 95 % of individuals are heterozygous at one or more sites, and haplotypes can also be assigned to them. The most conservative estimate of recombination frequency between G8 and HD is 6 %, with a 95 % confidence interval of 0–12 % (Folstein *et al.*, 1985). The error rate of genotype assignment thus excludes G8 segregation analysis from genetic counselling practice.

The discovery of this DNA marker is, nevertheless, already applicable to HD research. For example, the fact that some linkage relationships were found in HD families from different ethnic groups and with different clinical manifestations, strengthens the assumption of genetic homogeneity in HD. Physical mapping of the HD locus will focus the search on the short arm of chromosome 4 in order to find additional DNA markers closer to the disease locus, or flanking it.

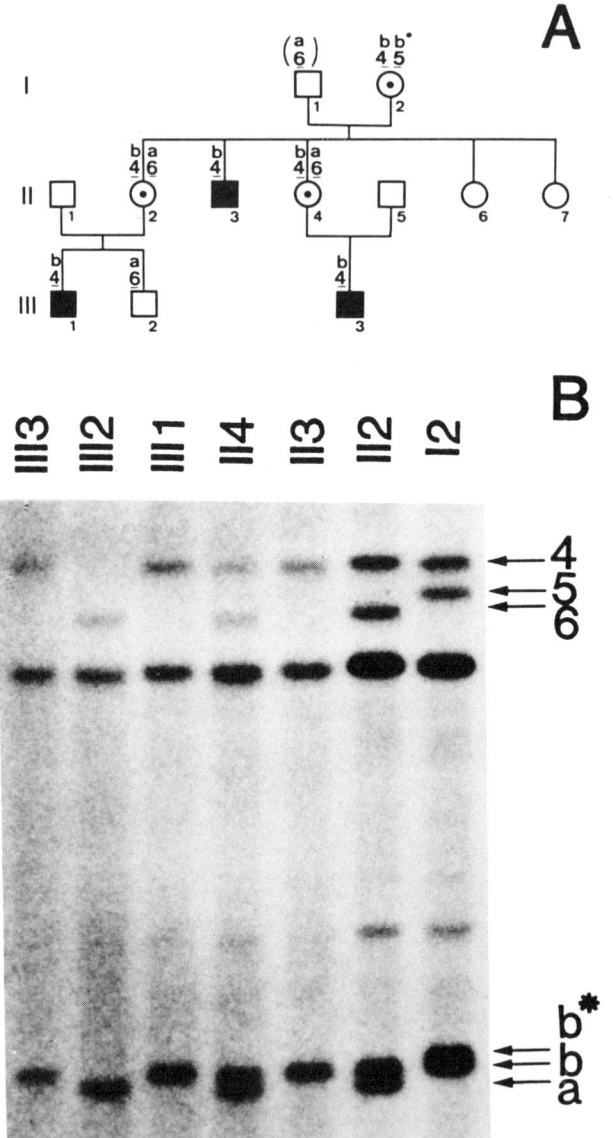

Fig. 17.4 Example of linkage analysis between haemophilia A and an anonymous probe, St14. (A) Pedigree of the family. The open squares denote normal males, the closed squares affected males and the dotted circles obligate female carriers. The underlined numbers refer to the individual genotypes at the St14 locus (alleles detected by St14 in TaqI digests). The genotype of the grandfather (I1) was deduced from the gentoype of II2 and II4. (B) Southern-blot analysis of TaqI-digested DNAs from members of the family. Fragments corresponding to alleles 4, 5 and 6 are indicated on the right. Another polymorphism revealed by St14 was detected in this family (allles a, b and b*). It also shows concordant segregation with haemophilia A.

If DNA markers very closely linked to HD are identified, cloning and characterisation of the abnormal gene on the basis of its map location can be anticipated (Gusella *et al.*, 1984). This would imply a chromosome-walking procedure
which uses the closest linked marker as a starting probe for the isolation of
neighbouring DNA sequences. This walking strategy has been proved effective
in *Drosophila* (Bender *et al.*, 1983; Haenlin *et al.*, 1985), but its application to
the human genome could be more difficult due to its complexity (twenty times
that of *Drosophila*) and due to the abundance of interspersed, repetitive
sequences. Two other problems will be encountered: how to estimate the length
and the direction of the 'walk'; and how to know that one has 'arrived'. It
should indeed be remembered that, on average, 1 % of recombination corresponds to 1,000 kb of DNA sequences, and that genetic distances are very
roughly estimated (the G8 probe may be separated from the HD locus by 500,
5,000 or even 12,000 kb!). Nevertheless, as proposed by Gusella *et al.* (1984),
linkage analysis will provide milestones during the chromosome walking: as the
walk proceeds towards the disease locus, recombination events, which were
revealed with the G8 probe will disappear from segregation analysis with new
probes generated along the walk.

In conclusion, HD was the first neurogenetic disorder to be mapped by linkage analysis to DNA markers. In the human genome, over 450 loci are already
assigned to a specific chromosome. 115 among these loci were confirmed as
X-linked traits (McKusick, 1983). It is rather simple to identify the X-linked
segregation pattern of a disease since, although they are usually recessive disorders, X-linked diseases behave as dominant traits in male progeny. This
chromosome was, therefore, the first target for the construction of a genetic
map including disease loci (Drayna *et al.*, 1984). In the following two examples
of X-linked neurogenetic disorders, subchromosomal location of the disease
locus afforded help in the screening of probes to be tested for linkage analysis.

17.3.3.2 Duchenne Muscular Dystrophy

Duchenne muscular dystrophy (DMD) is one of the most frequent, fatal X-linked
diseases (1 in 3–4,000 live male births), leading to death by about twenty years
of age. The very high rate of new mutations (nearly one-third of the cases) has
led investigators to suggest that either the gene is very large, or it lies in a site
prone to chromosomal rearrangements or recombinations. The DMD gene has
been mapped to the short arm of the X chromosome, in the p21 cytogenetically-
defined region. This mapping results from the cytogenetic analysis of the rare
females who expressed the DMD phenotype because their active X chromosome
was disrupted in p21 by X-autosome translocations (Verellen Dumoulin *et al.*,
1984; Worton *et al.*, 1984). This mapping was confirmed by cases in which cytogenetically visible deletions involving at least this region were detected in a
woman (Francke, 1984) and in a boy (Francke *et al.*, 1985).

Molecular biologists began to clone X-specific DNA markers and to screen them for their subchromosomal localisation (*see* Section 17.3.1). The first two probes reported as flanking markers of DMD were too far away and not informative enough to be accurate tools for diagnosis or for walking purposes (Davies *et al.*, 1983). Nevertheless, their linkage data were consistent with the assignment of DMD to the Xp21. Such linkage analyses were performed with Becker muscular dystrophy, a milder form of muscle degenerative disorder, which suggested that Becker muscular dystrophy and DMD may be allelic (Kingston *et al.*, 1984).

The use for diagnostic purposes of eleven polymorphic probes has recently been proposed (Bakker *et al.*, 1985), but the successful cloning of DNA fragments detecting deletions in or very near the DMD gene is the major breakthrough towards more accurate detection of females carrying the gene, and prenatal diagnosis. After cloning DNA sequences absent from one of the deletions responsible for DMD, Kunkel *et al.* (1985a) generated probes which detected deletions in 10 % of DMD-affected males (Monaco *et al.*, 1985). These probes will help delineate the extent of the DMD locus and are the best foreseeable starting points for chromosome walking. (The historical account of the rapid progress towards the cloning of the DMD gene has been very recently reviewed (Kedes, 1985) but is already outdated).

17.3.3.3 Fragile X-mental Retardation

The fragile X-mental retardation syndrome (Fra X) represents a complex and confusing situation for genetic counselling. It is a very prevalent X-linked disorder (1 in 1,500 newborn males), with pleiotropic traits consisting of: (a) the presence of a fragile site on the X chromosome at the q27-q28 interface, induced *in vitro* by conditions which impair thymidylate synthesis; (b) a variable (moderate to severe) degree of mental retardation in hemizygous males, usually accompanied by characteristic physical features; and (c) a 35 % risk of mental impairment in heterozygous females (for reviews see Turner and Jacobs, 1983; Sutherland, 1985). The genetics of the Fra X syndrome depart from classical X-linked inheritance in several respects. The Fra X gene does not appear to be fully penetrant in males: apparently normal males (cytogenetically and/or clinically) can transmit the disease. The percentage of clinically expressing females is much higher than in other sex-linked diseases. The diagnosis of carrier females is difficult, however, since only about one half of females who carry the Fra X mutation can be detected by their phenotype (mental retardation and/or fragile site expression (Sherman *et al.*, 1984)).

Probes mapping in Xq27-q28 were used for linkage analysis. Practically, two probes detecting TaqI RFLPs have been used: the coagulation factor IX gene (Camerino *et al.*, 1984), and the anonymous St14 probe (Oberlé *et al.*, 1985a). In a three-point linkage analysis (Lathrop and Lalouel, 1984; Oberlé *et al.*, 1986a) as well as by *in situ* hybridisation (Mattei *et al.*, 1985a), the Fra X locus was placed between the two marker loci. This supports further the notion that the mutation is located in the same region as the cytogenetically demonstratable fragile site. The estimate of the recombination fraction for the linkage factor IX-XFra was 0.12 (90 % confidence interval: 0.044-0.225) and 0.10 for St14-XFra (90 % confidence interval: 0.040-0.185). Several other estimates of the genetic distance between factor IX and the Fra X locus yield higher recombination fractions. Discrepancies between linkage data may result from heterogeneity among families, but statistical tools sensitive enough are rather difficult to devise for data samples as small as those provided by linkage analysis (see, however, Brown et al., 1985).

17.3.4 Linkage Analysis and Diagnosis

Diagnostic use of RFLPs linked to a disease has the same advantages and limitations as previously noticed (see Sections 17.2.6 and 17.3.2.1) for RFLPs within or near a gene. However, the estimated genetic distance between the DNA markers and the disease introduces a systematic error in diagnoses (confidence limits of this recombination fraction must also be taken into account).

In order to limit the diagnostic errors, it is important to use at least two markers which flank the disease locus. Indeed, if the two DNA markers are within 10 % recombination units from the disease locus, the probability of misdiagnosis due to a double recombination will only be 1 %. DMD and the Fra X mental retardation are examples where such diagnosis is presently possible (Bakker et al., 1985; Oberlé et al., 1985c). A single linked marker may also be used if the data suggest very close linkage (i.e. with narrow 95 % confidence limits) and/or if combined with information from other types of assay (i.e. biological dosages such as coagulating activity for haemophilia, creatine kinase for DMD, cytogenetic analysis for Fra X, etc.). Computer programs have been designed to calculate risks which combine data from segregation analysis and quantitative biological assays (Lathrop and Lalouel, 1984; and, for applications, Oberlé et al., 1985b).

17.3.5 Linkage to 'Candidate' Genes

An alternative to the random search for linked markers is the testing of 'candidate' genes when they have been cloned and when they are polymorphic. RFLPs in or near the gene would mark the inheritance of specific alleles of the gene in an affected family. If the tested gene is responsible for the disease we would expect a complete co-segregation of one allele with the affected phenotype. Of course, such positive findings are only strong evidence for a causal role of the gene, but lack of cosegregation is sufficient to exclude the tested gene as the primary defect in the families analysed. The latter restriction refers to the possible genetic heterogeneity of the disease, which could complicate such an approach (since different families having different forms of a disorder could yield different segregation data with a given candidate gene).

Positive results were obtained in osteogenesis imperfecta with type I collagen genes (Chu *et al.*, 1983; Pihlajaniemi *et al.*, 1984) and with probes for the α antithrombin III gene in a family with hereditary thrombosis (Prochownick *et al.*, 1983). Congenital adrenal hyperplasia results from a deficiency of 21-hydroxylase. Because of an intriguing close linkage between this recessive disorder and the major histocompatibility complex, White *et al.* (1984) tested cDNA clones of P-450 C_{21} as candidate gene and demonstrated its involvement in this disease. Another successful strategy was illustrated by the study of familial amyloidotic polyneuropathy in Japan. This autosomal dominant disease is characterised by systemic accumulation of amyloid fibrils and progressive disorder of peripheral nerves. In the Japanese type, amyloid fibril protein isolated from patients and has been shown to react with an antiserum to normal plasma prealbumin. An amino acid substitution (Met → Val) at position 30 in this protein is closely related to the disease and is thought to lead to amyloid fibril formation (Kametani *et al.*, 1984). The cloning and sequencing of the cDNA for normal human prealbumin (Sasaki *et al.*, 1984) demonstrated the presence of the expected mutation in the DNA of affected patients and provided a tool for presymptomatic diagnosis of familial amyloidotic polyneuropathy (Sasaki *et al.*, 1985). This recent example illustrates one important point to remember when one 'chooses' candidate genes for testing. One might think that, in a disease which affects a particular organ, the causative gene should be expressed more specifically in that organ. However, a mutation in a plasma protein is responsible for the Japanese type of familial amyloidotic polyneuropathy, and other neurological diseases such as Lesch–Nyhan and phenylketonuria are due to deficiencies in a housekeeping gene and in a liver-specific gene, respectively. Transgenic mice are being used to assess the molecular basis of the cell-specific expression of the disease in the case of the Lesch–Nyhan disease (Stout *et al.*, 1985).

Segregation analysis did not support the involvement of the β-nerve growth factor in hereditary neurofibromatosis (Darby *et al.*, 1985). This approach can be applied to more complex situations, such as polygenic diseases or genetic predisposition to diseases. Negative results have so far excluded the Harvey Ras and Kirsten Ras oncogene loci as the cause of Gardner syndrome in families with this genetic predisposition to colon cancer (Barker *et al.*, 1983). Many genes involved in lipid metabolism and transport are being cloned, and linkage analysis is being performed in families with hyperlipidaemia. At present, it has been shown that different mutations in the LDL receptor gene can cause familial hypercholesterolaemia, an autosomal dominant trait (Tolleshaug *et al.*, 1983; Lehman *et al.*, 1985), and RFLPs within its cDNA should allow presymptomatic diagnosis (Humphries *et al.*, 1985).

Population analysis offers an alternative to familial segregation analysis: one compares the frequency of a given allele, or haplotype, in the normal and affected population in search of linkage disequilibrium. This could be used to look for a genetic predisposition to trisomy 21 (Antonarakis *et al.*, 1985b). Some controversial results have also been reported concerning the association of specific alleles at the insulin locus with insulin-dependent or -independent diabetes (Rotwein *et al.*, 1981; Owerbach *et al.*, 1982a,b; Mandrup-Poulsen *et al.*, 1984).

17.4 Conclusion

What could be the impact of DNA recombinant technology in the study of Alzheimer's disease? In the families where typical Mendelian segregation of the disease has been identified, linkage analysis might facilitate chromosomal location or even gene isolation. Linkage analysis could be first attempted with DNA markers belonging to the candidate chromosome (the chromosome 21) or candidate genes (CAT, amyloid plaque core proteins, etc.). Besides helping diagnostic medicine, identification of the mutant gene should provide new insights into the pathogenesis of the disease and lead to a more logical pharmacological and therapeutic approach. Furthermore, it might yield information concerning genetically programmed functions of the human nervous system.

Acknowledgements

I am grateful to C. Kister, A. Marrell and C. Werlé for their help with the preparation of the mansucript.

References

Alter, B. P. (1981). *The Lancet*, **ii**, 1152–5.
Antonarakis, S. E., Kazazian, H. H., and Orkin, S. H. (1985a). *Hum. Genet.*, **69**, 1–14.
Antonarakis, S. E., Phillips, J. A., and Kazazian, H. H. (1982). *J. Pediatr.*, **100**, 845–56.
Antonarakis, S. E., Kittur, S. D., Metaxotou, C., Watkins, P. C., and Patel, A. S. (1985b). *Proc. Natl Acad. Sci. USA*, **82**, 3360–4.
Athwal, R. S., Smarsh, M., Searle, B. M., and Deo, S. S. (1985). *Somat. Cell. Mol. Genet.*, **11**, 177–82.
Baas, F., Bikker, H., Van Ommen, G. J. B., and De Vijlder, J. J. M. (1984). *Hum. Genet.*, **67**, 301–5.
Bakker, E., Hofker, M. H., Goor, N., Mandel, J. L., Wrogeman, K., Davies, K. E., Kunkel, L. M., Willard, H. F., Fenton, W. A., Sandkuyl, L., Majoor-Krakauer, D., Essen, A. J. V., Jahoda, M. G. J., Sachs, E. S., Van Ommen, G. J. B., and Pearson, P. L. (1985). *Lancet*, **i**, 655–8.
Barker, D., McCoy, M., Weinberg, R. (1983). *Mol. Biol. Med.*, **1**, 199–206.
Barsh, G. S., Roush, C. L., Bonadio, J., Byers, P. J., and Gelinas, R. E. (1985). *Proc. Natl Acad. Sci. USA*, **82**, 2870–4.
Bell, G. I., Selby, M. I., and Rutter, W. J. (1982). *Nature*, **295**, 31–5.
Bender, W., Arkam, M., Karch, F., Beachy, P. A., Peifer, M., Spierer, P., Lewis, E. B., and Hogness, D. S. (1983). *Science*, **221**, 23–9.

Benedict, W. F., Murphee, A. L., Banerjee, A., Spina, C. A., Sparkes, Ma., and Sparkes, R. S. (1983). *Science*, 219, 973–5.

Botstein, D., White, R. L., Skolnick, M., and Davis, R. W. (1980). *Am. J. Hum. Genet.*, 32, 314–31.

Boué, J., Oberlé, I., Heilig, R., Mandel, J. L., Moser, A., Moser, H., Larsen, J. W., Dumez, Y., and Boué, A. (1985). *Hum. Genet.*, 69, 272–4.

Brown, W. T., Gross, A. C., Chan, C. B., and Jenkins, E. C. (1985). *Hum. Genet.*, 71, 11–18.

Camerino, G., Oberlé, I., Drayna, D., and Mandel, J. L. (1985). *Hum. Genet.*, 71, 79–81.

Camerino, G., Grzeschick, K. H., Jaye, M., De La Salle, H., Tolstoshev, P., Lecocq, J. P., Heilig, R., and Mandel, J. L. (1984). *Proc. Natl Acad. Sci. USA*, 81, 498–502.

Capon, D. J., Chen, E. Y., Levinson, A. D., Seeburg, P. H., and Goeddel, D. V. (1983). *Nature*, 302, 33–7.

Carrano, A. V., Gray, J. W., Langlois, R. G., Burkhart Schulz, K. J., and Van Dullo, M. A. (1979). *Proc. Natl Acad. Sci. USA*, 76, 1382–4.

Cavanee, W. K., Leach, R., Mohandas, T., Pearson, P., and White, R. L. (1984). *Am. J. Hum. Genet.*, 36, 10–24.

Chandhari, N., and Hahn, W. E. (1983). *Science*, 220, 924–8.

Cheah, K. S. E. (1985). *Biochem. J.*, 229, 287–303.

Chu, H. L., Williams, C. J., Pepe, G., Hirsch, J. L., Prockop, D. J., and Ramirez, F. (1983). *Nature*, 304, 78–80.

Church, G., and Gilbert, W. (1984). *Proc. Natl Acad. Sci. USA*, 81, 1991–5.

Conneally, P. M. (1984). *Am. J. Hum. Genet.*, 36, 506–26.

Conner, B. J., Reyes, A. A., Morin, C., Itakura, K., Teplitz, R. L., and Wallace, R. B. (1983). *Proc. Natl Acad. Sci. USA*, 80, 278–82.

Cooper, D. N., Smith, B. A., Cooke, H. J., Niemann, S., and Schmidtke, J. (1985). *Hum. Genet.*, 69, 201–5.

Cox, D. W., Woo, S. L. C., and Mansfield, T. (1985). *Nature*, 316, 79–81.

Darby, J. K., Feder, J., Selby, M., Riccardi, V., Ferrell, R., Siao, D., Goslin, K., Rutter, W., Shooter, E. M., and Cavalli-Sforza, L. L. (1985). *Am. J. Hum. Genet.*, 37, 52–9.

Davies, K. E., Young, B. D., Elles, R. G., Hill, M. E., and Williamson, R. (1981). *Nature*, 293, 374–6.

Davies, K. E., Pearson, P. L., Harper, P. S., Murray, J. M., O'Brien, T., Sarfarazi, M., and Williamson, R. (1983). *Nucl. Acids Res.*, 11, 2303–12.

De Martinville, B., Kunkel, L. M., Bruns, G., Morlé, F., Koenig, M., Mandel, J. L., Horwich, A., Latt, S. A., Gusella, G. F., Housman, D., and Francke, U. (1985). *Am. J. Hum. Genet.*, 37, 235–49.

Drayna, D., Davies, K., Hartley, D., Mandel, J. L., Camerino, G., Williamson, R., and White, R. (1984). *Proc. Natl Acad. Sci. USA*, 81, 2836–9.

Folstein, S. E., Phillips, J. A. III, Meyers, D. A., Chase, G. A., Abbott, M. H., Franz, M. L., Waber, P. G., Kazazian, H. H., Conneally, P. M., Hobbs, W., Tanzi, R., Faryniarz, A., Gibbons, K., and Gusella, J. (1985). *Science*, 229, 776–9.

Francke, U. (1984). *Cytogenet. Cell Genet.*, 38, 298–307.

Francke, U., Holmes, L. B., Atkins, L., and Riccardi, V. M. (1979). *Cytogenet. Cell Genet.*, 24, 185–92.

Francke, U., Ochs, H. D., De Martinville, B., Giacolone, J., Lindgren, V., Disteche, C., Pagon, R. A., Hofker, M. H., Van Ommen, G. J. B., Pearson, P. L., and Wedgwood, R. J. (1985). *Am. J. Hum. Genet.*, 37, 250–67.

Gerhard, D. S., Kawasaki, E. S., Bancroft, F. C., and Szabo, D. (1981). *Proc. Natl Acad. Sci. USA*, 78, 3755–9.

Giannelli, G., Choo, K. H., Rees, D. J. G., Boyd, Y., Rizza, C. R., and Brownlee, G. G. (1983). *Nature*, 303, 181–2.

Gitschier, J., Wood, W. I., Tuddenham, E. G. D., Shuman, M. A., Goralka, T. M., Chen, E. Y., and Lawn, R. M. (1985a). *Nature*, 315, 427–30.

Gitschier, J., Drayna, D., Tuddenham, E. G. D., White, R. L., and Lawn, R. M. (1985b). *Nature*, 314, 738–40.

Goodbourn, S. E. Y., Higgs, D. R., Clegg, J. B., and Weatherall, D. J. (1983). *Proc. Natl Acad. Sci. USA*, 80, 5022–6.

Goss, S. J., and Harris, H. (1975). *Nature*, 255, 680–4.

Grunebaum, L., Cazenave, J. P., Camerino, G., Kloepfer, C., Mandel, J. L., Tolstoshev, P., Jaye, M., De la Salle, H., and Lecocq, J. P. (1984). *J. Clin. Invest.*, 73, 1491-5.

Gusella, J. F., Tanzi, R. E., Anderson, M. A., Hobbs, W., Gibbons, K., Raschtchian, B., Gillian, T. C., Wallace, M. R., Wexler, N. S., and Conneally, P. M. (1984). *Science*, 225, 1320-6.

Gusella, J. F., Wexler, N. S., Conneally, P. M., Naylor, S. L., Anderson, M. A., Tanzi, R. E., Watkins, P. C., Ottina, K., Wallace, M. R., Sakaguchi, A. Y., Young, A. B., Shoulson, I., Bonilla, E., and Martin, J. B. (1983). *Nature*, 306, 234-8.

Haenlin, M., Steller, H., Pirrotta, V., and Mohier, E. (1985). *Cell*, 40, 827-37.

Heilig, R., and Mandel, J. L. (1986). *Experientia* (in press).

Housman, D., Kidd, K., and Gusella, J. F. (1982). *Trends Neurosci.*, 5, 320-3.

Humphries, S. E., Kessling, A. M., Horsthemke, B., Donald, J. A., Seed, M., Jowett, N., Holm, M., Galton, D. J., Wynn, V., and Williamson, R. (1985). *Lancet*, i, 1003-5.

Jeffreys, A. J. K. (1979). *Cell*, 18, 1-10.

Jeffreys, A. J., Wilson, V., and Thein, S. L. (1985a). *Nature*, 314, 67-73.

Jeffreys, A. J., Wilson, V., and Thein, S. L. (1985b). *Nature*, 316, 76-9.

Kaartinen, M., Griffiths, G. M., Markham, A. F., and Milstein, C. (1983). *Nature*, 304, 320-4.

Kametani, F., Tonoike, H., Hoshi, A., Shinoda, T., and Kito, S. (1984). *Biochem. Biophys. Res. Comm.*, 125, 622-8.

Kan, Y. W., and Dozy, A. H. (1979). *Proc. Natl Acad. Sci. USA*, 75, 5631-5.

Karathanasis, S. K., Zannis, V. I., and Breslow, J. L. (1983). *Nature*, 305, 323-5.

Kazazian, H. H. Jr, Orkin, S. H., Markham, A. F., Chapman, C. R., Youssoufian, H. A., and Weber, P. G. (1984). *Nature*, 300, 152-4.

Kedes, L. H. (1985). *Trends Genet.*, 1, 205-9.

Kidd, V. J., Golbus, M. S., Wallace, R. B., Itakyra, K., and Woo, S. L. C. (1984). *New Eng. J. Med.*, 310, 639-41.

Kingston, H. M., Sarfarazi, M., Thomas, N. S. T., and Harper, P. S. (1984). *Hum. Genet.*, 67, 6-17.

Klobutcher, L. A., and Ruddle, F. H. (1981). *Ann. Rev. Biochem.*, 50, 533-54.

Krumlauf, R., Jeanpierre, M., and Young, B. D. (1982). *Proc. Natl Acad. Sci. USA*, 79, 2971-5.

Kunkel, L. M., Monaco, A. P., Middlesworth, W., Ochs, H. D., and Latt, S. A. (1985a). *Proc. Natl Acad. Sci. USA*, 82, 4778-82.

Kunkel, L. M., Lalande, M., Monaco, A. P., Flint, A., Middlesworth, W., and Latt, S. A. (1985b). *Gene*, 33, 251-8.

Kurachi, K., Chandra, T., Friezner Degen, S. J., White, T. T., Marchioto, T. L., Woo, S. L. C., and Davie, E. W. (1981). *Proc. Natl Acad. Sci. USA*, 78, 6826-30.

Lathrop, G. M., and Lalouel, M. (1984). *Am. J. Hum. Genet.*, 36, 460-5.

Leary, J. J., Brigati, D. J., and Ward, D. G. (1983). *Proc. Natl Acad. Sci. USA*, 80, 4045-9.

Ledbetter, D. H., Mascarello, J. T., Riccardi, V. M., Harper, V. D., Airhart, S. D., and Strobel, R. J. (1982). *Am. J. Hum. Genet.*, 34, 278-85.

Lehman, M. A., Schneider, W. J., Sudhof, T. C., Brown, M. S., Goldstein, J. L., and Russel, D. W. (1985). *Science*, 227, 140-6.

Lewin, B. (1985). In *Genes II*. J. Wiley & Sons, New York, pp. 67-84 and 281-303.

Lindgren, V., De Martinville, B., Horwich, A. L., Rosenber, L. E., and Francke, U. (1984). *Science*, 226, 698-700.

Little, P. F. R. (1981). In Williamson, R. (ed.), *Genetic Engineering* Vol. 1. Academic Press, London, pp. 61-102.

McAlpine, P. I., Shows, T. B., Miller, R. L., and Pakstis, A. J. (1985). *Cytogen. Cell Gen.*, 40 8-66.

McKusick, V. A. (1983). *Mendelian inheritance in man*, 6th ed. Johns Hopkins University Press, Baltimore.

Mandrup-Poulsen, T., Owerbach, D., Mortensen, S. A., Johansen, K., Meinertz, H., Sørensen, H., and Nerup, J. (1984). *Lancet*, i, 250-2.

Maniatis, T., Fritsch, E. F., and Sambrook, J. (1982). *Molecular Cloning: A Laboratory Manual*. Cold Spring Harbor Laboratory, New York.

Maniatis, T., Hardison, R. C., Lacy, F., Lauer, J., O'Connell, C., Quon, D., Sim, G. K., and Efstratiadis, A. (1978). *Cell*, 15, 687-91.

Mattei, M. G., Baeteman, M. A., Heilig, R., Oberlé, I., Davies, K., Mandel, J. L., and Mattei, J. F. (1985a). *Hum. Genet.*, 69, 327–31.
Mattei, M. G., Philip, N., Passage, E., Moisan, J. P., Mandel, J. L., and Mattei, J. F. (1985b). *Hum. Genet.*, 69, 268–71.
Miller, C. L., and Ruddle, F. H. (1978). *Proc. Natl Acad. Sci. USA*, 75, 3346–50.
Monaco, A. P., Bertelson, C. J., Middlesworth, W., Colletti, C. A., Aldridge, J., Fishbeck, K. H., Bartlett, R., Pericak-Vance, M. A., Roses, A. D., and Kunkel, L. M. (1985). *Nature*, 316, 842–5.
Murray, J. G., Demopoulos, C. M., Lawn, R. M., and Motulsky, A. G. (1983). *Proc. Natl Acad. Sci. USA*, 80, 5951–5.
Myers, R. M., Lumelsky, N., Lerman, L. S., and Maniatis, T. (1985). *Nature*, 313, 495–8.
Oberlé, I., Drayna, D., Camerino, G., White, R., and Mandel, J. L. (1985a). *Proc. Natl Acad. Sci. USA*, 82, 2824–8.
Oberlé, I., Camerino, G., Heilig, R., Grunebaum, L., Cazenave, J. P., Crapanzano, C., Mannucci, P. M., and Mandel, J. L. (1985b). *New Engl. J. Med.*, 312, 682–6.
Oberlé, I., Mandel, J. L., Boué, J., Mattei, M. G., and Mattei, J. F. (1985c). *Lancet*, i, 871.
Oberlé, I., Heilig, R., Moisan, J. P., Kloepfer, C., Mattei, M. G., Mattei, J. F., Boué, J., Froster-Iskenius, U., Jacobs, P. A., Lathrop, G. M., Lalouel, J. M., and Mandel, J. L. (1986a). *Proc. Natl Acad. Sci. USA*, 83, 1016–20.
Oberlé, I., Camerino, G., Kloepfer, C., Moisan, J. P., Grzeschick, K. H., Hellkuhl, B., Hors-Cayla, M. C., Van Cong, N., Weil, D., and Mandel, J. L. (1986b). *Hum. Genet.*, 72, 43–9.
Olsen, A. S., McBride, O. W., and Otey, M. C. (1980). *Biochemistry*, 19, 2419–28.
Orkin, S. H. (1984). *Blood*, 63, 249–53.
Orkin, S. H., and Kazazian, H. H. (1984). *Ann. Rev. Genet.*, 18, 131–71.
Orkin, S. H., Kazazian, H. H., Antonarakis, S. E., Goff, S. C., Boehm, C. D., Sexton, J. P., Waber, P. G., and Giardina, P. V. J. (1982). *Nature*, 296, 627–31.
Owerbach, D., Poulsen, S., Billesbølle, P., and Nerup, J. (1982a). *Lancet*, i, 880–3.
Owerbach, D., Billesbølle, P., Schroll, M., Johansen, K., Poulsen, S., and Nerup, P. (1982b). *Lancet*, ii, 1291–3.
Phillips, J. A. III, Hjelle, B. L., Seeburg, P. M., and Zachman, M. (1981). *Proc. Natl Acad. Sci. USA*, 78, 6372–5.
Pihlajaniemi, T., Dickson, L. A., Pope, F. M., Korhonen, V. R., Nicholls, A., Prockop, D. J., and Myers, J. C. (1984). *J. Biol. Chem.*, 259, 12941–4.
Piratsu, M., Kan, Y. W., Cao, A., Conner, B. J., Teplitz, R. L., and Wallace, R. B. (1983). *New Engl. J. Med.*, 309, 284–7.
Prochownik, E., Antonarakis, S., Bauer Rosenberg, R., Fearon, E., and Orkin, S. H. (1983). *New Engl. J. Med.*, 308, 1549–52.
Reeders, S. T., Breuning, M. H., Davies, K. E., Nicholls, R. D., Jarman, A. P., Higgs, D. R., Pearson, P. L., and Weatherall, D. J. (1985). *Nature*, 317, 542–4.
Rotwein, R., Chyn, R., Chirgwin, J., Cordell, B., Goodman, H., and Permutt, M. (1981). *Science*, 213, 1117–20.
Rozen, R., Fox, J., Fenton, W. A., Horwich, A. L., and Rosenberg, L. E. (1985). *Nature*, 313, 815–17.
Ruddle, F. H. (1981). *Nature*, 294, 115–20.
Sasaki, H., Sakaki, Y., Matsuo, H., Goto, I., Kuroiwa, Y., Sahashi, I., Takahashi, A., Shinoda, T., Isobe, T., and Takagi, Y. (1984). *Biochem. Biophys. Res. Comm.*, 125, 636–42.
Sasaki, H., Sakaki, Y., Takagi, Y., Sahashi, K., Takahashi, A., Isobe, T., Shinoda, T., Matsuo, H., Goto, I., and Kuroiwa, Y. (1985). *Lancet*, i, 100.
Saxon, P. J., Srivatsan, E. S., Leipzig, G. V., Sameshima, J. H., and Stanbridge, E. J. (1985). *Mol. Cell. Biol.*, 5, 140–6.
Schmidtke, J., and Cooper, D. (1985). *Gene Communications Newsletter*, I.3 (updated listing available upon request from Dr. Schmidtke).
Sherman, S. L., Morton, N. E., Jacobs, P. A., and Turner, G. (1984). *Ann. Hum. Genet.*, 48, 21–37.
Silhavy, T., Berman, M. L., and Enquist, W. (1984). *Experiments with Gene Fusions*. Cold Spring Harbor Laboratory, New York.
Southern, E. M. (1980). In Wu, R. (ed.), *Methods in Enzymology*, Vol. 68. Academic Press, New York, pp. 152–76.

Steel, C. M. (1984). *Lancet*, ii, 908–11 and 966–8.

Stout, J. T., Chen, H. Y., Brennand, J., Caskey, C. T., and Brinster, R. L. (1985). *Nature*, **317**, 250–2.

Sutherland, G. R. (1985). *Trends Genet.*, **1**, 108–12.

Tchen, P., Fuchs, R. P. P., Sage, E., and Leng, M. (1984). *Proc. Natl Acad. Sci. USA*, **81**, 3466–70.

Tolleshaug, H., Hobgood, K. K., Brown, M. S., Goldstein, M. S., and Goldstein, J. L. (1983). *Cell*, **32**, 941–51.

Tønnesen, T., Søndergaard, F., Güttler, F., Oberlé, I., Moisan, J. P., Mandel, J. L., Hauge, M., and Damsgaard, E. M. (1984). *Lancet*, ii, 932.

Treisman, R., Proudfoot, N. J., Shander, M., and Maniatis, T. (1982). *Cell*, **29**, 903–11.

Turner, G., and Jacobs, P. A. (1983). In Harris, H., and Hirschorn, K. (eds.), *Advances in Human Genetics*. Plenum Press, New York, pp. 83–112.

Verellen-Dumoulin, C., Freund, M., De Meyer, R., Laterre, C., Frédéric, J., Thompson, M. V., Markovic, V. D., and Worton, R. G. (1984). *Hum. Genet.*, **67**, 115–19.

Vogel, F., and Motulsky, A. G. (1979). In *Human Genetics: Problems and Approaches*. Springer-Verlag, Berlin, pp. 293–309.

Watson, J. D., Tooze, J., and Kurtz, D. T. (1983). *Recombinant DNA: A Short Course*. Scientific American Books, New York.

White, P. G., New, M. I., and Dupont, B. (1984). *Proc. Natl Acad. Sci. USA*, **81**, 7505–9.

Willard, H. F., Skolnick, M. H., Pearson, P. L., and Mandel, J. L. (1985). *Cytogenet. Cell Genet.*, **40**, 360–489.

Williamson, R. (1981–3). *Genetic Engineering*, Vol. I–IV, Academic Press, London.

Winship, P. R., Anson, D. S., Rizza, C. R., and Brownlee, G. G. (1984). *Nucl. Acids Res.*, **12**, 8861–72.

Worton, R. G., Duff, C., Sylvester, J. E., Schmickel, R. D., and Willard, H. F. (1984). *Science*, **224**, 1447–9.

Wyman, A., and White, R. (1980). *Proc. Natl Acad. Sci. USA*, **77**, 6754–8.

Yang, T. P., Patel, P. I., Chinault, A. C., Stout, J. T., Jackson, L. G., Hildebrand, B. M., Caskey, C. T. (1984). *Nature*, **310**, 412–14.

18

Genetics of Alzheimer's Disease: A Large Kindred with Apparent Mendelian Transmission: Possible Implications for a Linkage Study

J.-F. Foncin, D. Salmon and A. C. Bruni

18.1 Introduction

The introduction of genetics into a collection of contributions dedicated to new concepts in Alzheimer's disease (AD) may seem a paradox at many levels. First, the importance of genetic factors in the determination of AD is not a new concept, since it has been surmised almost from the first description of the disease. It was indicated by a number of reports (not reviewed in this present paper) of relatively small familial groups in which a few cases of AD were clustered. Second, with therapy at the legitimate foreground of our concerns, the genetic code (as a symbol of fixed fate impervious to medical influence) would, at least until recent times, have seemed a barrier to any practical use of genetic studies. Third, the Parkinson paradigm and the ensuing focus on neurotransmitters, and hence on therapy aimed at the mechanisms, as distinct from the causation, of disease, has directed much of the recent AD research effort towards neuro-pharmacology.

The L-DOPA story itself, however, reminds us that this class of therapeutic agents has at best a limited span of usefulness in progressive disease. Knowledge of aetiology is a prerequisite for rational, long-term therapy or prevention, according to the paradigm of what had been called the general paresis of the insane (GPI), which was as much a mystery in the nineteenth century as AD now is, and which is, of course, dementia due to late syphilis of the brain. Establishing working concepts for research in this direction has long been made difficult by the attribution of AD to 'degenerescence' or 'premature ageing', untestable *obscurum per obscurius* explanations devoid of predictive value. Strictly speaking, the occurrence of AD at a given age ought to be ascribed to factors present in the zygote (genetic factors *sensu lato*) and/or to factors intervening during life (environmental factors). The latter, mainly involving metals, have recently been the object of much research and speculation (Gajdusek, 1984a,b). We are going to outline problems concerning the former, taking the opportunity presented by a study in progress which focusses on a large kindred of Italian origin (Foncin *et al.*, 1985).

18.2 Methods

18.2.1 Early Investigations

The study of a kindred in which early-onset presenile AD is remarkably frequent, thereafter to be called the "N" kindred from the initial of the historical name of its place of origin, was initiated more than twenty-three years ago in the USA (Feldman *et al.*, 1963). L. E. Nee (NINCDS, Bethesda) has recently carried on the study of this branch. In 1972, one of the present authors (J.-F. Foncin) independently established the diagnosis of AD through classical and electron-microscopic study of a right-frontal cortical biopsy taken at the occasion of trephination for diagnostic aeric ventriculography on a 42-year-old woman directed to the neurosurgery department of La Salpètrière Hospital for suspected brain tumor. Familial history obtained from the husband revealed that the father of the patient had been affected by a similar condition and had died in a mental hospital near their common place of origin in southern Italy. The results of a preliminary survey were presented at the Barcelona World Congress of Neurology (Foncin and Supino-Viterbo, 1973), and investigations have been carried on since that time.

18.2.2 Data Collection

Investigations using three different methods were pursued simultaneously in the region of origin of the "N" kindred:

(a) The homes of members of the proband's family (including those of first cousins) were visited. Available persons were examined and the history of absent or deceased relatives was noted.

(b) Municipal records (birth, marriage and death registers) were systematically surveyed, copies being taken of certificates in which one of the cited patronymics was known from previous steps of the investigation. Municipal records in the former Kingdom of the Two Sicilys start in 1809, and spot investigations only were made of the anteceding parish records. Investigations were made with the objective of minimising ascertainment bias by following maternal as well as paternal ancestry of apparently spared as well as apparently affected branches. This rule was less rigorously adhered to in the first stages of the investigation, that is for the generation immediately preceding the one clinically affected in 1973.

(c) The archives (starting at 1880) of the provincial mental hospital were surveyed, copies being taken of case histories clinically compatible with AD which pertained to patients with patronymics known from steps (a) and (b).

Data pertaining to neuropsychic disorders other than presenile dementia were recorded if readily available, but were not systematically sought for. Specifically, only one instance of Down's syndrome has been recorded (a granddaughter of the proband) and no instance of senile dementia which could be ascribed to the Alzheimer type (SDAT).

In 1981, it occurred to us by serendipity (actually in the form of an official bearing an Italian-sounding name who is acknowledged at the end of the paper) that the American AD family with a similar clinical picture which was described by Feldman *et al.* (1963) might be a branch of the one we were studying. In fact, comparison of original data (provided through the courtesy of Dr Feldman) showed that subjects I-1 and I-2 (Feldman *et al.*, 1963), common ancestors of the American patients, were identical to those bearing serial numbers 17 and 18, respectively, in our own files. Doctor Feldman kindly made his data available, and American and European data are now listed in one file, which is constantly being updated.

18.2.3 Data Implementation

All the subjects identified through the above-mentioned procedures, and linked to the American or the European proband through the transitive (consanguinity, marriage) relationship, are listed in a computer file. The two probands are equivalent from this point of view, since they are themselves linked through their common ancestors, subjects 17 and 18. For each subject there is a chain of 80 alphanumeric characters, comprising: arbitrary serial number; patronymic and given name (abbreviated to 12 characters); gender; date of birth; age at death; serial number and given name of the father; serial number, patronymic and given name of the mother; and a three-figure code number indicating the diagnostic status and the mode of ascertainment of that status. An auxiliary file comprises at most 50 characters with free-form commentary. Linear sorting produces alphabetical lists of subjects or sibships: the corresponding printouts are used in further stages of data collection, in order to assess the potential relationship to the kindred of a newly ascertained subject. Demography may be studied through sorting according to date of birth, age at death and gender. Cross-sorting according to diagnostic status coupled with any other characteristic leads to correlation studies. Software developed by Landre *et al.* (1972) enables one first to detect inconsistencies, and then to group and class sib-ships, to establish their filiation, to optimise their placing on a classical gene-logical tree, to calculate their coordinates, and finally to trace automatically, with the aid of a Benson tracer, the complete tree (or any one corresponding to a previously defined subset). Inbreeding coefficient was calculated as the probability that at a given locus the homologous genes of the same individual would be identical by descent (Malecot, 1948), i.e. originate from the same common ancestor through different paths.

18.3 Results

18.3.1 Overall Figures

About 1,600 subjects linked to the histologically proven AD probands by the transitive (filiation, marriage) relationship are listed: 138 derive from the study of the American branch, and the remainder derive from the European survey. Ten subjects are illegitimate with both parents unknown; 522 are founders, that is to say that their parents are as yet unidentified (as distinct from illegitimate children known as such). Founders are only known, as a rule, through a mention in a certificate primarily concerning one of their children or a spouse. Forty-eight patients are identified (22 males and 26 females): 13 by history; 21 by medical record; 14 by personal examination (either by Dr Feldman and his team or by one of the present authors). Neuropathological confirmation has been obtained in four instances in the American branch (Feldman *et al.*, 1963; Krigman *et al.*, 1965; additional cases have come to autopsy, but diagnoses are not avail-able) and in two instances, through biopsies, in the European branch (Foncin and Supino-Viterbo, 1973; Foncin *et al.*, unpublished). As we are not going to further discuss neuropathological problems relevant to the genetics of AD, let us briefly state that the AD diagnostic triad, consisting of plaques, tangles and, in cases in which Ammons's horn could be examined, granulovacuolar degeneration, was abundantly represented, and that a diagnosis of Cruetzfeldt–Jakob disease (CJD) could not be entertained from a neuropathological standpoint, neither at the light microscopic nor at the electron microscopic level.

18.3.2 Clinical Neurology

It is of course impossible to transcribe here the record of each and every affected member of the "N" kindred; as of June 1984, they may be found in the speciality thesis of the junior author (Bruni, 1984). However, in order to help assign a place among the many clinical variants of AD, to the form which has been con-sistently observed in the "N" kindred, we think it useful to synthesise briefly its clinical picture. In view of the heterogeneous sources of clinical data, it would be preposterous to calculate the proportion of cases in which any given symptom may be present.

The condition affects persons who, before the onset of disease, were often intellectually gifted and well-adapted and, especially in the USA, had reached positions of responsibility. Apparent onset of symptoms usually takes place in the early forties, but is difficult to ascertain, being aspecific and marked mainly by memory loss. The symptoms are easier to pinpoint in subjects in intellectual professions and are often apparent, in such cases, in the late thirties; this is more often the case in the American branch than in the European. In women, symptoms are often noticed for the first time at the occasion of the birth of a child, and are marked by their inability to care for the newborn. Later on, they are manifested in professional life by disinterest and aberrant conduct: for instance, a taxi driver lets his charge down in open country. Unlawful behaviour, such as sexual offences or embezzling (often associated with inappropriate euphoria) sometimes evoked a diagnosis of GPI. More often, in older mental hospital records, we find 'depression' or 'schizophrenia' as an initial diagnosis, but the corresponding symptomatology is only vaguely indicated. Hallucinations are sometimes mentioned.

Dementia rapidly becomes obvious. The patient becomes incapacitated for daily life, verbal contact is reduced and later absent, with palilalia and echolalia. The latter symptom is often very marked, and may be the first pathognomic one in at-risk subjects when diagnosis is obscured by associated conditions, e.g. alcoholism or reactive depression. Neurological symptoms then become manifest; akinesia stands in the foreground with amimia. The latter is interrupted from time to time by facial expressions of pain or terror, which may be in relationship with underlying hallucinations. Gait is slow, with the body slanted forwards; motor initiative is absent. Neurological examination shows hypertonia, both plastic and oppositional; a slight cog-wheel phenomenon may occasionally be found at the upper extremities. We never observed any true tremor, although tremor is reported in some older clinical charts, but this may correspond to the myoclonus we observed in most patients at a later stage. Myoclonus is irregular and asymetric, often triggered by external stimuli. It is more frequent at the proximal segment of extremities, which may be slightly displaced, but it may also occur in the facial or truncal muscles. Midline and deep reflexes are brisk, plantar reflexes are flexor. Grand mal epilepsy may occur at a late stage, and seems to herald the terminal period. Dementia evolves into a purely vegetative state, and death intervenes in cachexy, often with bronchopneumonia or urinary tract infection; it may be deferred for some time by the loving home care provided by Italian families. Total duration of illness is approximately ten years, but is difficult to ascertain in many instances due to difficulties in determining a precise onset age. No affected subject was found to have died older than 66, with a majority dying in the years 45 to 54 (see Section 18.3.3).

Laboratory investigations did not bring additional information. Liquor was normal. Air encephalography or ventriculography and, more recently, CT scan evidenced, in demented patients, enlarged ventricles and sulci, mainly in the frontal region. Non-specific changes may be observed on the electroencenphalogram (EEG) after onset of the first clinical symptoms, with theta waves and, later, slow bitemporal bursts. Intermittent polymorph spike-and-wave discharge has been recorded at a late stage, particularly in the interval between convulsive seizures. An important negative finding was the absence of permanent periodic paroxystic activity at all stages of disease evolution, even when myoclonus had been observed during EEG recording.

Within the limits of available documents, we were not able to delineate variants of clinical presentation which could be interpreted as characteristic of different groups within the "N" kindred. On the contrary, two patients with strikingly similar conditions who were examined by the same investigator (ACB) shared a nearest possible common ancestor situated in the middle eighteenth century, eighteen generations up and down: fixity of phenotype appears to be a characteristic of transmission in the "N" kindred. Specifically, we could not evidence the so-called anticipation phenomenon, that is earlier age of onset in successive generations: whatever difference we could find could be ascribed to earlier detection in a medically more developed society which, on the other hand, puts more strain on its members.

18.3.3 Demography

It became apparent at an early stage of our work that the age at death was to be an important discriminating factor in our retrospective studies, and one which could enable us to explore the transmission of disease in periods of time for which no clinical data would be available. A first study showed that the mortality rate did not significantly differ according to gender or birth year for the cohorts, whose fate could be completely determined, that is essentially those born in the nineteenth century. As a result, we were entitled to treat all demographic data as a whole.

Infant mortality has been very high in southern Italy in the nineteenth and early twentieth centuries; moreover, relative mortality is probably overestimated in the younger classes due to an important emigration trend. Comparative study of mortality was done on five-year classes, starting at age 15, of affected and control subjects. Control subjects were the subjects not at risk (assuming negligible incidence in the general population and dominant transmission with complete penetrance), such as spouses and their relatives, 'escapers' and their descendants. Affected groups for the classes too young for AD to be manifest were calculated, assuming the same mortality for AD carriers and controls in these classes. Results showed a significant ($p < 0.05$, Kolmogorov–Smirnov test) difference between the two groups. The theorem of Bayes (1763) then enables us to estimate the probability for a subject to have been affected, given his age at death and an estimate of the *a priori* risk. Under the same assumptions, subjects at first-degree risk (*a priori* risk = 0.5) carry a 0.89 or 0.87 probability of having been affected if they died aged 45 to 49 or 50 to 54, respectively, and a null probability if they died aged 70 or older.

As is often the case with Bayesian probabilities, the main difficulty lies in estimating *a priori* risk. An estimate has been obtained taking the opportunity of the heredity of surnames (Crow and Mange, 1965). The surname M . . ., that of subject number 18 (the common ancestor of the American and European probands), is borne by 33 sibships in the file, of which 3 are affected and 20 are control, as defined above, the remainder being of undefined status. The *a priori* risk for an M . . . sibship may then be estimated at 3/23 = 0.13. Applying Bayes' theorem and compound probability axioms to the sibship born of subject number 1259 (M . . . Giuseppe) in the second quarter of the nineteenth century, we found a 0.70 probability for that sibship to have been affected. Although no confidence interval could be given for this result, given the type of assumptions made in the first place, it has later been confirmed through the identification of an affected sibship (with one examined patient and with two siblings and the mother known by history to have been affected) in descent of subject number 1259.

18.3.4 Genealogy

The pedigree, with ascending *and* descending indefinite ramifications, comprises about 1,600 connected subjects in 11 generations. It is of course impossible to reproduce in print even a significant fragment of the corresponding computer-generated genealogical tree. The most ancient subject with known date of birth was born in 1745 and is part of the second generation. The most ancient affected subjects known as such (two by medical record and one by history) are part of a sibship in the fifth generation, born between 1832 and 1842 of subject number 18 (M . . . Pietro Salvatore) who was born in 1803 and died aged 45, and his wife, subject number 17 (C . . . Rosa) who was born in 1809 and died aged 50. Bayesian probabilities as applied to demographic data (*see* Section 18.3.3) do not allow us to decide which of the parents had been the (affected, *see* Section 18.3.5) carrier. However, remote hearsay evidence obtained by Feldman *et al.* (1963) tended to show that C . . . Rosa had been unaffected; this indication is supported by recent results showing that the surname M . . . was associated in at least another instance with familial AD in the first half of the nineteenth century (*see above*).

The pedigree shows only three inbred unions, all belonging to the next to last generation. No affected subject was found to be in descent from an inbred union known as such, and no instance of possible homozygocity for the AD trait was found. These results are the more remarkable in view of the fact that methods followed in data collection, as well as computer tracing of the extended genealogical tree and calculation of inbreeding coefficients, would tend to detect any instance of even remote inbreeding. Inbred unions are in fact frequent in the region of origin of the "N" kindred, as evidenced by the Parma University data base which is drawn from Catholic Church dispensation registers (Moroni and Mariotti, personal communication). From indications given by subject number 236 who was a member of an affected sibship but was herself 68 years old and consequently an 'escaper', the taboo against inbred unions had been a conscious one in the "N" kindred, and our informant was deploring the fact that the 'young ones' were now marrying cousins.

18.3.5 Transmission

A large majority of known, affected subjects have another known, affected subject as a parent, almost all of the remainder have a parent who was probably affected (as deduced from his age at death), and for none do we find both parents unaffected, as could possibly have been demonstrated by their age at death (see Section 18.3.3). We may validly conclude that only affected subjects transmit the condition to their children. Further study of the mode of transmission is made easier in the "N" kindred by its fecundity, sibships with ten or more children being the rule. The proportion of affected children is not significantly different whether the transmitter is the father or the mother: there is no maternal effect. We did not detect any effect of the birth order of the at-risk child.

Segregation ratio is notoriously difficult to calculate in human genetics, due to ascertainment bias. In an earlier stage of the study, it was planned to test various hypotheses on segregation with the aid of complex segregation analysis software (Lalouel and Morton, 1981). Later on, drawing of the pedigree appeared to strongly favour autosomal dominant inheritance, so that costly computer evaluations were avoided. We have chosen instead to do calculations by hand, taking into account solely those sibships the status of the members of which was exhaustively known (or nearly so). Bias was minimised by the systematic incorporation of subjects into the file through municipal records survey (see Section 18.2), a method we think does not favour the inclusion of affected subjects. In this way, we drew information from nine sibships with a total of 55 subjects remaining after elimination of probands and of subjects who died before minimum AD age of onset in the "N" kindred. Among these 55 subjects, 36 are affected, 6 are 'escapers', 13 are of unknown status. If we account the subjects with unknown status as unaffected, together with the 'escapers', we may calculate a minimum segregation ratio of 0.65, a figure significantly superior ($p < 0.05$) to the 0.5 ratio expected in the elementary hypothesis of Mendelian dominant monogenic inheritance.

18.4 Discussion

18.4.1 Transmission

It is prudent not to hastily conclude Mendelian dominant transmission from the sole fact of transmission by affected subjects of both sexes (Harper, 1977). A discussion of transmission mode is therefore warranted.

Environmental factors appear to play a negligible role in the determination of AD in the "N" kindred: there is no significant difference in incidence, age of onset, clinical picture or evolution between branches living in Italy or in the USA in vastly different circumstances (the migration having taken place at the end of the nineteenth century). Vertical non-genetic transmission is highly unlikely: there is no maternal effect, no birth order effect, and no cluster effect; some affected American subjects have been separated at birth from their natural family and raised in foster homes. Cytoplasmic heredity is ruled out by the fact that fathers transmit the condition with the same segregation ratio as do mothers.

We are then brought back to the Mendelian hypothesis. It might well be said that all the results point to classical monogenic autosomal dominant inheritance with complete penetrance, with the exception of the 0.65 segregation ratio. A discussion of this finding is, in consequence, of central importance. First, it may be that bias has been introduced in spite of the methodological care taken. It could not have been introduced significatively at the internal level of sibships, since these are large and exhaustively described; what is more, subjects of uncertain status were counted as unaffected. The choice of exhaustively described sibships may have been biased by the presence of numerous affected subjects.

If, nevertheless, we accept a 0.65 segregation ratio as reflecting reality, two explanations may be advanced. One could be polygenic inheritance. In order to entail a segregation ratio greater than 0.5, it would involve a degree of homozygocity. We could not find any consanguinity in the sample subjects, except thrice in the more recent generation, and that was in not-at-risk subjects. However, due to its stability and high fecundity, this population may be considered as having been an isolate for a long time. Even in the absence of local inbreeding, the effect of gene frequency differentiation caused by random genetic drift is important (Kimura and Ohta, 1971). Studying the frequency of isonymous marriages in Hutterites, Crow and Mange (1965) showed that more than half of the total inbreeding effect in that population is attributable to a remote common ancestry. We might well be in a comparable situation concerning the "N" kindred, which shows a considerable degree of isonymy. Further study of eighteenth- and seventeenth-century parish records may help in pinpointing common ancestors of the present 'founders'.

Another possible cause for a segregation ratio greater than 0.5 could be greater resistance of AD carriers during their early life (as indicated above, we did not take into account, in calculating the segregation ratio, siblings who died before minimum age of onset of familial AD in the "N" kindred). A model for this hypothesis could be afforded, at the population genetics scale, by the sickle-cell trait or, nearer to the birthplace of most of the included sibships, thalas-saemia. Such a phenomenon could have been very discriminating, in view of the high infant mortality in the population under study.

In conclusion, we think that the null hypothesis of classical Mendelian mono-genic autosomal dominant transmission has not been disproved for the transmis-sion of AD in the "N" kindred, in spite of extensive testing of other hypotheses made possible by the large numbers involved.

18.4.2 Relevance

The next issue to be discussed is whether our findings represent an isolated instance or may have bearing to more general problems in AD.

The first point, of course, is whether the cases of presenile dementia occurring in the "N" kindred really represent instances of AD. This is primarily a matter of nosological definition in respect of the five cases for which neuropathological confirmation has been obtained, inasmuch they presented the clinico-patho-logical association of dementia with the triad consisting of plaques, tangles and granulo-vacuolar degeneration. The question of whether this association defines AD as a unique and only nosological entity is going to be approached later. Concerning "N" kindred cases without neuropathological confirmation, the paucity of clinical data concerning some of the retrospective cases does not seriously interfere with diagnosis: death in the 45–54 years range by itself entails a near 0.9 probability for AD in subjects at first degree risk; the additional notion of preceding dementing illness, in view of the rarity of dementia in that age range, ought to bring the probability to practical certitude.

A far more important and complicated issue is whether the condition trans-mitted within the "N" kindred and, more generally, familial AD, is representative of AD in general. This issue is linked with that of unity against multiplicity of nosological entities within AD. On the clinical side, the question arises of the sig-nificance of neurological symptoms observed at a late phase of evolution in most of the AD cases in the "N" kindred, mainly myoclonus, rigidity and convulsive seizures. Although myoclonus might point to an association of AD with CJD (Gaches et al., 1977; Masters et al., 1981), it is frequently observed in typical AD (Terry, 1970); it is more frequent in familial forms of AD, but is found also in apparently sporadic instances (Jacob, 1970). Other neurological symptoms have been observed in exceptional AD kindreds, for instance paraplegia in the cases described by Van Bogaert et al. (1940).

On the epidemiological side, the central question is the relative numerical importance of familial AD. Difficult as it is with the presenile forms of AD, it is almost impossible to address AD directly in late forms by means of methods involving retrospective surveys (the only ones which may produce extended pedigrees). Dementia arising later in life did not use to attract much medical attention and went (and still, in many parts, goes) unrecorded or misdiagnosed, often as cerebrovascular disease. The prototype of studies addressing this question is that by Sjögren *et al.* (1952), who traced affected relatives of probands with presenile AD. Ten % of the probands led to familial cases and the pattern was consistent with autosomal dominant transmission, but the overall picture was interpreted as suggesting multifactorial heredity. The work of Constantinidis *et al.* (1965) proceeded from a similar approach, but with a method based on the comparison of the brains of relatives examined in the same neuropathological laboratory. Taking into account both presenile and senile AD, they found a 'familial risk' comparable to that found by Sjögren *et al.* (1952); they interpreted their failure to find senile AD in two successive generations as an indication of recessive transmission of the senile forms, as distinct from the dominant transmission of presenile forms. However, their finding of both presenile and senile forms in the same families might, on the contrary, be interpreted in favour of the genetic unity of both forms.

More recently, the Folstein group (Chase *et al.*, 1983; Breitner and Folstein, 1984) has refined the approach of Sjögren *et al.* (1952) by applying actuarial methods in order to estimate the 'true' number of secondary cases among first-degree relatives of AD patients. The unselected index cases were identified in nursing homes by score evaluation, and were mostly late forms. The obvious principle is that, especially in late forms, a number of AD carriers can never be clinically identified, because they die of other causes before AD age of onset. In that way, they were able to calculate a segregation ratio, within a narrow confidence interval, to 0.5 and to conclude that the generality of AD instances represents manifestations of a Mendelian dominant autosomic disease with complete penetrance. This is not the place for a discussion of these conclusions, which have been a matter of dispute. If warranted, they would greatly enhance the relevance of large pedigrees with apparently Mendelian AD. The establishment of such pedigrees would not be dependent on basic problems, but would only be a matter of favourable conditions for investigation, namely: early onset and uniform expression of the disease; fecundity and cooperation of the family; existence and accessibility of civil and medical archives; and good luck and hard work on the side of investigators.

18.4.3 Beyond Formal Genetics

The methodologies to be followed in order to increase our fundamental knowledge of AD depend on the paradigm which is considered the most fruitful. With the exception of the Parkinson paradigm alluded to in the introduction, most have a relationship with genetics.

18.4.3.1 The Down's Syndrome (DS) Paradigm

The relevance of this paradigm to AD stems from two factors: the first is the long-known early occurrence of AD in DS victims (Bertrand and Koffas, 1946), more recent is the awareness that most, if not all, patients with DS who survive into their third or fourth decades develop AD (for a review see Lott, 1982); the second is the concentration of DS cases, along with AD, in relatives of AD probands (Heston and Mastri, 1977). A logical consequence of this paradigm is research on AD cytogenetics. Early claims of increased 'aneuploidy' in AD patients, particularly in familial cases, have been disputed, and the AD 'microtubular' unifying hypothesis (Cook *et al.*, 1979) is weakened by the total absence of any morphological and chemical relationship between microtubules and the paired helical filaments of AD. A remaining interest of this paradigm is of course to make chromosome 21 the leading contender as carrier of an AD 'gene'.

18.4.3.2 The CJD Paradigm

This is a particularly tantalising paradigm, especially at the genetics level, given the many analogies between AD and CJD (for a review see Foncin and Supino-Viterbo, 1983). The position of familial as against sporadic CJD is very much comparable with that of the respective forms of AD (Masters *et al.*, 1981), with the important difference that familial instances of CJD are transmissible to animals in the same manner as sporadic instances are. What is lacking here is a clear demonstration, through quantitative study of large pedigrees, that CJD familial forms are indeed genetically transmitted and are not instances of vertical, Kuru-style transmission. This hypothesis is, *a priori*, much more plausible in this case than the corresponding one we have discussed and eliminated for AD in the instance of the "N" kindred. Although earlier claims of transmission of familial AD to primates have practically been abandoned (Goudsmit *et al.*, 1980), new hints of relationship between AD and CJD keep arising. Scrapie-associated fibrils, which are also present in CJD and may represent the infectious agent (Merz *et al.*, 1984), are similar to amyloid fibrils found in AD (Merz *et al.*, 1983). The problem of possible integration of a transmissible agent into the genome is clearly one which transcends the question of AD genetics, but which should be kept in the background of our reflections on that subject.

18.4.3.3 The Huntington Paradigm

This paradigm was born from the epoch-making 'new biology' work of Gusella *et al.* (1983), leading to the discovery of a DNA marker genetically linked to the Huntington disease (HD) locus and assigned to chromosome 4, which has immediately led the same authors to speculate that AD might be amenable to identical methods (Gusella *et al.*, 1984; Wexler *et al.*, 1985). Any linkage, as distinct from association, study necessitates as a starting material a large and accessible kindred, a remarkable example of which was the Venezuelian kindred, living near Lake Maracaibo, which was studied by Gusella *et al.* (1983). However, AD pedigrees large enough to be informative are very few in comparison with HD pedigrees. To our knowledge, besides the "N" kindred, only the New Brunswick kindred studied by Nee *et al.* (1983) with 51 affected members, and the Askhenase kindreds studied by Goudsmit *et al.* (1981), with 37 affected members in two probably related branches, are of a size which may yield enough information for restriction fragment length polymorphism (RFLP) linkage studies. Linkage with phenotypically detectable polymorphism, as detected qualitatively and tested with the lod score method, would seem to require less extensive material. In fact, no such linkage has yet been found. Absence of linkage with HLA phenotypes has been demonstrated in the "N" kindred (Muller *et al.*, in preparation). Other polymorphous markers, either normal or disease marker, are yet to be studied. This type of study could be fruitful with genetically determined endemic conditions detectable by blood screening, for instance the highly polymorph thalassaemia group, which is well-represented in parts of southern Italy. We are not going to discuss association studies, which have a bearing on statistical association at the population level of a given genetic characteristic (for instance one HLA allele or group of alleles) with AD. They refer to the rather vague notion of susceptibility, a quite different one from the hypothesis of genetic determination postulated by the HD paradigm. RFLP studies seem for the time being, in our opinion, the best bet for progress in AD research. Gathering of material for DNA production has been started on the "N" kindred, in collaboration with the French Blood Transfusion Organisation (CNTS) and the NINCDS – NIH (Bethesda). In view of the enormous task ahead, it is our own intention to make material available to qualified investigators, care being taken to avoid duplication of effort: the comparative speed with which one team   (Gusella *et al.*, 1983) managed to detect RFLP linkage in HD through virtually 'blind' studies may not be repeated.

Lastly, we may be allowed to speculate on the possible outcomes from linkage, and particularly RFLP, studies. First, let us acknowledge that clear-cut and generally applicable results are far less likely to be obtained with AD than with HD. If indeed genetically determined, AD is likely to be highly polymorphic, according to the thalassaemia model. The first application is likely to be a diagnostic one. However, apart from the obvious ethical problems involved, difficulties, due in particular to recombination, encountered with HD (Gusella *et al.*, 11.cc.) remind us that this first target may be remote.

Far more important, but even more remote, is the insight which will be afforded by direct molecular access to the AD 'gene(s)', and thence to molecular mechanisms of AD. In this case, too, the HD model is going to be too simple in view of the polymorphism of AD. An interesting model could be the Sinc gene controlling the scrapie incubation period (Dickinson and Miekle, 1971). This model would integrate the CJD paradigm in a particularly interesting way, in view of the importance of age at onset in the epidemiology of AD. This condition would be interpreted as due to universal infection (as were measles before vaccination), the genetic variable being the incubation period. What is more, Sinc has recently been shown (Bruce and Dickinson, 1985) to be implicated in the production of plaques in scrapie-infected mice. It is our hope that our own pedigree tracing work may contribute in the future to such developments.

References

Bayes, T. (1763). Essay toward solving a problem in the doctrine of chances. *Phil. Trans. (London)*, in *Biometrika*, 45, 293–315 (1958).

Bertrand, I., and Koffas, D. (1946). Cas d'idiotie mongolienne adulte avec nombreuses plaques séniles et concrétions calcaires pallidales. *Rev. neurol. (Paris)*, 78, 338–45.

Breitner, J. C. S., and Folstein, M. F. (1984). Familial nature of Alzheimer's disease. *N. Engl. J. Med.*, 14, 63–80.

Bruce, M. E., and Dickinson, A. G. (1985). Genetic control of amyloid plaque production and incubation period in Scrapie-infected mice. *J. Neuropath. Exp. Neurol.*, 44, 285–94.

Bruni, A. C. (1984). Studio di una popolazione afetta da una malattia di Alzheimer Familiare. *Tesi di Specializzazione*, Università degli Studi di Napoli, pp. 131.

Chase, G. A., Folstein, M. F., Breitner, J. C. S., Beaty, T. H., and Self, S. G. (1983). The use of life tables and survival analysis in testing genetic hypotheses, with an application to Alzheimer's disease. *Am. J. of Epidemiology*, 117, 590–7.

Constantinidis, J., and Ajuriaguerra, J. de (1965). L'incidence familiale des plaques séniles. *Confin. Psychiat.*, 8, 130–7.

Constantinidis, J., Garrone, G., Tissot, R., and Ajuriaguerra, J. de (1965). L'incidence familiale des altérations neurofibrillaires corticales d'Alzheimer. *Psychiat. Neurol. (Basel)*, 150, 237–47.

Cook, R. H., Ward, B. E., and Austin, J. H. (1979). Studies in aging of the brain. IV. Familial Alzheimer's disease: relation to transmissible dementia, aneuploidy, and microtubular defects. *Ne rology*, 29, 1402–12.

Crow, J. F and Mange, A. P. (1965). Measurement of inbreeding from the frequency of marria s between persons of the same surname. *Eugenics Quarterly*, 12, 199–203.

Dickinson, A. G., and Miekle, V. M. H. (1971). Host-genotype and agent effects in scrapie incubation: Change in allelic interaction with different strains of agent. *Mol. Gen. Genet.*, 112, 73–9.

Feldman, R. G., Chandler, K. A., Levy, L. L., and Glaser, G. H. (1963). Familial Alzheimer's disease. *Neurology*, 13, 1402–12.

Foncin, J. F., and Supino-Viterbo, V. (1973). Maladie d'Alzheimer familiale: histopathologie ultrastructurale, étude généalogique. *Excerpta Medica*, International Congress Series, 296.

Foncin, J. F., and Supino-Viterbo, V. (1983). La maladie d'Alzheimer et ses formes familiales. Leurs rapports avec les encéphalopathies spongiformes transmissibles. In Court, L., and Cathala, F. (eds.), *Virus non conventionnels et affections du système nerveux central*. Masson & Cie, Paris, pp. 248–58.

Foncin, J. F., Salmon, D., Supino-Viterbo, V., Feldman, R. G., Macchi, G., Mariotti, P., Scoppetta, C., Caruso, G., and Bruni, A. C. (1985). Démence présénile d'Alzheimer transmise dans une famille étendue. *Rev. Neurol. (Paris)*, 141, 194–202.

Gaches, J., Supino-Viterbo, V., and Foncin, J. F. (1977). Association de maladies d'Alzheimer et de Creutzfeldt-Jakob. *Acta Neurol. Belg.*, 77, 202–12.

Gajdusek, D. C. (1984a). Interference with axonal transport of neurofilaments: the underlying mechanism of pathogenesis in Alzheimer's disease, amyotrophic lateral sclerosis, and many other degenerations of the CNS. *The Merrimon Lecture*. The School of Medicine, The University of North Carolina at Chapel Hill, 1–14.

Gajdusek, D. C. (1984b). Environmental factors provoking physiological changes which induce motor neurone disease and early neuronal ageing in high incidence foci in the Western Pacific. In Clifford Rose, F. (ed.), *Research Progress in Motor Neuron Disease.* Pitman, London, 44–69.

Goudsmit, J., White, B. J., Weitkamp, L. R., Keats, B. J. B., Morrow, C. H., and Gajdusek, D. C. (1981). Familial Alzheimer's disease in two kindreds of the same geographic and ethnic origin. A clinical and genetic study. *J. Neurol. Sci.*, 49, 79–89.

Goudsmit, J., Morrow, C. H., Asher, D. M., Yanaghiara, R. T., Masters, C. L., Gibbs Jr, C. J., and Gajdusek, D. C. (1980). Evidence for and against the transmissibility of Alzheimer's disease. *Neurology*, 30, 945–50.

Gusella, J. F., Tanzi, R. E., Anderson, M. A., Hobbs, W., Gibbons, K., Raschtchian, R., Gilliam, T. C., Wallace, M. R., Wexler, N. S., and Conneally, P. M. (1984). DNA markers for nervous system diseases. *Science*, 225, 1320–5.

Gusella, J. F., Wexler, N. S., Conneally, P. M., Naylor, S. L., Anderson, M. A., Tanzi, R. E., Watkins, P. C., Ottina, K., Wallace, M. R., Sakaguchi, A. Y., Young, A. B., Shoulson, I., Bonilla, E., and Martin, J. B. (1983). A polymorphic DNA marker genetically linked to Huntington's disease. *Nature*, 306, 234–8.

Harper, P. S. (1977). Mendelian inheritance or transmissible agent? The lesson of Kuru and the Australia antigen. *J. Med. Genetics*, 14, 389–98.

Heston, L. L., and Mastri, A. R. (1977). The genetics of Alzheimer's disease. Associations with hematologic malignancy and Down's syndrome. *Arch. Gen. Psychiatry*, 34, 976–81.

Jacob, H. (1970). Muscular twitching in Alzheimer's disease. In Wostenholme and O'Connor (eds.), *Alzheimer's Disease and Related Conditions*. Churchill, London, 75–89.

Kimura, M., and Ohta, T. (1971). *Theoretical Aspects of Population Genetics.* Princeton University Press, Princeton, New Jersey, p. 118.

Krigman, M. R., Feldman, R. G., and Bensch, K. (1965). Alzheimer's presenile dementia. A histochemical and electron microscopic study. *Lab. Invest.*, 14, 381–96.

Lalouel, J. M., and Morton, N. E. (1981). Complex segregation analysis with pointers. *Human Hered.*, 31, 312–21.

Landre, M. F., Valat, M. T., and Jutier, P. (1972). Reconnaissance automatique des liens de parenté. Tracé automatique d'arbre généalogique. *M.I.S.*, 10, SIMEP, Villeurbanne.

Lott, I. T. (1982). Down's syndrome, aging and Alzheimer's disease: a clinical review. In Sinex, E. M., and Merril, C. R. (eds.), *Alzheimer's Disease, Down's Syndrome and Aging*. Annals NY Academy of Sciences, 396, 15–27.

Malecot, G. (1948). *Les Mathématiques de l'Hérédité.* Masson, Paris.

Masters, C. L., Gajdusek, D. C., and Gibbs Jr, C. J. (1981). The familial occurrence of Creutzfeldt–Jakob disease and Alzheimer's disease. *Brain*, 104, 535–58.

Merz, P. A., Rohwer, R. G., Kascsak, R., Wisniewski, H. M., Sommerville, R. A., Gibbs, C. J., and Gajdusek, D. C. (1984). An infection specific particle from the unconventional slow virus diseases. *Science*, 225, 437–40.

Merz, P. A., Sommerville, R. A., and Wisniewsky, H. M. (1983). Abnormal fibrils in scrapie and senile dementia of the Alzheimer type. In Court, L. and Cathala, F. (eds.), *Virus non conventionnels et affections du système nerveux central.* Masson & Cie, Paris, pp. 259–81.

Nee, L. E., Polinsky, R. J., Eldridge, R., Weingartner, J., Smallberg, S., and Ebert, M. (1983). A family with histologically confirmed Alzheimer's disease. *Arch. Neurol.*, 40, 203–8.

Sjogren, T., Sjogren, H., and Lindgren, H. (1952). A genetic study of Morbus Alzheimer and Morbus Pick. *Acta Psychiat. Scand.*, 82, Suppl. 9.

Terry, R. D. (1970). Discussion. In Wostenholme and O'Connor (eds.), *Alzheimer's Disease and Related Conditions.* Churchill, London, 91.

Van Bogaert, L., Maere, M., and de Smedt, E. (1940). Sur les formes familiales précoces de la maladie d'Alzheimer. *Monatschr. Psychiat. Neurol.*, 102, 247–301.

Wexler, N. S., Conneally, P. M., Houseman, D., and Gusella, J. F. (1985). A DNA polymorphism for Huntington's disease marks the future. *Arch. Neurol.*, 42, 20–4.

19

DNA Markers in Familial Alzheimer's Disease

P. H. St. George-Hyslop, R. Tanzi, W. Hobbs, K. Gibbons, J. F. Gusella,
L. Nee, R. Polinsky, J. Haines and P. M. Conneally

19.1 Introduction

Several biochemical abnormalities have been described in Alzheimer's disease
(AD) (Whitehouse *et al.*, 1981; Lewis *et al.*, 1984; Sajdel-Sulkowska and Marrotta,
1984; Morrison *et al.*, 1985; St George-Hyslop and Crapper McLachlan, 1985).
However, it currently seems likely that all of these abnormalities are secondary
events in the pathogenesis of AD, and consequently the primary aetiologic event
in most forms of AD remains elusive. The only form of AD for which the
primary event is known is familial Alzheimer's disease (FAD), which results from
a dominantly inherited autosomal gene defect. Although FAD is undoubtedly a
special form of AD, it is probable that an understanding of the nature of the
gene dysfunction which causes FAD, and knowledge of the mechanism by which
this defective gene causes Alzheimer's disease, will shed light upon the molecular
abnormalities causing the more common sporadic forms of AD.

Unfortunately, neither the nature of the gene defect which causes FAD, nor
even the chromosomal location of this defective gene, is known. We are currently
attempting to define the chromosomal location of the FAD gene by employing a
modification of classical gene-linkage studies. Simply stated, this gene-linkage
strategy attempts to show that a genetic marker whose chromosomal location is
known, is co-inherited with, and is thus located near, the FAD gene. From this,
the chromosomal location of the FAD gene can then be inferred. Knowledge of
the location of the FAD gene could lead to attempts to isolate and characterise
the normal and disease alleles from the FAD locus.

19.2 Principles of DNA Markers and Genetic Linkage Studies

Gene linkage studies are based on the observation that there is a relationship between the distance separating any two genes on a given chromosome and the probability that they will be separated by recombination events with the sister chromosome during meiosis. Thus genes situated close together will virtually always be inherited together in the offspring. Genes less closely linked will tend to be inherited more frequently than by chance alone, but will occasionally be separated by crossover events. Genes situated far apart will frequently be separated by crossover events, and therefore will be co-inherited 50 % of the time by chance alone, as will genes on separate chromosomes. Consequently, by examining the co-inheritance of two genes one may determine whether they are linked. This is judged by calculating a 'lod score' (logarithm of the odds score), which is expressed as the ratio of the likelihood that the observed pattern of inheritance of the two genes occurred because they are linked, against the probability that the observed pattern of inheritance occurred by chance alone. Generally, genes are considered linked if the lod score is greater than 3 (i.e. 1000:1 odds in favour of linkage). Lod scores of less than -2 (100:1 odds in favor of random association) are taken to imply absence of linkage. Lod scores between -2 and $+3$ are indeterminate, neither confirming nor excluding linkage.

Clearly, in order to show that a marker gene and a disease gene are inherited together, one must be able to distinguish the marker gene on the disease-bearing chromosome, from the same gene on the non-disease chromosome. Classically, this has been done by employing as markers genes which are expressed, such as the ABO blood group and HLA transplantation antigens. These marker genes display a natural variation (polymorphism) which can be used to identify the alleles on each of the two chromosomes. Recently, it has been observed that DNA itself contains polymorphisms which can be used as genetic markers (Botstein et al., 1980). These DNA polymorphisms result from naturally occurring nucleotide differences as small as a single base change in the genomic DNA. The substitution of a single nucleotide may alter the recognition sequence for one of several enzymes which cleave DNA at very specific DNA nucleotide sequences (restriction endonucleases). The creation or loss of these cleavage sites will result in the generation of a shorter or longer than usual fragment of DNA when genomic DNA is cleaved by that restriction endonuclease (restriction fragment length polymorphisms RFLPs). This polymorphism can be recognised by cleaving the subject's genomic DNA with the restriction endonuclease, separating the resulting DNA fragments according to size by agarose gel electrophoresis, and then transferring these fragments to a nylon filter by Southern blotting. A radiolabelled DNA probe, which has a known, unique chromosomal location is then applied to the filter. The radiolabelled probe will anneal only with complementary sequences in the digested genomic DNA on the filter to produce a hybrid molecule (DNA hybridisation). At a restriction enzyme site which displays nucleotide sequence variations, and which is located close to the sequence complementary to that of the applied DNA probe, the result will be as follows. If the recognition sequence is altered by a nucleotide substitution, the subject's genomic DNA will not be cleaved, and consequently the probe will hybridise to a single long fragment. Conversely, if the cleavage site is present, the probe will hybridise to two small fragments. One can then use the presence of a single long fragment, or of two smaller fragments, to distinguish two otherwise identical genes on the sister chromosomes and thus follow their inheritance.

The advantage of employing DNA polymorphisms rather than the classical protein markers is threefold. First, the technology is relatively simple and is the same for all probes. Second, DNA sequence polymorphisms occur at a frequency of approximately 1 in 250-500 bases and occur both in protein coding sites and in non-coding sites, thus dramatically increasing the number of potential markers (Murray et al., 1984). Third, many DNA probes detect independent polymorphisms for more than one restriction endonuclease. As mentioned, a basic principle of linkage analysis is that the marker genes must be different on the two chromosomes (heterozygous) in order to follow the inheritance of the two chromosomes. Clearly, if the marker locus is identical on both sister chromosomes (homozygous) it is not possible to determine which chromosome bears the disease gene. Most classical protein markers have only a single variable characteristic, and thus if an individual is homozygous for that marker no further information can be gained. DNA probes which demonstrate RFLPs with more than one restriction endonuclease, on the other hand, are likely to be heterozygous for at least one restriction site, and therefore to be informative. The use of RFLPs as genetic markers has already permitted localisation of the genes causing Huntington's chorea and Duchenne dystrophy, and is being applied to a number of other neurodegenerative diseases (Gusella et al., 1984).

19.3 Genetic Linkage Studies in Familial Alzheimer's Disease

We are currently attempting genetic linkage studies using DNA restriction fragment length polymorphisms in a large kindred with pathologically confirmed FAD (Fig. 19.1) (Nee et al., 1983). Bearing in mind the association of Down's syndrome with Alzheimer's disease (Jervis, 1948; Crapper et al., 1975; Heston, 1982), our initial studies are designed to determine if the FAD gene also resides on chromosome 21. The same strategy can, however, be extended to other chromosomes as well.

In order to pursue the question of linkage of FAD to a DNA marker on chromosome 21, a series of single-copy human chromosome 21 DNA probes were generated from a phage library constructed from a human–mouse hybrid cell line (Gusella et al., 1985). A large reference pedigree was then used to determine which restriction endonucleases produce RFLPs with each of these probes, and to construct a genetic linkage map displaying the order of these probes on chromosome 21 (Fig. 19.2).

260

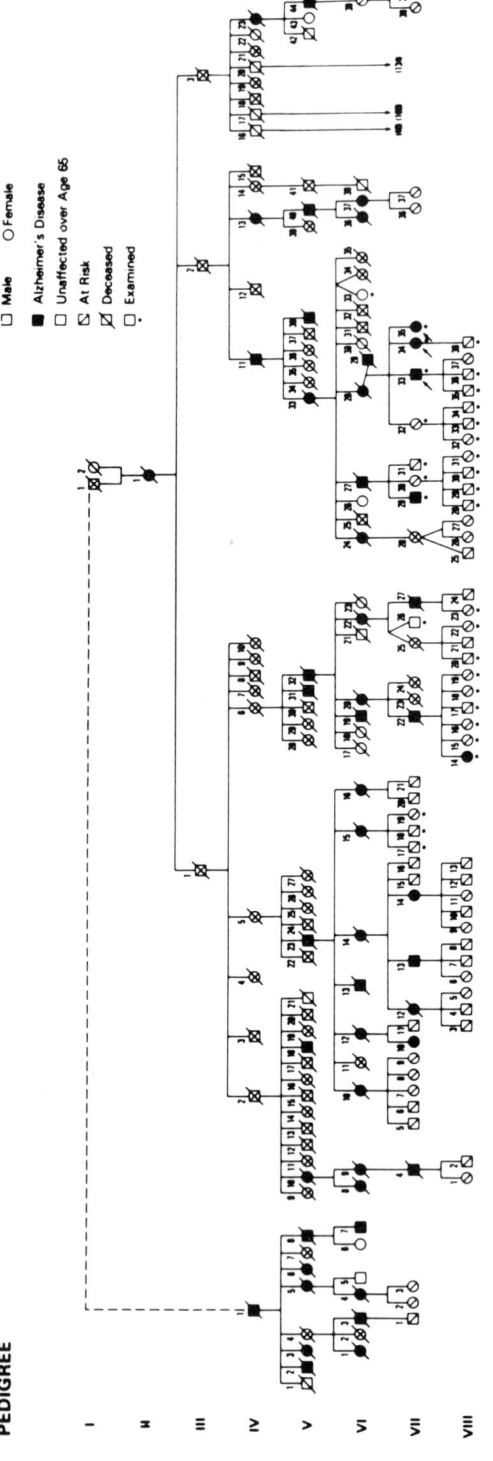

Fig. 19.1 Familial Alzheimer's disease pedigree.

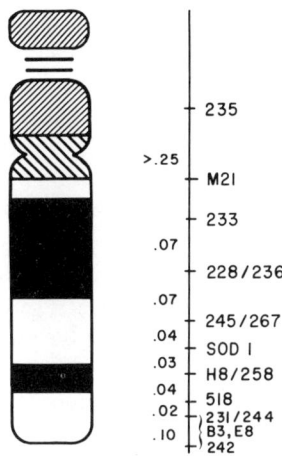

Fig. 19.2   Chromosome 21 linkage map.

Genomic DNA from all available family members was isolated either directly from the buffy coat of blood samples, or from lymphocyte cultures immortalised with Epstein–Barr virus. Each subject's genomic DNA was digested with various restriction endonucleases, and the resulting DNA fragments were separated according to size by agarose gel electrophoresis, and then transferred to a nylon filter by Southern blotting. The previously prepared single copy chromosome 21 probes were hybridised to the genomic DNA on the filter, revealing the polymorphisms present in each individual, and permitting computation of the individual's genotype for each probe. Once the genotype of each available individual was determined for each probe site, the linkage of that probe with FAD gene was tested using two-point linkage analysis (FAD against marker)

The preliminary results from the first four probes yielded maximum lod scores within the indeterminate range (-2 to $+3$), which neither confirms nor refutes the possibility of linkage of FAD to these chromosome 21 probes. The primary reason that a more decisive result has not been generated from these preliminary studies is the natural history of FAD. The clinical course typically followed by patients with FAD in this, and probably most other pedigrees, is one of a prolonged asymptomatic period, with onset of symptoms in the fifth and sixth decades. After the onset of symptoms, there is a rapid decline to death within six years (Nee *et al.*, 1983). This type of clinical course has two effects. First, it is unlikely that there will be large numbers of affected members alive at any given time, although there will be many members alive who are at 50 % risk. Second, it is even more unlikely that an effected parent and an affected offspring will be alive at the same time. Furthermore, the later onset of symptoms in the affected offspring makes it probable that the unaffected parent will also have died, so rendering it impossible to reconstruct the probable genotype of the deceased affected parent. The absence of affected individuals in two contiguous generations, and the frequent inability to even reconstruct the genotype of individuals in two contiguous generations makes it then difficult to directly test the hypothesis of co-inheritance of the marker and the FAD gene from affected parent to affected child, a feature which dramatically reduces the information content of the pedigree. Instead, one must rely on concordance of genotype between affected individuals who may be separated by several generations. Unfortunately, this strategy permits two sources of loss of information. First, if affected individuals are separated by several generations, even a closely linked marker may occasionally be separated from the disease gene by crossover events, resulting in apparent non-linkage. This source of error is accounted for in the computer analysis which can assume different degrees of linkage. The second, and more damaging factor causing loss of information, is the effect of the genotype of deceased 'married-in' members of the pedigrees. If these 'married-in' relatives have died, their probable genotypes must be estimated from those found in the general population. This produces an effect which, at first glance, seems paradoxical. DNA markers usually give greatest information if the marker is frequently polymorphic in the population (i.e. the alleles of the marker have approximately equal frequencies), giving a high incidence of heterozygosity with which to distinguish the two chromosomes. In the current context, however, where two affected members are separated by several generations, the significance of apparent concordance for a high-frequency allele of the marker is diluted by the high probability that such an allele could have been acquired instead from a 'married-in' family member. On the other hand, a marker which is infrequently polymorphic in the general population, and which is usually of low information value since it results in a high incidence of homozygous × homozygous matings, may paradoxically be of greater benefit in this situation if it is segregating with the disease state in the family. Under these conditions, if several distantly related affected individuals can be shown to be concordant for the infrequent allele of the marker, it is extremely unlikely that it could have been acquired in all the affected individuals by inheritance from 'married-in' members.

To illustrate this point further, we have modelled these two possibilities, using our pedigree. We have assigned the heterozygous state to all affected members, and to 50 % of 'at risk' offspring, in order to simulate a hypothetical probe with the '1' allele close to the FAD gene on the disease-bearing chromosome, and the '2' allele on the normal counterpart, to give a gentotype of '1, 2' (Fig. 19.3). We assigned the homozygous state for the '2' allele (genotype '2, 2') to all living non-affected members, and to all living 'married-in' members. We then performed the linkage analysis using LIPED 3, but varied the frequency with which the '1' allele occurs in the general population. For the reasons stated above, when the frequency of the '1' allele was set at 50 % in the general population, which under most circumstances would give a highly informative marker,

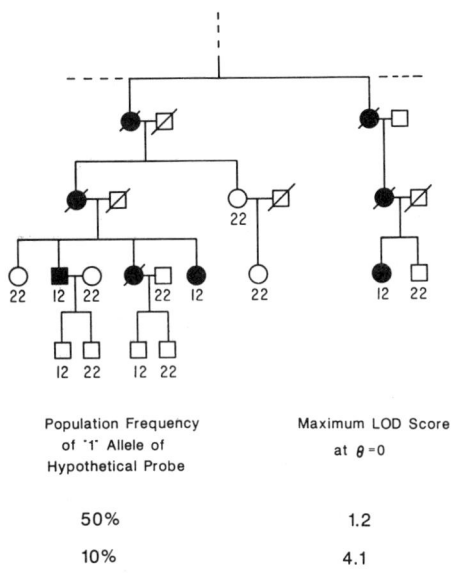

Population Frequency of '1' Allele of Hypothetical Probe	Maximum LOD Score at $\theta = 0$
50%	1.2
10%	4.1

Fig. 19.3   Effect of varying population frequency of an allele of a marker linked to FAD.

the maximum achieveable lod score was only 1.2 assuming no recombination ($\theta = 0$). However, when the '1' allele was assigned a frequency of 10 % (a frequency which would ordinarily make such a marker quite uninformative), the '1' allele 'observed' in all affected individuals, and in 50 % of at-risk individuals, would then be very unlikely to have been consistently inherited from 'married-in' members in previous generations. Consequently, the lod score rises to 4.1 assuming no recombination ($\theta = 0$).

19.4 Conclusions

The implications of our preliminary results are that linkage analysis is capable of localising the FAD genes, but that the natural history of FAD will make this analysis difficult, and special strategies will therefore be required. Two strategies will be of particular value. First, if it is assumed that two families with FAD have a similar defect at the same locus, then the lod scores gained independently for each family are additive, thus allowing linkage to be detected more easily. We are therefore currently examining a second pedigree, and we are actively seeking out other kindreds. This strategy, however, does expose the analysis to the risk of including phenotypically similar, but genotypically heterogeneous diseases with different gene defects at different loci, which would generate a false negative result. The second strategy we are pursuing is to identify markers with multiple alleles, each allele having a low incidence in the population. For the reasons noted above this type of marker may be a more efficient tool for linkage analysis in the situation when it is segregating in the family.

References

Botstein, D., White, R. L., Skolnick, M., and Davis, R. (1980). Construction of a genetic linkage map in man using restriction fragment length polymorphisms. *Am. J. Hum. Gen.*, **32**, 314-31.

Crapper, D. R., D'Alton, A. J., Skoptiz, M., Scott, J. W., and Hachinski, V. L. (1975). Alzheimer degeneration in Down's syndrome. *Arch. Neurol.*, **32**, 618-23.

Gusella, J. F., Tanzi, R. E., Anderson, M. A., *et al.* (1984). DNA markers for nervous system diseases. *Science*, **225**, 1320-6.

Gusella, J. F., Tanzi, R. E., Watkins, P., *et al.* (1985). Isolation of polymorphic DNA segments from human chromosome 21. *N.A.R.*, **13**, 6075-88.

Heston, L. L. (1982). Alzheimer's disease and Down's syndrome: evidence suggesting an association. In Sinex, F. M., and Merrill, C. R. (eds.), *Alzheimer's Disease, Down's Syndrome, and Aging.* Ann. N.Y. Acad. Sci., **396**, 3-13.

Jervis, G. A. (1948). Early senile changes in mongoloid idiocy. *Am. J. Psychiat.*, **105**, 102-6.

Lewis, P. N., Lukiw, W. J., DeBoni, U., Crapper McLachlan, D. R. *et al.* (1984). Changes in chromatin structure associated with Alzheimer's disease. *J. Neurochem.*, **37**, 1193-202.

Morrison, J. H., Rogers, J., Scherr, S., Benoit, R., and Bloom, F. E. (1985). Somatostatin immunoreactivity in neuritic plaques of Alzheimer's patients. *Nature*, **314**, 90-2.

Murray, J. C., Milles, K. A., Demopoulos, C. M., Hornung, S., and Motulsky, A. (1984). Linkage disequilibrium and evolutionary relationships of DNA variants (RFLPs) at the serum albumin locus. *Proc. Natl Acad. Sci. USA*, **81**, 3486-90.

Nee, L. E., Polinsky, R. J., Eldridge, R., Weingartner, H., Smallberg, S., and Ebert, M. (1983). Family with histologically confirmed Alzheimer's disease. *Arch. Neurol.*, **40**, 203-23.

St George-Hyslop, P. H., and Crapper McLachlan, D. R. (1985). Brain phosphofructokinase in Alzheimer's disease, Down's syndrome, and other dementia associated disease. (In press).

Sajdel-Sulkowska, E. M., and Marrotta, C. A. (1984). Alzheimer's disease brain: alterations in RNA levels and in a ribonuclease inhibitor complex. *Science*, **225**, 947-9.

Whitehouse, P. J., Price, D. L., Clark, A. W., Coyle, J. T., and DeLong, M. R. (1981). Alzheimer's disease: Evidence of loss of cholinergic neurons in the nucleus basalis. *Ann. Neurol.*, **10**, 122-6.

20

Behavioural Recovery Following 6-OHDA Lesions of the Nucleus Accumbens and Intra-accumbens Implantation of Dopaminergic Grafts

K. Choulli, J. P. Herman, D. Nadaud, K. Taghzouti, H. Simon and M. Le Moal

20.1 Introduction

The technique of neural grafting, although relatively old (Björklund and Stenevi, 1985), has gained a new impetus in the last few years, mainly due to the development of transplantation techniques more effective than those existing previously. Another factor which explains the recent development of this field is that it has been realised that the approach of grafting into the central nervous system can give useful information concerning different problems which became ripe for investigation in the course of the development of neuroscience during the late seventies: the mechanisms of development and plasticity of neuronal circuitries in the CNS; the problem of functional repair following central lesions; and the role of identified neuronal subsystems, etc.

One of the best-known transmitter systems in the mammalian CNS, in term of anatomy, physiology and functional role, is the central dopaminergic system. This fact explains why dopaminergic grafts have been among the most studied and why the first example of functional intracerebral neural transplants concerned the intrastriatal implantation of dopaminergic neurons (Björklund et al., 1980b). This and subsequent studies (Freed et al., 1980; Dunnett et al., 1983a,b, 1984; Nadaud et al., 1984) have shown that dopaminergic grafts can restore functional deficits resulting from previous lesions of the host's dopaminergic neurons. These deficits mainly concerned relatively simple sensorimotor responses (Björklund *et al.*, 1980b; Dunnett *et al.*, 1983a,b), or pharmacologically induced behaviours such as rotation (Björklund *et al.*, 1980a,b; Freed *et al.*, 1980; Dunnett *et al.*, 1983a) or locomotion (Dunnett *et al.*, 1984; Nadaud *et al.*, 1984). However, few data are available concerning the capabilities of neural grafts to restore more complex behaviours. In the case of the nigrostriatal dopaminergic system there are relatively few experimental models for testing such behaviours. Therefore, we addressed ourselves to the mesocorticolimbic dopaminergic system, the lesion of which provokes deficits of more complex emotional and cognitive responses, as previously described by Le Moal *et al.* (1977), Simon and Le Moal (1984), Kelley and Stinus (1985) and Taghzouti *et al.* (1985).

Our first study concerning mesocorticolimbic grafts involved the destruction of the dopaminergic neurons localised in the ventral mesencephalic tegmentum, or A10 area, followed by the implantation of dopaminergic neurons into the nucleus accumbens, one of the regions innervated by these neurons. One of the consequences of such a lesion is the abolition of the locomotor stimulation brought about by amphetamine, an indirect dopaminergic agonist (Kelly *et al.*, 1977). This deficit was, indeed, restored by an intra-accumbens dopaminergic graft (Nadaud *et al.*, 1984). As a next step we wanted to extend this study to deficits in more complex behaviours. But instead of performing the lesion in the A10 area and thereby destroying the dopaminergic innervation of virtually the whole forebrain (with the exception of the striatum innervated by A9 neurons), we chose to lesion more selectively a given terminal area, namely the nucleus accumbens. The reason for adopting this procedure was that it was hoped that with such a more circumscribed lesion, leading to a better characterised and less multifactorial behavioural syndrome than with the A10 lesion (Simon and Le Moal, 1984), the possible restorative capabilities of dopaminergic grafts would be more apparent. The results presented here indicate that such graft-induced functional recovery can indeed be demonstrated. It will also be shown that the comparison of the details of spontaneous behavioural recovery (occurring in lesioned, non-grafted animals) and of the graft-induced functional repair can give some useful hints as to the mechanism of action of such neural grafts.

20.2 Methodological Aspects

Experimental subjects were female Wistar rats, weighing 200 g at the beginning of the experiment. The animals were housed individually in plastic cages with food and water freely available.

The dopaminergic innervation of the nucleus accumbens was lesioned by bilateral stereotaxic injections of 6-hydroxy-dopamine (6-OHDA, 4 μg/μl; 8 and 4 μg being injected at two different vertical coordinates on each side) into this region. Two-thirds ($n = 20$) of the lesioned animals were grafted four weeks later with a dopaminergic neuronal suspension implanted bilaterally into the nucleus accumbens. Briefly, the technique, based on that described by Björklund *et al.* (1980a), was as follows. Mesencephali from rat embryos (ED 14) were dissected out under phosphate-buffered saline and were collected into the same solution supplemented with glucose. The tissue fragments were briefly trypsinised (8 min at 20 °C), washed, and mechanically dissociated by repeated aspiration through a small-bore Pasteur pipette in a synthetic culture medium (S-MEM-HEPES, Gibco) containing DNAase and a trypsin inhibitor. The suspension was centrifuged and the pellet resuspended in the same culture medium. This suspension, which contained 170 000 viable cells/μl, was kept on ice and 2 × 3 μl was injected into each nucleus accumbens. Behavioural testing was conducted two weeks before, and at different times after, grafting. Locomotor activity was measured in a circular corridor (10 cm wide, 140 cm long with walls 50 cm high) equipped with four photocells. Open-field behaviour was tested by putting the animals in a 1 m × 1 m white, illuminated arena, the floor of which was divided into 16 squares and by recording for 10 min the number of squares crossed and rearing scores. Exploratory activity was also tested by recording the number of holes visited in a 1 m × 1 m dimly illuminated arena in the corners of which were four holes. Hoarding behaviour was examined after having placed the animals on a restricted diet so that their body weight was approximately 85 % of their free-feeding weight. The hoarding arena consisted of a dimly illuminated 1 m × 1 m open field, one corner of which was cut away to accommodate the home cage of the animal. The number of pellets (out of 60 pellets placed into the arena) brought by the animals into its home cage over 90 min was taken as the hoarding score.

At the end of the experience, approximately ten months after grafting, the endogenous dopamine system of the grafted animals was destroyed by an injection of 6-OHDA into the lateral hypothalamus. One week later the animal were sacrificed by intracardiac perfusion of a fixative, the forebrain was cut into 50 μm thick serial sections and immunohistochemical staining was performed using a dopamine-specific antiserum (Geffard *et al.*, 1984).

20.3 Results

20.3.1 Influence of Transplants on Amphetamine-induced Locomotor Activation

As expected (Kelly *et al.*, 1977), the lesion abolished totally the stimulating effect of the drug when tested three weeks after lesion. There was a total restoration of this deficit nine weeks after the implantation of the dopaminergic neurons in the nucleus accumbens (Fig. 20.1(A)). Two phenomena must be noted. First, some improvement could also be seen in the lesioned, non-grafted controls, although their activity remained well below that of the non-lesioned controls. Second, the locomotor activity evoked by amphetamine in the grafted

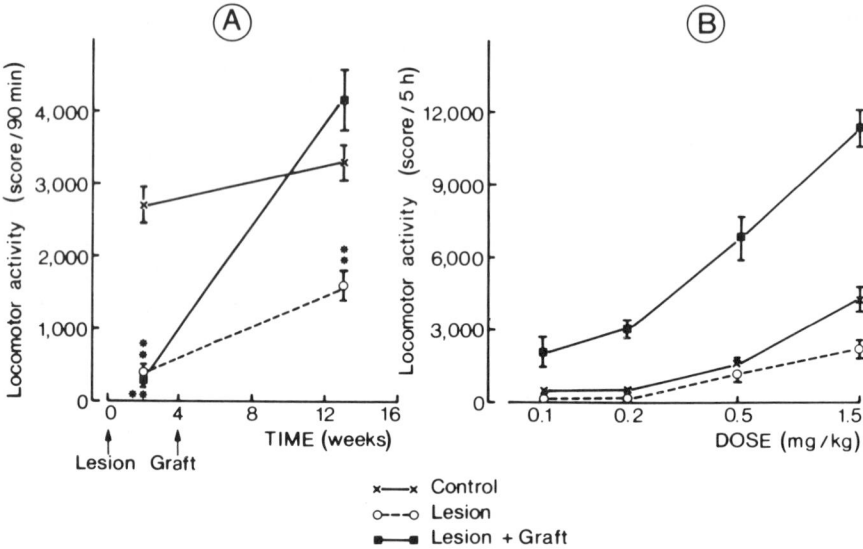

Fig. 20.1 Locomotor activation by amphetamine in intact, lesioned and lesioned and grafted animals. (A) The effect of 1.5 mg/kg i.p. d-amphetamine before and after grafting. Here, and on subsequent figures, results are mean ± S.E.M., n = 10-20. *: $p < 0.05$, **: $p < 0.01$ compared to intact controls. (B) Locomotor activation induced by different doses of d-amphetamine. Dose–response relationship has been established between 5 and 7 months after grafting.

animals seemed to be higher than that in the intact controls. This last observation prompted us to later examine in detail the amphetamine-induced locomotor activity of grafted animals. It appeared that the grafted animals were much more responsive, both in terms of sensitivity (Fig. 20.1(B)), and duration of action, to amphetamine than normal controls. The reason for the increased response of the grafted animals as compared to that of the controls is not yet understood but could reflect a general property of grafted dopaminergic neurons, as we (Herman *et al.*, 1985b), as well as others (Dunnett *et al.*, 1983a), have found the same hyper-responsiveness for striatal grafts.

This experiment indicated that the grafted neurons were indeed present in the nucleus accumbens and, furthermore, that their stimulation could evoke the same sort of behavioural response as the stimulation of the normal mesolimbic dopaminergic system. The next question was to ask whether they would also be able to repair deficits of spontaneous, non-pharmacologically-induced behaviour.

20.3.2 *Influence of Transplants on Spontaneous Behaviours: Short-term Study*

The 6-OHDA lesion of the nucleus accumbens is known to induce several modifications in the behaviour of the rat placed into an open-field: increase of start-latency, and decrease of locomotor activity and number of rearings (Taghzouti *et al.*, 1985). The same type of deficits (increase of start latency, decrease of the number of hole-visits) can be observed in the so-called four-hole box test, which measures exploratory behaviour more explicitly (Taghzouti *et al.*, 1985). Hoarding is also disrupted as a consequence of the lesion: while in the test conditions normal animals usually bring all of the pellets into their home cage within 15–20 min, lesioned animals do not hoard at all during the whole test period (Kelley and Stinus, 1985). We decided, therefore, to test the influence of the graft on these behavioural impairments. In order to see a possible time-dependent evolution of the graft's action, the tests were repeated several times. A summary of the main results of this study is given on Figs. 20.2 and 20.3.

The results from the open-field and four-hole box tests are depicted in Fig. 20.2. It is apparent that the lesion did indeed decrease both locomotor activity in an open field and exploration, while increasing start-latency, as tested two weeks after the initial lesion. The results were quite different when tested shortly after the grafting procedure, i.e. around the twelfth week post-lesion. Paradoxically, while the grafted animals still presented the same deficits as they did immediately after the lesion, the lesioned controls displayed a clear-cut trend toward recovery from the initial locomotor and exploratory deficits, although the increased start-latency was still present in this group, too.

One of the reasons for the grafts not to produce recovery from the deficits could be that, due to their unphysiological location, the activity of the grafted dopaminergic neurons might not have been high enough (and/or was not modulated sufficiently) to spontaneously sustain a function. In order to test this hypothesis the same tests were repeated four weeks later. In this case, however, half of the animals were pre-treated with a small dose (0.1 mg/kg i.p.) of d-amphetamine given ten minutes before the tests. The results are shown on Fig. 20.2. They indeed fulfilled our expectation, in that following amphetamine treatment the locomotor and exploratory deficits of the grafted animals were completely abolished. However, the increase in start-latency was not reversed by the treatment (results not shown). On the other hand, independently of the pre-treatment, the behavioural scores of the lesioned controls were similar to those from the first tests, i.e. not different statistically from those of the intact controls (except, again, for the latencies).

The short-term results concerning hoarding behaviour followed roughly the same pattern (Fig. 20.3), except that in this case no tendency for recovery could be seen in the lesioned controls, be it with or without pre-treatment. The grafted animals again displayed the hoarding deficit when tested without pre-treatment. However, when the test was repeated after having pre-treated them with a small dose (0.2 mg/kg) of d-amphetamine, the hoarding score of the grafted animals was greatly increased, and for half of them (9/20), reached the level of the controls. Although the same dose of amphetamine also increased the locomotor activity of the grafted animals (Fig. 20.1(B)), there was no correlation between the degree of locomotor activity and the reversal of the hoarding deficit for the

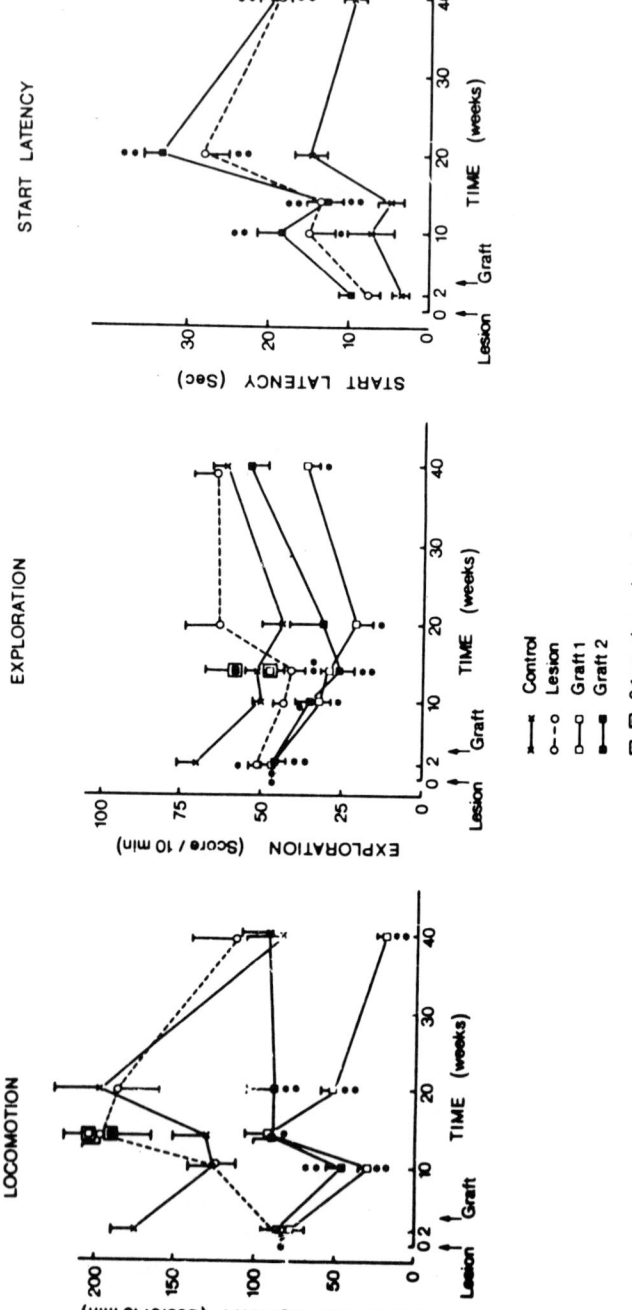

Fig. 20.2 Evolution of: locomotor activity in an open-field; number of hole visits in the four-hole box test (exploration); and start-latency in an open field in intact, lesioned and grafted animals. The grafted group was subdivided *a posteriori* into G1 and G2 subgroups, based on the presence of spontaneous recovery in locomotor activity and exploration.

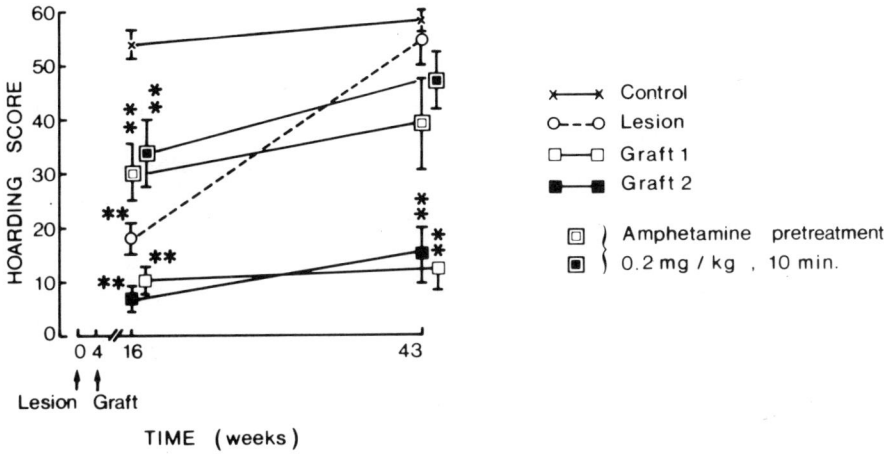

Fig. 20.3   Evolution of hoarding behaviour. Groups are the same as in Fig. 20.2.

individual animals. Furthermore, the hoarding deficit in lesioned animals was not affected at all by a similar pre-treatment with amphetamine.

Two features were therefore apparent shortly after grafting. First, the grafted animals seemed to recover the majority of the deficits tested. However, this recovery was not displayed spontaneously but required the stimulation of the graft by a small dose of d-amphetamine. Second, there was an apparent tendency of the lesioned, non-grafted control subjects to spontaneously recover from part of the initial deficits three months after the lesion.

20.3.3 Influence of Transplants on Spontaneous Behaviours: Long-term Study

When studied at longer time after grafting, the characteristics of the recovery seen previously in the experimental groups were somewhat modified. The recovery of the lesioned controls presented a further evolution: while open-field activity was, as before, at the level of intact controls, their exploratory score increased further and reached the control level around five months post-lesion (Fig. 20.2). Furthermore, hoarding, which was still totally depressed at three months post-lesion, had recovered by ten months post-lesion (Fig. 20.3). The evolution of the grafted animals was again different. While at three months post-lesion they were totally deficient on all the behavioural tests examined, some of them (subgroup G2) presented a progressive recovery in the open-field and four-hole box test at later times and reached the level of controls seven months later (Fig. 20.2). However, the other half of the grafted group (subgroup G1) still presented the original deficits. Hoarding presented a different evolution. While spontaneous hoarding was still not observed in any of the grafted animals, amphetamine again reversed this deficit in almost all of the grafted animals (independently of their belonging to the G1 or G2 subgroups (Fig. 20.3)). An evolution could be seen in this respect too, however, in that this ameliorating effect of the drug could also be observed at that time in grafted subjects which were previously unaffected by the drug.

In summary, three types of recovery pattern were apparent from this long-term follow-up. For the first type (start-latency in open-field or an exploratory task) there was no recovery in either of the groups even ten months after the lesion. In the second type (exemplified in Fig. 20.3 by the results concerning hoarding) the recovery pattern at ten months was the same as that seen at three months post-lesion for locomotion and exploration, i.e. spontaneous recovery in the lesioned animals; amphetamine-dependent recovery in the grafted animals. Finally, spontaneous recovery from the initial deficit for both experimental groups was apparent in exploratory and open-field behaviour (Fig. 20.2).

In order to test whether the behavioural recovery seen in the lesioned, non-grafted controls could be related to some reinnervation by catecholaminergic fibres of the lesioned structures, half of the animals of this group were re-lesioned ten months after the first lesion, using the same procedure of intra-accumbens 6-OHDA injection as before. The animals were submitted to the behavioural tests two weeks later. It appeared (Fig. 20.4) that the recovery seen in the non-grafted animals was, indeed, abolished by the second lesion.

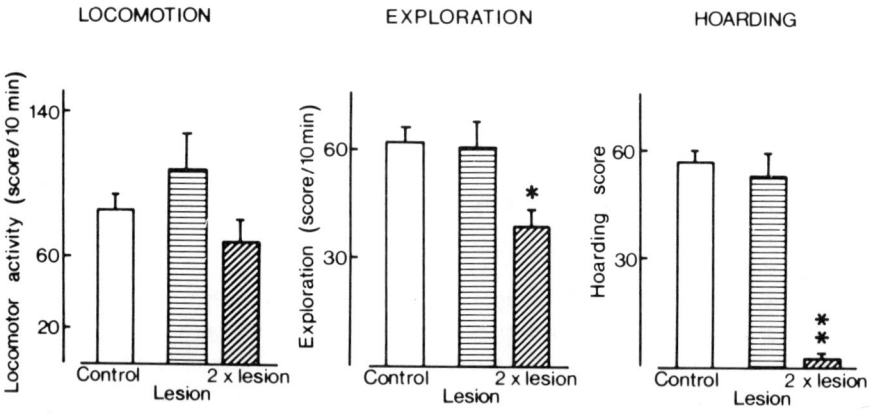

Fig. 20.4 Behavioural effects of a second nucleus accumbens lesion. Half of the lesioned animals were submitted to the same 6-OHDA lesion procedure as ten months before and the animals were tested two weeks after this second lesion.

20.3.4 Immunohistochemical Study

The anatomical study of the grafted and of the lesioned, non-grafted animals was performed between 40 and 44 weeks after the grafting procedure. The lesioned animals displayed an almost total depletion of dopaminergic fibres in the nucleus accumbens and in the anteromedial striatum, although some occasional fibres could be detected in the nucleus accumbens. Furthermore, no dopaminergic fibres could be seen either in the medial frontal cortex or in the septum. This pattern of denervation is demonstrated in Fig. 20.5(a). On the other hand, a massive reinnervation of these structures by the graft could be observed in the grafted animals, as depicted schematically in Fig. 20.5(b).

The graft itself, localised in the anteromedial striatum and in the nucleus accumbens, had the appearance of an undifferentiated tissue mass intercalated in the host structure with the dopaminergic cells localised, in the vast majority, either at the periphery of the graft in close vicinity with, or directly within, the host parenchyma. Counting the number of dopaminergic neurons in the grafts gave a figure between 1800 and 7200 per animal, the average being around 4000. However, due to the poor penetration of antibodies during the immunohisto-chemical procedure, this figure is most certainly an underestimation of the real number of dopaminergic neurons implanted. Although dopaminergic fibres could only rarely be seen within the graft itself, they could be seen in great density innervating the host nucleus accumbens as well as the anteromedial striatum. Furthermore, in almost all of the grafted animals a dopaminergic innervation of near-normal density could also be seen in the anteromedial cortex. Sometimes, a few grafted neurons could be seen stuck to one corner of the anterior septum, and in these animals a reinnervation of the ipsilateral posterior medial and lateral septum could also be seen. A characteristic feature of the reinnervation in all these structure was that its pattern was strongly reminiscent of the pattern seen in normal animals: while in the cortex this reinnervation had the appearance of a loose mesh of fibres, in the nucleus accumbens (Fig. 20.6(a))

a)

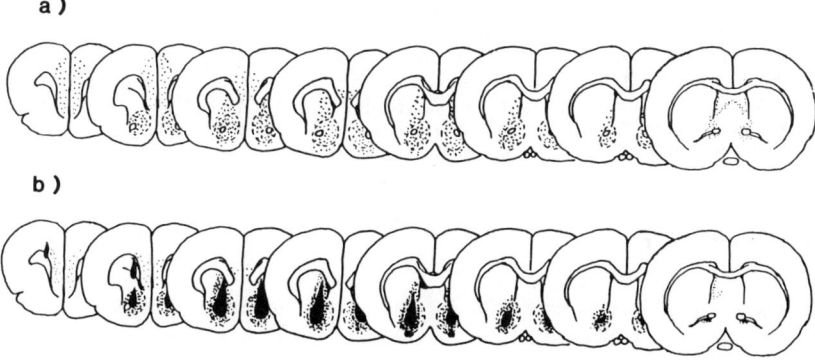

b)

Fig. 20.5   Average extent of depletion of dopaminergic innervation after the intra-accumbens injections of 6-OHDA (dotted area in (a)) and of the reinnervation provided by the dopamin-ergic grafts implanted into the nucleus accumbens (dotted area, in (b)). The black area in (b) corresponds to the central mass of the transplant.

and striatum there was a dense, homogenous reinnervation. When graft-derived dopaminergic fibres could be detected in the septum they were localised in the very same part of the septum where normal dopaminergic innervation is usually seen and, furthermore, the formation of basket-like innervation around septal perikarya, similar to that described by Moore (1978) for the normal septal innervation, could also frequently be seen in these cases (Fig. 20.6(b)).

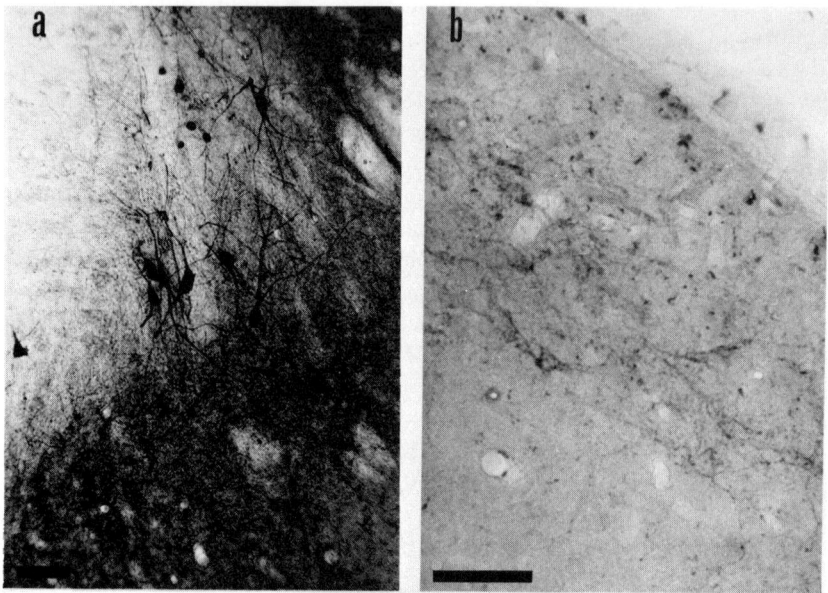

Fig. 20.6 Dopaminergic reinnervation provided by the grafts, as detected by immunohistochemistry using anti-dopamine antibody. Bars represent 50 μm. (a) Appearance of the graft (upper left corner) with dopaminergic neurons aligned along its periphery. The densely reinnervated anteromedial nucleus accumbens is seen on the right side of the picture. (b) Reinnervation of the lateral septum by implanted dopaminergic cells stuck to the ipsilateral upper corner of the anterior septum. The lateral ventricle is seen at the upper right corner. Several basket-like innervation patterns can be distinguished.

20.4 Conclusion

One of the main questions raised by the results related above concerns the mechanism by which the functional recovery observed in these experiments was attained. This question is related to the general hypothesis concerning the role of central ascending dopaminergic systems. These systems are considered not so much as conveying specific information to diverse forebrain regions but rather as having a general 'enabling' or 'tuning' function for their target structures (Simon and Le Moal, 1984). The dopaminergic stimulation of, for example the nucleus accumbens, would render this latter able to perform its specific role corresponding to the actual incoming specific informations. According to this hypothesis, functional recovery following a lesion of dopaminergic systems could be attained just by restoration of a minimal degree of general dopaminergic stimulation of the denervated target structures. This could explain, for example, the reinstatement of hoarding behaviour in rats bearing a lesion of the dopaminergic innervation of the nucleus accumbens, or even the beneficial effect of L-DOPA after the same lesion (Kelley and Stinus, 1985) or in Parkinson's disease.

How could such a restoration of dopaminergic stimulation, thus leading to functional recovery, be brought about in the lesioned, non-grafted animals? As described by various authors (Ungerstedt, 1971; Agid et al., 1973; Björklund and Stenevi, 1979) the lesion of central dopaminergic terminals induces various compensatory changes, such as supersensitivity of post-synaptic receptors, hyperactivity of remaining terminals and regeneration or sprouting of dopaminergic fibres. All these processes presumably occur in the lesioned animals considered in our experiments. Supersensitivity of the receptors is evidenced by the increased behavioural action (locomotor activation) of apomorphine seen in these animals (Herman et al., 1985c); an increase of dopamine turnover in the spared striatal terminals has been measured in animals bearing lesion of the nigrostriatal system (Herman et al., 1985a). The functional manifestation of these processes requires the presence of some dopaminergic innervation. The presence of dopaminergic neurons remaining in the A10 area, as well as of fibres grown into the denervated area, has indeed been observed in the animals of the present lesioned control group, and the reappearance of the deficits following the re-lesion of the nucleus accumbens indicates the involvement of these fibres in the functional recovery seen in our experiments. The overall result of these changes could be an increase of the dopaminergic stimulation of the previously lesioned structures thus leading to the functional recovery seen in these animals. It must be stressed, however, that this recovery was possible because of the experimental paradigm used, i.e. the use of a lesion of the dopaminergic terminals in the nucleus accumbens which spread not only striatal dopaminergic innervation but also part of the A10 mesocorticolimbic dopaminergic neurons, thus allowing collateral sprouting, as well as regeneration, to occur. In fact, no such recovery seems to exist in animals in which the lesion was performed by destroying the dopaminergic neurons themselves by injecting 6-OHDA directly into the A10 area (Herman et al., in preparation).

An interesting feature of the functional recovery seen in the lesioned controls was the non-simultaneous recovery of the different deficits. Thus, while hoarding was not restored at all 12–15 weeks after the lesion, open-field activity is totally recovered by this time and the exploratory deficit was significantly attenuated. In fact, these latter deficits, together with amphetamine-stimulated locomotion, began to recover around ten weeks after the lesion. Later on, ten months after the lesion, all of these deficits were completely abolished. This suggests that the recovery of different deficits could require a different degree of reinnervation.

The mechanism of the restoration of dopaminergic stimulation of the denervated structures (and thus of functional recovery) in the grafted animals seems to be attained mainly by an extensive reinnervation of the target tissue (see immunohistochemical results), while that of the other two processes (receptor supersensitivity and hyperactivity of dopaminergic terminals) seems to be less pronounced than in the lesioned animals (Herman et al., 1985a,c). The fact that this reinnervation is provided by dopaminergic neurons of exogenous origin implanted into the nucleus accumbens itself could, however, lead to differences in the recovery pattern of these animals as compared to that seen in the lesioned group and, in fact, such differences have indeed been observed. First, a very marked difference in the kinetics of spontaneous recovery in the grafted animals was noted which could be detected either much later than in lesioned controls (open-field behaviour or exploration), or not at all (hoarding). Furthermore, a total repair of the deficits in the grafted animals could be obtained provided that the graft was stimulated beforehand by a small dose of d-amphetamine, while this treatment was ineffective in ameliorating deficits (e.g. in hoarding) still present in the lesioned subjects.

The fact that a recovery can be evidenced following stimulation of the graft at a time when no recovery is yet seen in the lesioned controls indicates that the recovery seen at this time is indeed related to the presence of the graft in the nucleus accumbens. According to our present hypothesis, the differences observed between the recovery patterns of lesioned controls and of grafted subjects could reflect a difference in the mechanism of the recovery and be a consequence of the location of the implanted dopaminergic grafts. Due to their location in a terminal area, the implanted dopaminergic neurons lack the afferentation which impinges on mesencephalic dopaminergic neurons. As a consequence, either their activity could be too low to ensure a level of dopaminergic stimulation required for behavioural recovery or this activity could be non-modulated. This could explain the fact that spontaneous recovery was not seen with the graft despite a massive dopaminergic reinnervation of the target structures. Amphetamine could make up for the inputs and modulations which are lacking by increasing the apparent activity of the grafted neurons and could in this way reveal a behavioural action of the grafts. This hypothesis concerning such a reduced spontaneous physiological effectiveness of the grafted neurons is reinforced by the observation that behavioural recovery in the lesioned controls does not require a stimulation by amphetamine. The recovery in these animals seems to be mediated by the reinnervation of the nucleus accumbens which, although orders of magnitude weaker than the graft-derived one, could be more effective as it is provided by neurons having normal physiological locations and regulations. Additionally, the unphysiological location of the grafted neurons, which leads to a lack of regulation of their activity, could also explain their hypersensitivity to amphetamine (Fig. 20.1; see also Herman et al., 1985b) and, as a consequence, the behavioural action of doses of amphetamine which are too low to affect intact or lesioned controls.

The fact that no spontaneous recovery could be seen in the grafted animals, in contrast with the lesioned controls, seems to indicate that the graft could also inhibit normal processes which lead to a functional restoration after a lesion. Different mechanisms could explain this inhibitory action: the effect of the mechanical lesion due to the implanted tissue mass; or competition of the graft-derived fibres with regrowing endogenous fibres, etc. In fact, the mechanical lesion provoked by the graft could explain why the behavioural deficits are even potentiated shortly after the grafting procedure. On the other hand, it is also possible that this inhibition leads only to a slowing down of the ingrowth of endogenous fibres and that the late spontaneous recovery seen in the grafted animals on some tests could reflect a recovery mediated, not by the graft itself, but rather by these ingrown, regenerated fibres coming from the host's dopaminergic neurons. Experiments are under way in our laboratory aimed at clarifying these issues.

Another interesting aspect of the present results is the reinnervation pattern provided by the grafted dopaminergic neurons. This pattern is very much like the normal, endogenous innervation pattern, a result which is most conspicuous in the case of the reinnervation of the septum (*see* Fig. 20.6(b)). The formation of such a specific pattern has been previously documented for the reinnervation of the hippocampus by cholinergic grafts (Björklund *et al.*, 1983), but this is the first time that it has been observed for dopaminergic grafts. This phenomenon suggests that the ingrowth of dopaminergic fibres does not proceed randomly but is determined by some organising influence of the target tissues. Another result pointing towards an orienting influence of the target tissue during the development of the graft is the localisation of the implanted dopaminergic neurons at the periphery of the main body of the tissue mass representing the transplant. This characteristic localisation could be due to a migration of the dopaminergic neurons towards the target and/or the death of those located in the center of the implanted tissue mass, i.e. more distant from the target. The mechanism by which the target tissue exerts its influence on the development of the graft is as yet unknown, but could involve trophic factors originating in the target. Further studies should help understanding of the mechanisms of those processes.

References

Agid, Y., Javoy, F., and Glowinski, J. (1973). Hyperactivity of remaining dopaminergic neurons after partial destruction of the nigrostriatal dopaminergic system in the rat. *Nature (Lond.)*, **245**, 150–1.

Björklund, A., and Stenevi, U. (1979). Regeneration of monoaminergic and cholinergic neurons in the mammalian central nervous system. *Physiol. Rev.*, **59**, 62–100.

278   NEW CONCEPTS IN ALZHEIMER'S DISEASE

Björklund, A., and Stenevi, U. (1985). Intracerebral neural grafting: a historical perspective. In Björklund, A., and Stenevi, U. (eds.), *Neural Grafting in the Mammalian CNS*. Elsevier. Amsterdam, pp. 3–14.
Björklund, A., Schmidt, R. H., and Stenevi, U. (1980a). Functional reinnervation of the neostriatum in the adult rat by the use of intraparenchymal grafting of dissociated cell suspension from the substantia nigra. *Cell Tiss. Res.*, 212, 39–45.
Björklund, A., Gage, F. H., Stenevi, U., and Dunnett, S. B. (1983). Survival and growth of intrahippocampal implants of septal cell suspensions. *A. Physiol. Scand. Suppl.*, 522, 59–66.
Björklund, A., Dunnett, S. B., Stenevi, U., Lewis, M. E., and Iversen, S. D. (1980b). Reinnervation of the denervated striatum by substantia nigra transplants: functional consequences as revealed by pharmacological and sensorimotor testing. *Brain Res.*, 199, 307–33.
Dunnett, S. B., Bunch, S. B., Gage, F. H., and Björklund, A. (1984). Dopamine-rich transplants in rats with 6-OHDA lesions of the ventral tegmental area: I. Effects on spontaneous and drug-induced locomotor activity. *Behav. Brain Res.*, 13, 71–82.
Dunnett, S. B., Björklund, A., Schmidt, R. H., Stenevi, U., and Iversen, S. D. (1983a). Behavioural recovery in rats with unilateral 6-OHDA lesions following implantation of nigral cell suspension in different brain sites. *A Physiol. Scand. Suppl.*, 522, 29–37.
Dunnett, S. B., Björklund, A., Schmidt, R. H., Stenevi, U., and Iversen, S. D. (1983b). Behavioural recovery in rats with bilateral 6-OHDA lesion following implantation of nigral cell suspensions. *A. Physiol. Scand. Suppl.*, 522, 39–47.
Freed, W. J., Perlow, M. J., Karoum, F., Seiger, A., Olson, L., Hoffer, B., and Wyatt, R. J. (1980). Restoration of dopaminergic functions by grafting of fetal substantia nigra to the caudate nucleus: long-term behavioural, biochemical and histochemical studies. *Ann. Neurol.*, 8, 510–19.
Geffard, M., Buijs, R. M., Seguela, P., Pool, C. W., and Le Moal, M. (1984). First demonstration of highly specific and sensitive antibodies against dopamine. *Brain Res.*, 194, 161–5.
Herman, J. P., Choulli, K., and Le Moal, M. (1985a). Activation of striatal dopaminergic grafts by haloperidol. *Brain Res. Bull.*, 15, 543–6.
Herman, J. P., Choulli, K., and Le Moal, M. (1985b). Hyperreactivity to amphetamine in rats with dopaminergic grafts. *Expl. Brain Res.*, 60, 521–6.
Herman, J. P., Nadaud, D., Choulli, K., Taghzouti, K., Simon, H., and Le Moal, M. (1985c). Pharmacological and behavioral analysis of dopaminergic grafts placed into the nucleus accumbens. In Björklund, A., and Stenevi, U., (eds.), *Neural Grafting in the Mammalian CNS*, Elsevier, Amsterdam, 19–27.
Kelley, A. E., and Stinus, L. (1985). Disappearance of hoarding behavior after 6-hydroxydopamine lesion of the mesolimbic dopamine neurons and its reinstatement with L-DOPA. *Behav. Neurosci.*, 99, 531–45.
Kelly, P. H., Joyce, E. M., Minneman, K. J., and Phillipson, O. (1977). Specificity of 6-hydroxydopamine-induced destruction of mesolimbic or nigrostriatal dopamine containing terminals. *Brain Res.*, 122, 382–7.
Le Moal, M., Stinus, L., Simon, H., Tassin, J. P., Thierry, A. M., Glowinski, J., and Cardo, B. (1977). Behavioral effects of a lesion in the ventral mesencephalic tegmentum: evidence for involvement of A10 dopaminergic neurons. In Costa, E., and Gessa, G. L. (eds.), *Non-striatal Dopaminergic Neurons*. Raven Press, New York, pp. 237–45.
Moore, R. Y. (1978). Catecholaminergic innervation of the basal forebrain: the septal area. *J. Comp. Neurol.*, 177, 665–83.
Nadaud, D., Herman, J. P., Simon, H., and Le Moal, M. (1984). Functional recovery following transplantation of ventral mesencephalic cells in rats subjected to 6-OHDA lesions of the mesolimbic dopaminergic neurons. *Brain Res.*, 304, 137–41.
Simon, H., and Le Moal, M. (1984). Mesencephalic dopaminergic neurons: functional role. In Usdin, E., Carlsson, A., Dahlström, A., and Engel, J. (eds.), *Catecholamines. Neuropharmacology and Central Nervous System. Theoretical Aspects.* Alan R. Liss, New York, 293–307.

Taghzouti, K., Simon, H., Louilot, L., Herman, J. P., and Le Moal, M. (1985). Behavioral study after local injection of 6-hydroxydopamine into the nucleus accumbens in the rat. *Brain Res.*, **344**, 9–20.
Ungerstedt, U. (1971). Postsynaptic supersensitivity after 6-hydroxydopamine induced degeneration of the nigrostriatal dopamine system. *A. Physiol. Scand. Suppl.*, **367**, 69–93.

21

Transplantation of 5-HT Neurons to the Adult Rat Brain

A. Privat, H. Mansour, M. Geffard and M. Lerner-Natoli

21.1 Introduction

Transplantation of monoaminergic neurons has raised considerable interest since the advent of specific histochemical techniques which have permitted first, a precise anatomical mapping of noradrenergic, dopaminergic and serotonergic neurons and, second, an evaluation of their ability to regenerate, once severed, and to invade the host's tissue once transplanted (Gash, 1983). The usefulness of this new anatomical approach was exemplified by its showing that Parkinson's disease is the result of the lesion of dopaminergic neurons of the substantia nigra, leading itself to the depletion of striatal dopamine. It was soon found that drug treatment was able to partially reverse neurological symptoms, and one could anticipate that cell replacement could do as least as well as drug therapy, thus providing a rationale for neural transplants in the mammalian brain (Freed *et al.*, 1984).

An increasing body of evidence points to a multiple transmitter deficit in Alzheimer's disease (for a review see Bowen *et al.*, 1985). Although the cholinergic system seems to be the one most constantly and extensively involved, several reports have recently emphasised a serotonergic deficit (*see* Chapter 8; and Bowen *et al.*, 1983). It appears, then, appropriate to consider the studies of plasticity and repair of the serotonergic system as providing a potential contribution to the therapeutic strategies for Alzheimer's disease and related disorders. In contrast to the abundant literature on transplantation of catecholaminergic neurons, there exist relatively few reports on serotonergic transplants (Nygren *et al.*, 1977; Azmitia *et al.*, 1981, McRae Degueurce *et al.*, 1981, 1983). This reflects the absence, until recently (Steinbusch *et al.*, 1978; Lauder *et al.*, 1982), of specific immunological tools allowing the detection of these neurons and the tracing of their projections. In previous studies (McRae-Degueurce *et al.*, 1983, 1984), we have demonstrated with 5-HT antibodies the survival and integration into the host's brain of solid transplants of raphe nuclei from newborn rats injected into the fourth and lateral ventricles of adult recipients. The purpose of the present report is to describe the anatomical integration of cell suspensions obtained from foetal raphe nuclei injected under stereotaxic control into two target areas of the serotonergic system: the olfactory bulb and the spinal cord. The reasons for choosing these two regions are twofold. First, the anatomical organisation of the 5-HT projection is very different in the two structures. In the olfactory bulb, 5-HT terminals are concentrated in a discrete area, the glomerular layer (Anden *et al.*, 1966; Consolazion and Cuello, 1982), whereas the spinal cord projections are more widespread (Steinbusch, 1984). Second, the 5-HT innervation of these two regions can be monitored (Lerner-Natoli *et al.*, 1985; Privat *et al.*, 1985) with functional parameters, thus providing the potential control of the activity of the grafted neurons. These two models differ in an important respect: whereas the 5-HT innervation of the olfactory bulb is left intact before transplantation, that of the spinal cord is destroyed by complete section of the cord prior to the transplantation (which is performed into the distal segment). Thus, in one case transplanted neurones compete with intrinsic ones for specific synaptic sites, and in the other many synaptic sites, either specific to the 5-HT innervation or vacated by other boutons, are available.

21.2 Materials and Methods

21.2.1 Antibodies

Antibodies against 5-HT were prepared according to Geffard *et al.* (1985). They were used at a dilution of 20 000–30 000 times.

21.2.2 Transplant Preparation

Fourteen- to fifteen-day-old Sprague–Dawley rat foetuses, obtained by laparotomy, were transferred into Hanks' buffered solution, enriched with 5 % glucose, and the brain was dissected in order to isolate the region of the brain stem included between the pontine and mesencephalic flexures. The raphe region was then isolated with two parasagittal sections (Privat, 1982). Tissue blocks including the raphe nuclei were then mechanically dissociated by gentle pipetting in Ca^{++} Mg^{++} Free Puck saline, centrifuged and resuspended in the same vehicle in order to reach a concentration of 25–30 000 cells/μl.

21.2.3 Transplantation into the Olfactory Bulb

Adult Sprague–Dawley rats were anaesthetised with equithesin, and they were stereotaxically injected by Hamilton syringe with 1 μl of the above suspension in the medullary layer of the right olfactory bulb. They were then left to survive for three weeks to six months.

21.2.4 Transplantation into the Spinal Cord

Adult Sprague–Dawley rats anaesthetised with equithesin underwent a laminectomy at the lower thoracic level. The spinal cord was then sectioned, taking great care to minimise vascular damage, and a fragment 1 mm thick was excised. The muscles and skin were then sutured. Seven days later, half of the animals were re-anaesthetised, and injected with 2 to 5 μl of the cell suspension in the distal fragment of the spinal cord, just under the section. They were allowed to survive for two weeks to two months.

21.2.5 Preparation of the tissues

One-and-a-half hours prior to sacrifice, the animals were pre-treated with pargylin (100 mg/kg) and tryptophan (100 mg/kg). They were perfused with 5 % glutaraldehyde and 1 % sodium metabisulphite in 0.05 M Cacodylate buffer. The brain or spinal cord was then dissected and immersed for 1 h in the same perfusate. 50 μm thick vibratome sections were then collected, rinsed in tris buffer, reduced with 1 % sodium borohydride for 10 min, and reacted with the P.A.P. method (Privat *et al.*, 1986). After reaction with di-amino-benzidine, some of the sections were then mounted on slides for light microscopy while others were treated with osmium tetroxide and flat-embedded in araldite for electron microscopy. After re-embedding in gelatin capsules, 1 μm sections were stained with toluidin blue for light microscopy, and ultra-thin sections contrasted with uranyl and lead for electron microscopy.

21.3 Results

21.3.1 Olfactory Bulb

Serotonergic axons in the olfactory bulb course rostrally in the medullary layer, and distribute radially to the glomerular layer, where they end up as periglomerular varicose arborisations (Fig. 21.1). Ultrastructural examination after 5-HT immunocytochemistry (Privat, in preparation) has shown that 5-HT-positive boutons exclusively contact dendrites and axons in the glomerular layer and, to a limited extent, in the external plexiform layer. Specifically, no contacts were found on the perikarya of mitral, tufted or horizontal cells.

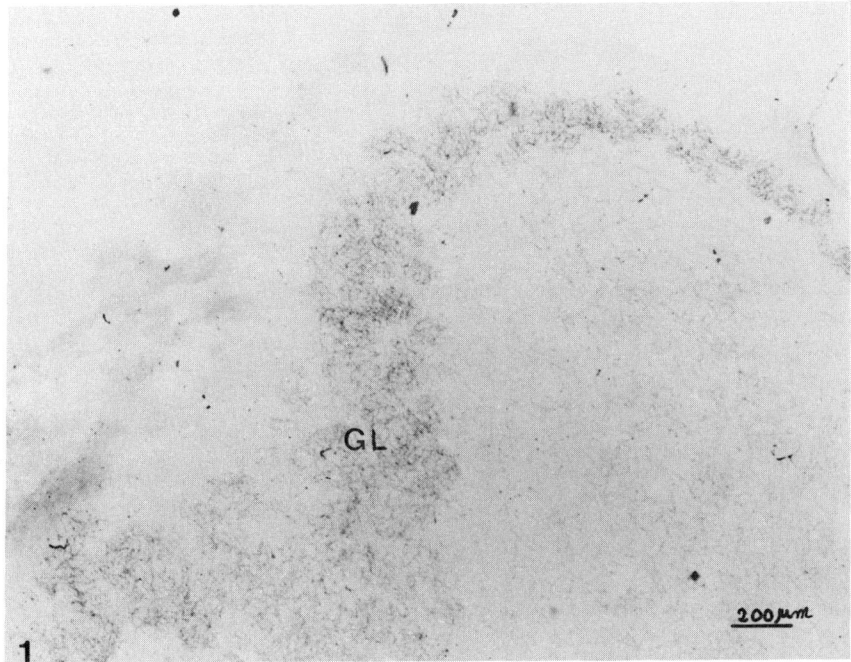

Fig. 21.1 Vibratome section of the olfactory bulb of a control rat, reacted with anti-5-HT antibodies: the glomerular layer (GL) is heavily labelled with 5-HT terminals.

In all of the 20 injected bulbs, 5-HT immunoreactive cells were found after the various survival intervals. They appeared most often clustered at the site of injection (Fig. 21.2), although in several cases isolated cells were seen at some distance from the bulk of immunoreactive perikarya (Fig. 21.5). Most of the perykarya appeared strongly immunoreactive, and they corresponded in shape and size to their counterparts in the raphe nuclei of the intact animal: we could see small round (Fig. 21.4), medium fusiform (Fig. 21.3), and large polygonal perikarya (Figs. 21.3 and 21.5). Dendrites displayed a large variety of shapes and sizes and, on rare occasions, could be seen extending over 150–200 μm. In most cases, however, they could be followed over 30–50 μm, as is the case *in situ* (Steinbusch, 1984). Axons could be seen arising either from the peri-karyon or from the initial segment of a dendrite. They immediately branch profusely, but frequently (Fig. 21.4) did not seem to invade the host tissue over large distances. In several instances, however, a large bundle of axons was directed to the surface of the bulb and the glomerular layer, and 'hyperinnervated' glo-meruli could be seen (Figs. 21.7 and 21.8).

284

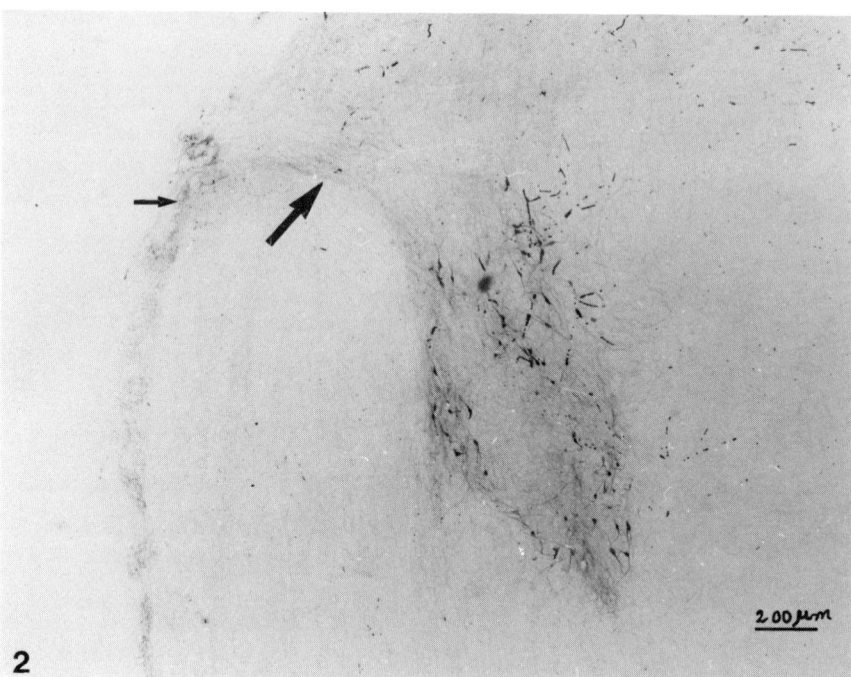

Fig. 21.2 Vibratome section of the olfactory bulb of a rat transplanted with raphe suspension one month before sacrifice. Many 5-HT immunoreactive perikarya can be seen in the centre of the picture. A bundle of axons (large arrow) is directed towards the glomerular layer, where some glomeruli are hyperinnervated (small arrow).

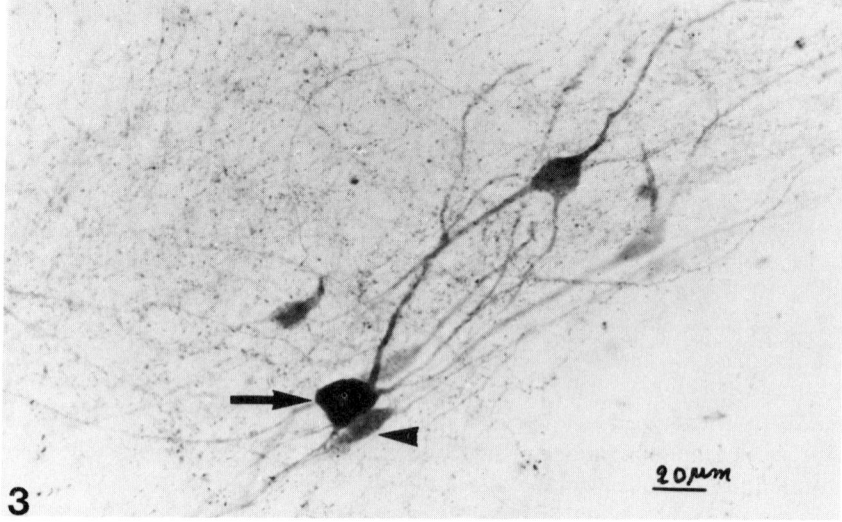

Fig. 21.3 High magnification of 5-HT immunoreactive neurons, one month after transplantation into the olfactory bulb. The arrow points to a large polygonal cell, and the arrowhead points to a small fusiform cell. In the upper right corner are other polygonal and fusiform cells. Notice the very dense immunoreactive neuropile.

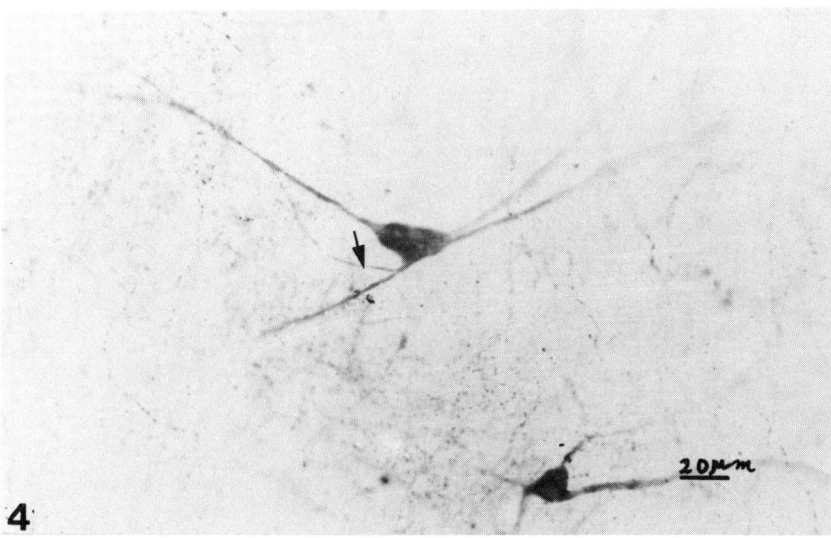

Fig. 21.4   Same as Fig. 21.3. The arrow points to an axon arising from the initial segment of a dendrite. In the lower part of the picture is a small round neuron.

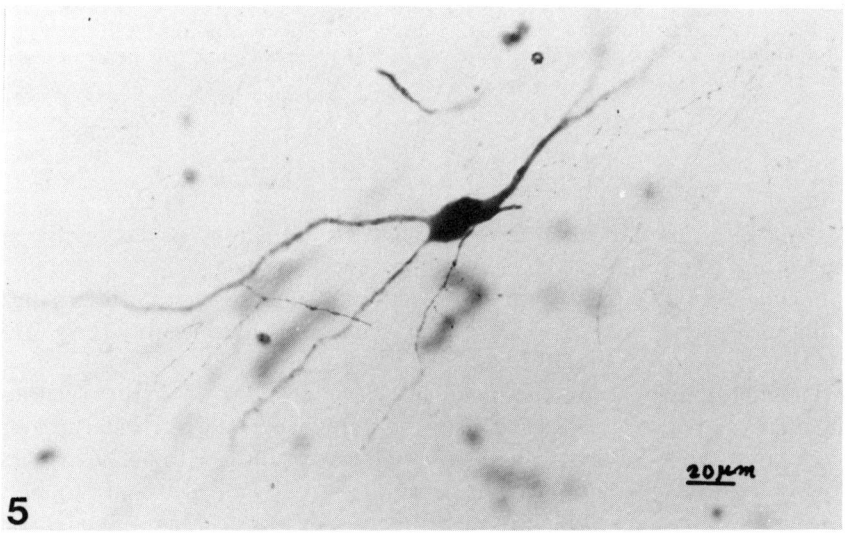

Fig. 21.5   Same as Fig. 21.3. A medium-sized fusiform neuron is located at some distance from the site of transplantation, as testified by the paucity of immunoreactive processes in its vicinity.

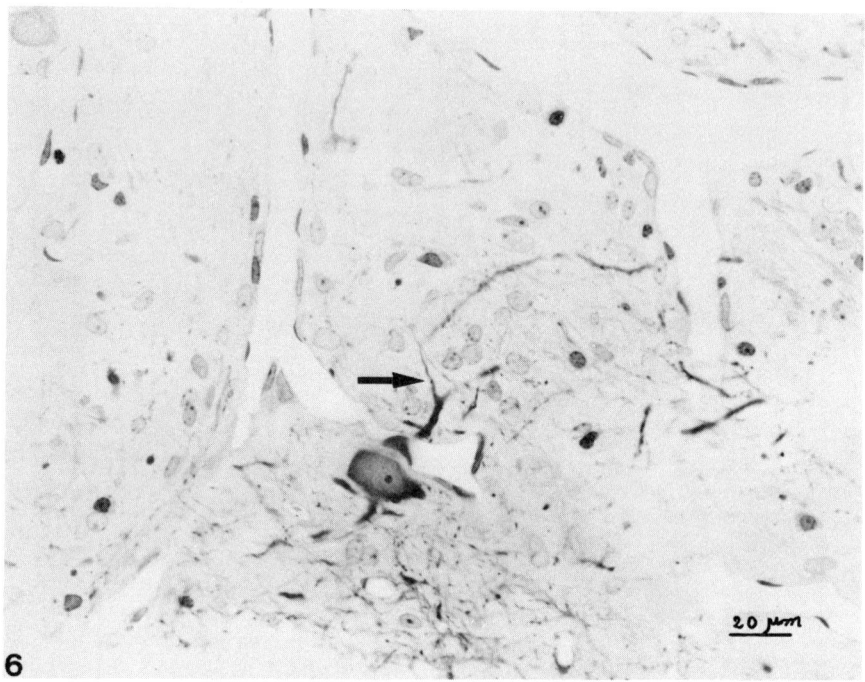

6

Fig. 21.6 1 μm plastic section counterstained with toluidin blue showing a large polygonal 5-HT immunoreactive neuron and its arborisation. The arrow points to the axon arising from a dendritic trunk.

At the ultrastructural level we could identify 5-HT neurons, and their afferent and efferent connections.

Immunoreactive perikarya and dendrites are contacted by numerous axonal boutons, displaying a large variety of morphological characteristics (Figs. 21.9 and 21.10).

Immunoreactive boutons are in contact with unlabelled perikarya, dendrites and axons, and in several instances make typical synapses (Fig. 21.11). However, we have frequently seen immunoreactive varicosites, filled with 40 nm vesicles, which were not facing post-synaptic densities (Fig. 21.12). Such configurations, suggestive of non-conventional synapses (Descarries *et al.*, 1975), were also seen in control animals in the glomerular layer (Fig. 21.13).

Finally, immunoreactive boutons were also seen facing immunoreactive dendrites (Fig. 21.14). The frequent close proximity of several immunoreactive 5-HT neurons precludes the identification of those contacts as autapses. It is more likely that the pre- and post-synaptic elements belong to different cells.

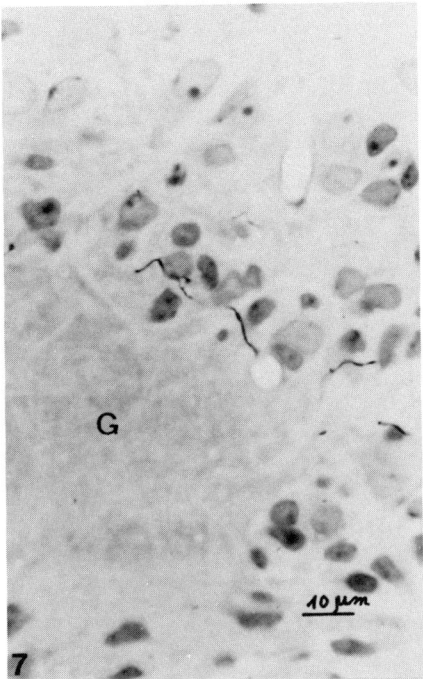

Fig. 21.7 Same as Fig. 21.6. Glomerular layer of a control rat showing 5-HT-immuno-reactive fibres at the periphery of a glomerulus (G).

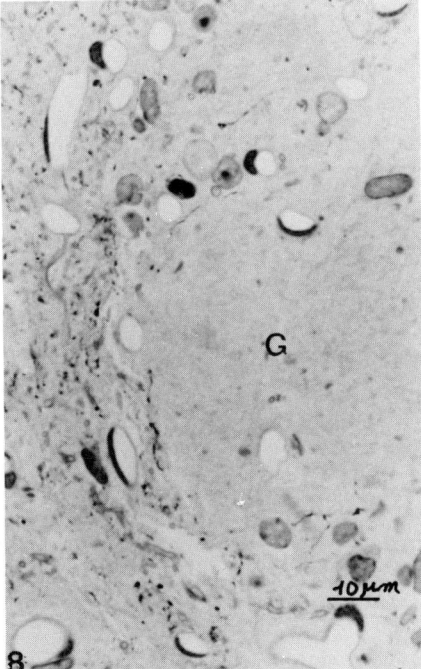

Fig. 21.8 Same as Fig. 21.6. Glomerular layer of a transplanted rat showing the dense innervation of the periphery of a glomerulus in the left of the picture, contrasting with the almost total absence of fibres in the glomerulus itself (G).

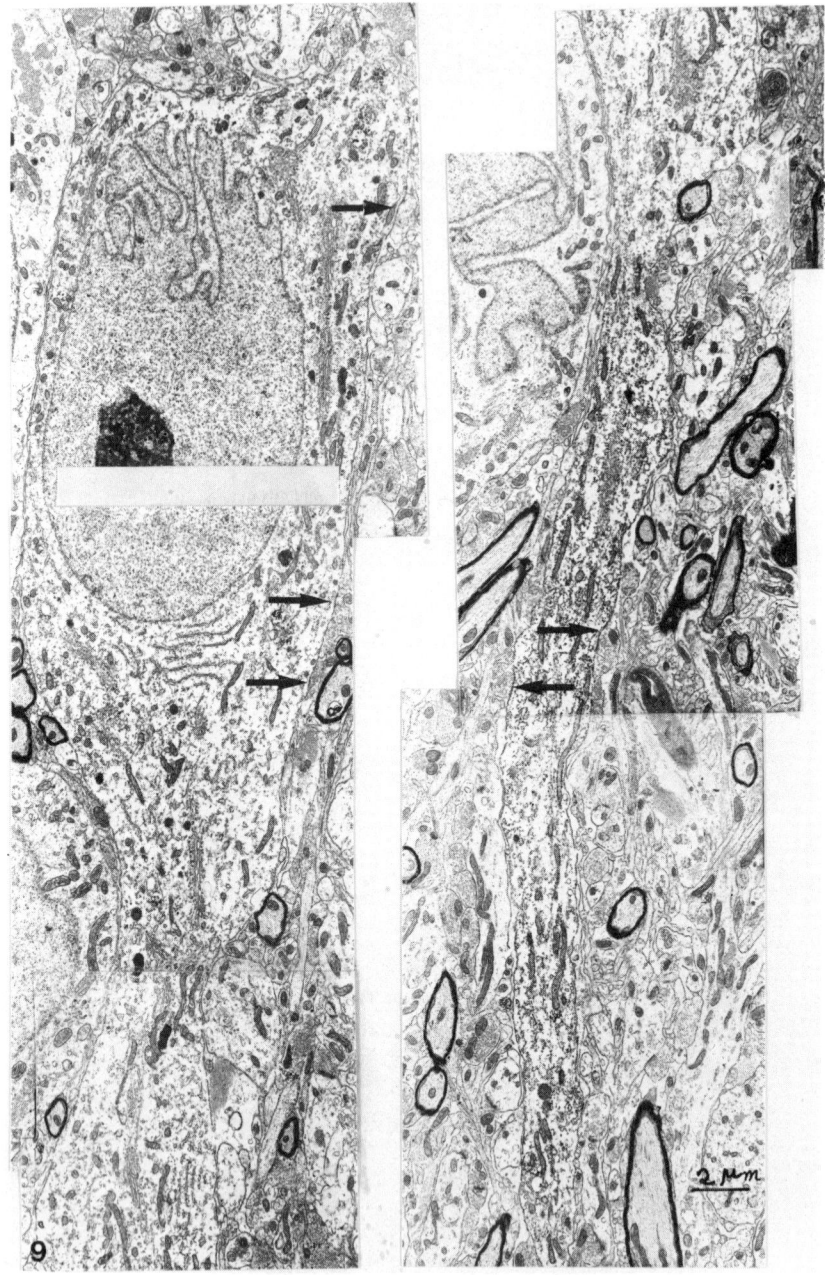

Fig. 21.9 Electron microscope 5-HT immunocytochemistry. A 5-HT immunoreactive neuron, two months after transplantation to the olfactory bulb, has been partially reconstructed. The dendrite extending below the nucleus in the left column can be followed throughout the right column. Arrows indicate afferent synapses.

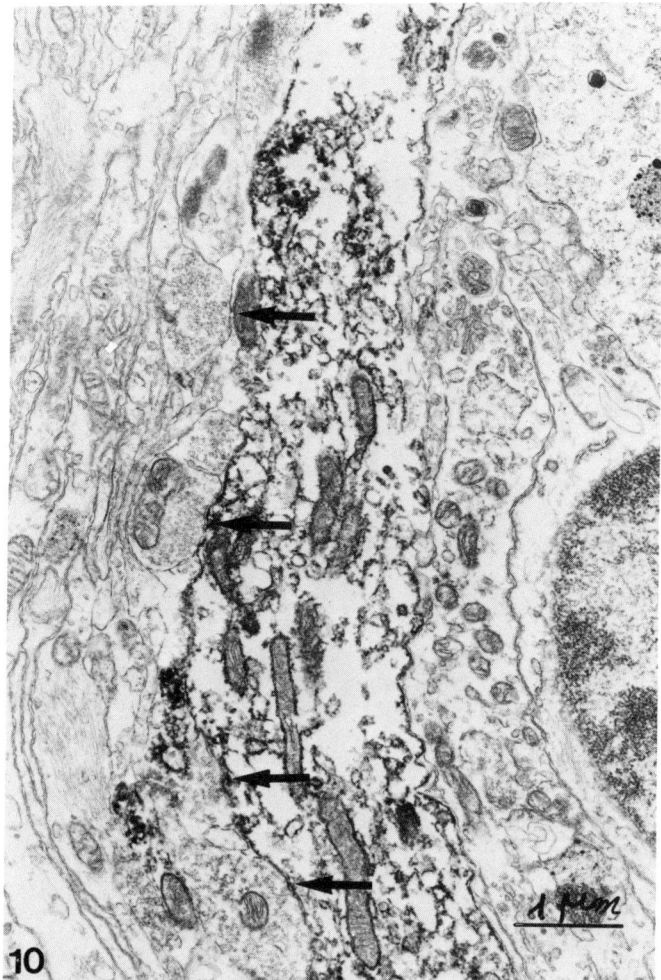

Fig. 21.10 Same as Fig. 21.9. A 5-HT immunoreactive dendrite is contacted by several afferent boutons (arrows).

21.3.2 Spinal Cord

The serotonergic innervation of the thoracic spinal cord is essentially concentrated in the anterior part of the ventral horn, around motoneurons, in the intermedio-lateralis horn and, to a lesser extent, in the most posterior part of the dorsal horn. This pattern is illustrated on Fig. 21.15, corresponding to a mid-thoracic level above the section of the spinal cord.

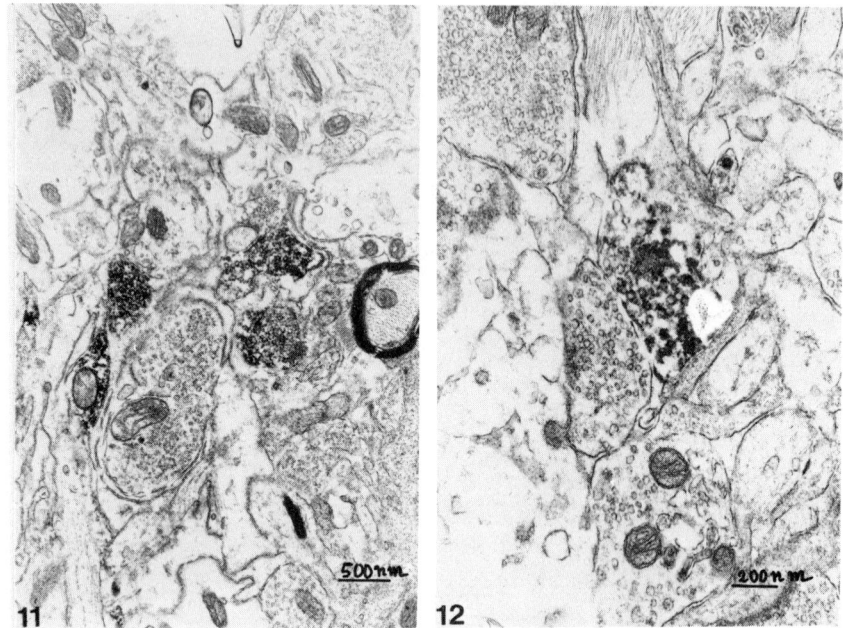

Fig. 21.11 Same as Fig. 21.9. 5-HT immuno-reactive boutons are in contact with un-labelled dendrites.

Fig. 21.12 Same as Fig. 21.9. An immuno-reactive bouton, filled with synaptic vesicles, is not accompanied by a post-synaptic density in the neighbouring profiles.

Control animals, which had their spinal cord sectioned, showed a total dis-appearance of 5-HT immunoreactivity below the section. Samples taken 5, 10 and 15 millimetres below the section did not show any immunoreactive profile 20 and 35 days after the surgery (Fig. 21.16).

Experimental animals show, ten days after transplantation, well-developed 5-HT perikarya and processes (Fig. 21.17). Perikarya display the variety of sizes and shapes already seen in olfactory bulb transplants (Figs. 18 and 19). In addition, and at variance with the latter, grafted cells were seen at large distances (up to 10 mm) from the level of the graft. The pattern of innervation is highly characteristic, with the higher density in the anterior horn (Figs. 21.20 and 21.22) and the intermedio-lateral horn (Fig. 21.23). With time, there is a pro-gressive increase in the extent of axonal growth; whereas, after ten days, axonal growth cones are seen 10 to 15 mm from the graft (Fig. 21.21), after 1 month, varicose endings can be seen as far as 20 mm below the graft. Again, they are concentrated in the anterior and intermediate horns (Figs. 21.22 and 21.23).

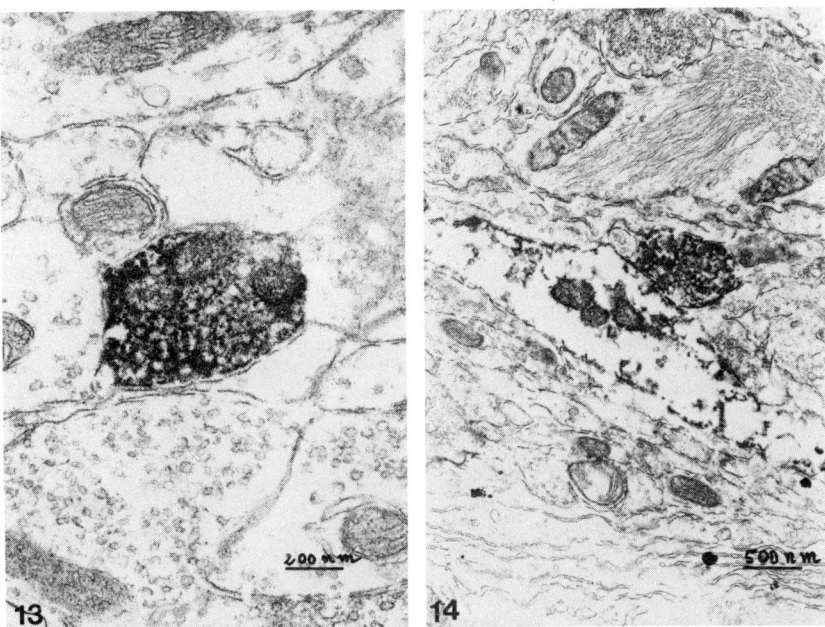

Fig. 21.13   Immunoreactive bouton in the glomerular layer of a control rat olfactory bulb. As in Fig. 21.12, this bouton does not correspond to a post-synaptic density.

Fig. 21.14   Same as Fig. 21.9. An immunoreactive bouton is in synaptic contact with an immunoreactive dendrite.

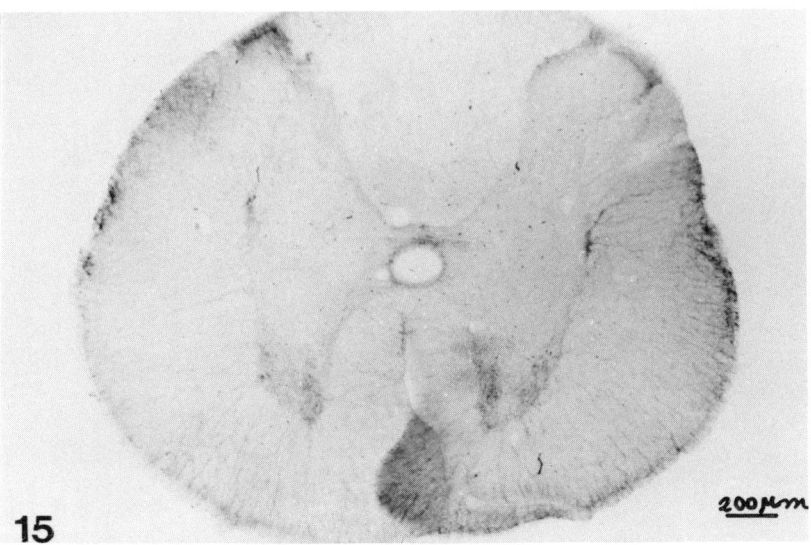

Fig. 21.15   Cross-section of thoracic spinal cord of an adult rat, reacted with 5-HT antibodies. Strong immunoreactivity is seen in the anterior portion of the ventral horn, in the intermedio-lateralis column, and in the most posterior part of the dorsal horn. Moderate immunoreactivity is seen in the white matter of the anterior and lateral funiculi.

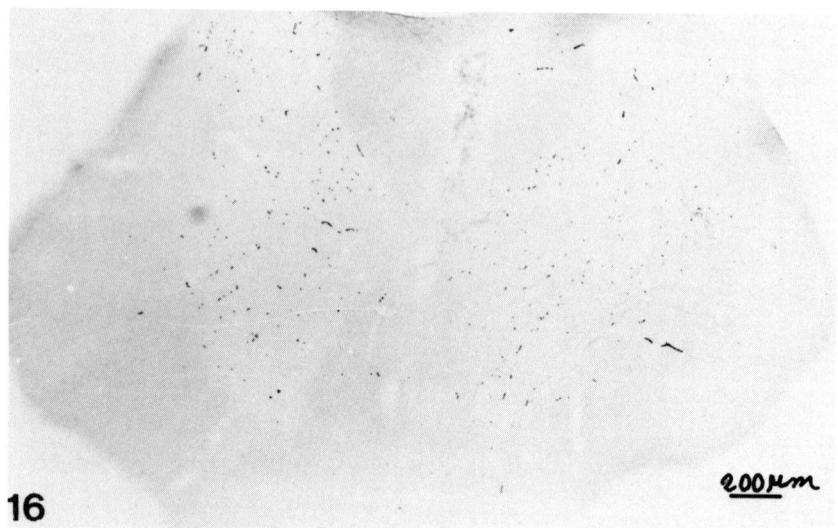

Fig. 21.16 Same as Fig. 21.15. This section has been performed below a spinal cord tran-
section, one month after surgery. No 5-HT immunoreactivity is present. The dark spots in
the picture correspond to capillaries infarcted with red blood cells.

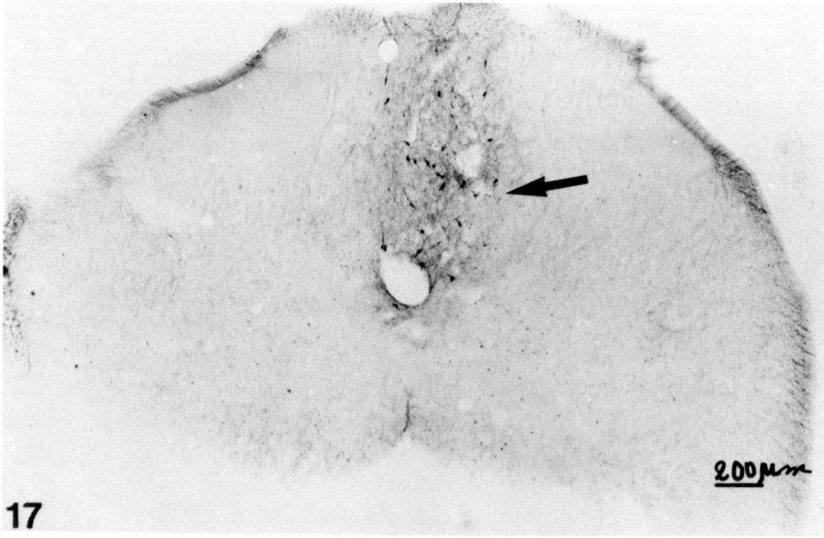

Fig. 21.17 Same as Fig. 21.15. Ten days after transplantation of raphe suspension many
5-HT immunoreactive perikarya are seen in the dorsal columns of the cord (arrow).

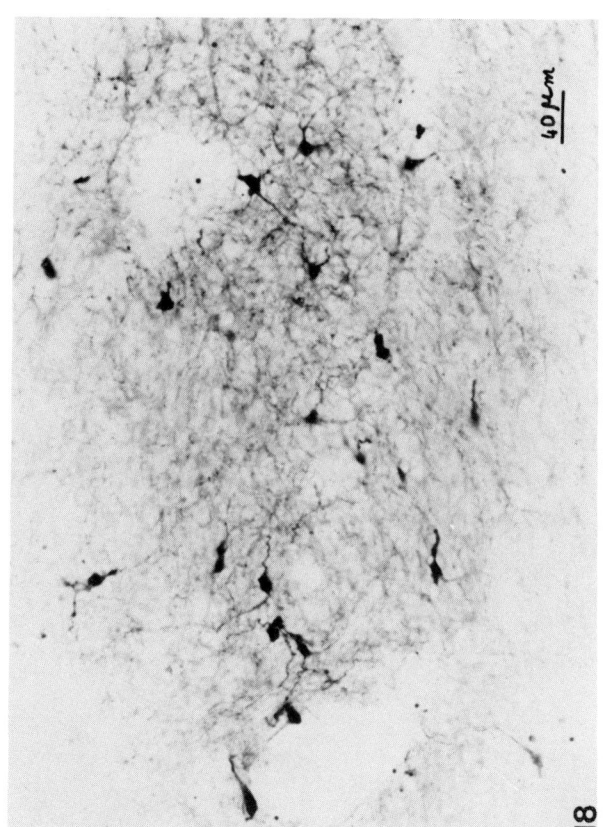

Fig. 21.18 Same as Fig. 21.17. In the area of the graft, 5-HT immunoreactive neurons display a large variety of shapes and sizes.

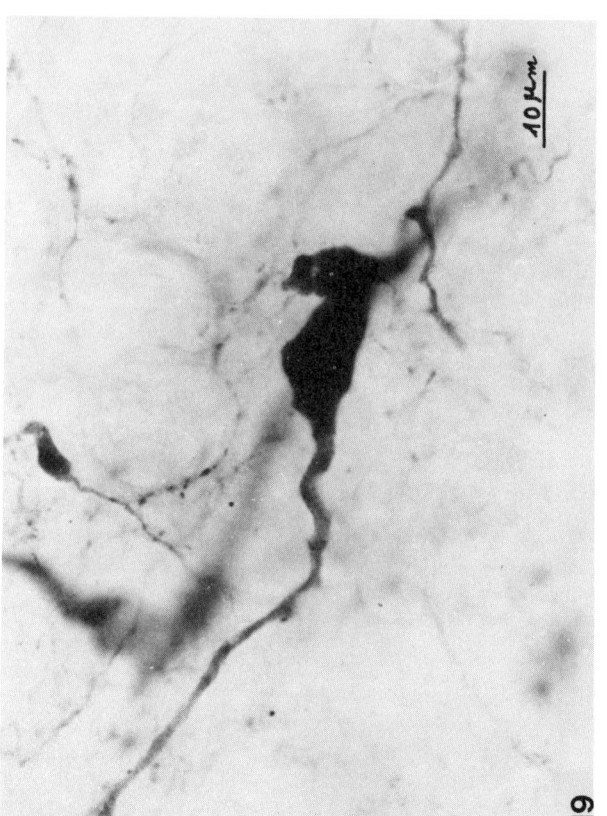

Fig. 21.19   Same as Fig. 21.17. A medium-sized 5-HT neuron is strongly immunoreactive.

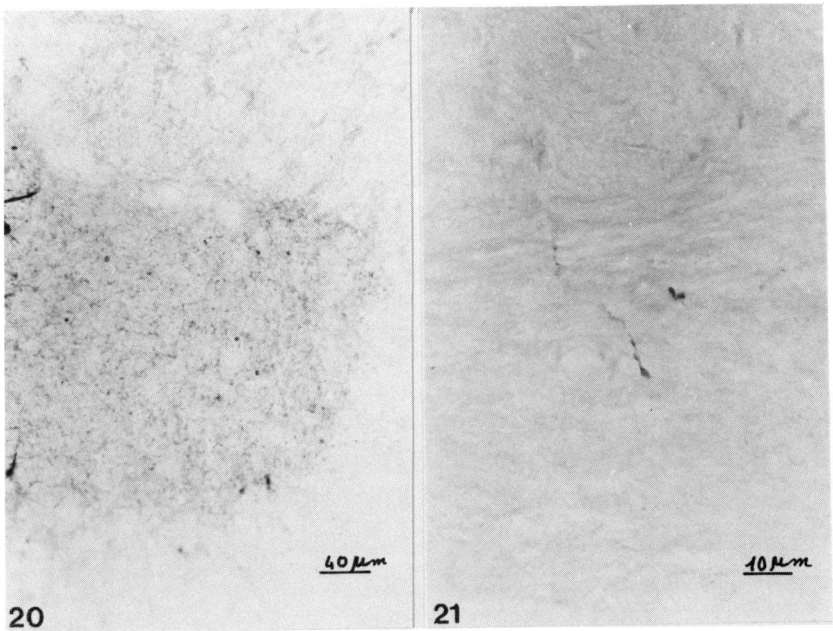

Fig. 21.20 Same as Fig. 21.17. The anterior horn contains a high density of 5-HT immunoreactive fibres.

Fig. 21.21 Same as Fig. 20.17. 10 mm below the level of the graft, 5-HT immunoreactive neurites endowed with growth cones are seen in the anterior horn.

21.4 Discussion

The present report has established that 5-HT foetal neurons transplanted into the olfactory bulb and the spinal cord of adult rats can survive, grow their axons and dendrites, and establish synaptic connections with the host neurons. However, the conditions were different in the two models. In the olfactory bulb the intrinsic 5-HT innervation was intact, and this condition is similar to that described already by Azmitia *et al.* (1981) in the hippocampus. However, these authors concluded that innervations provided by the transplant followed a pattern similar to that of intrinsic neurons. In the olfactory bulb, the results are slightly different, as neurons which are not normally contacted by 5-HT axons show afferent synaptic boutons filled with 40 nm vesicles. Nevertheless, axons which reached the normal target of 5-HT innervation, the glomerular layer, showed a strikingly similar pattern of innervation, i.e. large varicose fibres confined at the periphery of glomeruli (Fig. 21.8). This difference from the results of Azmitia *et al.* (1981) could be due to the fact that the hippocampus in the

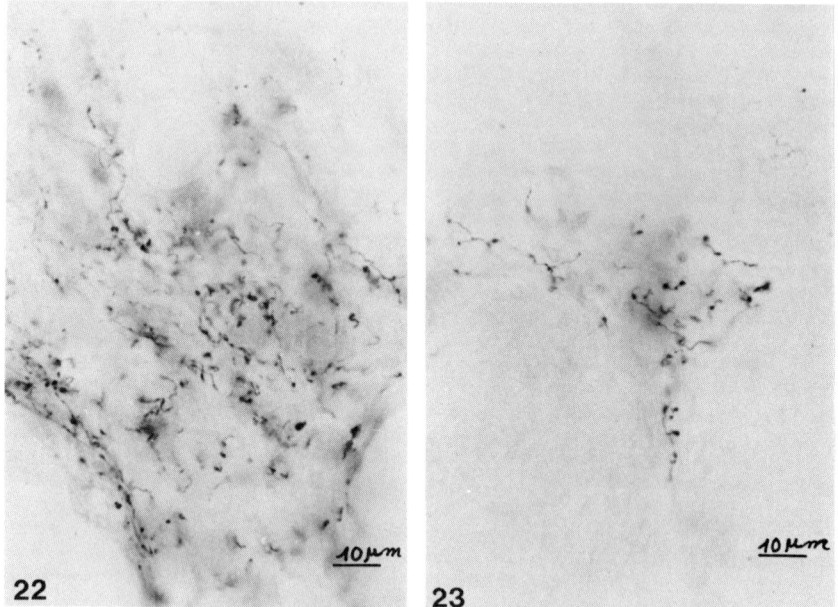

22

23

Fig. 21.22 One month after transplantation, the anterior horn contains a high
density of 5-HT immunoreactive varicose
fibres, 10 mm below the level of a graft.

Fig. 21.23 Same as Fig. 21.22. 5-HT immunoreactive varicose fibres concentrated
in the intermedio-lateralis column.

normal animal is profusely innervated with 5-HT fibres, whereas the innervation
of the olfactory bulb is very precisely limited to the glomerular layer. Thus,
5-HT neurons transplanted to the hippocampus may not have a chance to show
heterotopic innervation, at least at the light microscope level. Ongoing studies
in our laboratory are directed at clarifying this point at the ultrastructural level.

Similar ultrastructural studies have been carried out by Freund *et al.* (1985),
Mahalik *et al.* (1985) and Jaeger (1985) on dopaminergic neurons transplanted
into the striatum of adult rats. These authors identified in the grafted animals
synaptic arrangements which are normally never seen in the neostriatum, despite
the fact that the host's striatum had previously been deprived of intrinsic dopaminergic innervation.

Regarding the functional influence of these transplants, preliminary studies
(Lerner-Natoli *et al.*, in preparation) have shown that they could influence
electrical excitability of bulbar intrinsic neurons. We have shown recently
(Lerner-Natoli *et al.*, 1985) that destruction of 5-HT innervation of the bulb
with the neurotoxin 5-7 DHT induced a facilitation and acceleration of kindling
(Racine and Coscina, 1979) elicited from the bulb, suggesting that 5-HT exerts

an inhibitory tone upon bulbar neurons. Some of the grafted animals have been subsequently kindled, and it was found that the threshold for after-discharge triggering was significantly increased in contrast to non-grafted controls. Work is now in progress to decide whether this effect is specific for serotonergic neurons, or if it can be triggered by other transplanted neurons.

For the spinal cord, the only previous report of transplanted 5-HT neurons (Nygren et al., 1977) recorded a very limited outgrowth of axons outside of the graft. This study, as did those of Nornes et al. (1984) and Commissiong (1984) with noradrenergic neurons, made use of solid transplants and those, in our experience, are not as successful as cell suspensions. We have recorded, in the present study, the growth of axons over more than 20 mm in the grey matter of the cord. Cell migration was also found over at least 10 mm, but always occurred in close vicinity to the central canal, which was most often enlarged, thus providing a possible axis for migration. The pattern of innervation was strikingly similar to that of the intact cord, but again it must be noted that the thoracic cord is profusely innervated with 5-HT terminals, as is the hippocampus dentate gyrus (Azmitia et al., 1981). It was worth noting, however, the concentration of 5-HT varicose fibres in the anterior and intermediate horns, as described by Steinbusch (1984) for the thoracic cord. It may thus be hypothesised that grafted aminergic neurons show a relative specificity of connections, irrespective of the presence or absence of homologous intrinsic innervation. Besides their normal targets, they may innervate other structures, and possibly contribute through them to the reported functional restoration (Freund et al., 1985). Preliminary results indicate that, whereas sectioned-ungrafted rats showed absence of sphincteral control, which led in same cases to death secondary to acute urine retention, grafted animals seemed to have restored bladder control within one week after graft, and generally showed better recovery and greater spontaneous activity. Work is now in progress to objectively evaluate the influence of these grafts upon motor and visceral functions below the level of the section. In addition, we are currently evaluating the anatomical characteristics and functional consequences of grafts from other neuronal types.

21.5 Conclusion

This preliminary study with transplants of 5-HT neurons to the olfactory bulb and the spinal cord of adult rats shows that transplanted neurons are able to grow, differentiate the express their transmitter phenotype. Moreover, they establish synaptic contacts with the host neurons. These contacts differ in several cases from those of the corresponding intrinsic innervation, indicating a relative lack of specificity. Despite that, preliminary results indicate some functional influence of grafted neurons whose mechanism awaits further clarification.

Acknowledgement

This work has been supported by a DRET Grant no. 84-126. The authors acknowledge the help of Mrs F. Sandillon for histological techniques and Mrs V. Kimbor for typing of the manuscript.

References

Anden, N. E., Dahlström, A., Fuxe, K., Larsson, K., Olsen, L., and Ungerstedt, U. (1966). Ascending monoamine neurons to the telencephalon and diencephalon. *Acta Physiol. Scand.*, 67, 313-26.

Azmitia, E. C., Perlow, M. J., Brennan, M. J., and Lauder, J. M. (1981). Fetal raphe and hippocampal transplants into adult and aged C57BL/6N mice: a preliminary immunocytochemical study. *Brain Res. Bull.*, 7, 703-10.

Bowen, D. M., Davison, A. M., Francis, P. T., Palmer, A. M., and Pearce, B. R. (1985). Neurotransmitter and metabolic dysfunction in Alzheimer's dementia: relationship to histopathological features. *Interdiscipl. Topics Geront.*, 19, 156-74.

Bowen, D. M., Allen, S. J., Benton, J. S., Goodhardt, M. J., Haan, E. A., Palemr, A. M., Sims, N. R., Smith, C. C. T., Spillane, J. A., Esiri, M. M., Neary, D., Snowdon, J. S., Wilcock, G. K., and Davison, A. N. (1983). Biochemical assessment of serotoninergic and cholinergic dysfunction and cerebral atrophy in Alzheimer's disease. *J. Neurochem.*, 41, 266-72.

Commissiong, J. W. (1984). Fetal locus coeruleus transplanted into the transected spinal cord of the adult rat: some observation and implications. *Neurosci.*, 21, 839-53.

Consolazione, A., and Cuello, A. C. (1982). CNS serotonin pathways. In Osborne, N. N. (ed.), *Biology of Serotonergic Transmission*. Wiley, Chichester, 29-61.

Descarries, L., Beaudet, A., and Watkins, K. C. (1975). Serotonin nerve terminals in adult rat neocortex. *Brain Res.*, 100, 563-88.

Freed, W. J., Hoffer, B. J., Olsen, L., and Wyatt, R. J. (1984). Transplantation of catecholamine-containing tissues to restore the functional capacity of damaged nigrostriatal system. In Sladek, J. R., and Gash, D. M. (eds.), *Neural Transplants: Development and Function*. Plenum Press, New York, pp. 373-402.

Freund, T. F., Bolam, J. P., Bjordklund, A., Stenevi, U., Dunnet, S. B., Powel, J. F., and Smith, A. D. (1985). Efferent synaptic connections of grafted dopaminergic neurons reinnervating the host neostriatum: a tyrosin hydroxylase immunocytochemical study. *J. Neurosci.*, 5, 603-16.

Gash, D. M. (1983). Neural transplants in mammals. A historical overview. In: Sladek, J. R., and Gash, D. M. (eds.), *Neural Transplants: Development and Function*. Plenum Press, New York, 1-11.

Geffard, M., Henrich-Roch, A-M., Dulluc, J., and Seguela, P. H. (1985). Antisera against small neurotransmitter-like molecules. *Neurochem. Int.*, 7, 403-13.

Jaeger, C. B. (1985). Cytoarchitectonics of substantia nigra grafts: a light and electron microscopic study of immunocytochemically identified dopaminergic neurons and fibrous astrocytes. *J. Comp. Neurol.*, 231, 121-35.

Lauder, J. M., Wallace, J. A., Krebs, H., Peterusz, P., and McCarthy, K. (1982). *In vivo* and *in vitro* development of serotonergic neurons. *Brain Res. Bulletin*, 9, 605-25.

Lerner-Natoli, M., Rondouin, G., Malafosse, A., Sandillon, F., and Privat, A. (1986). Facilitation of olfactory bulb kindling after specific destruction of serotoninergic terminals in the olfactory bulb of rat. *Neurosci. Lett.*, 66, 299-304.

McRae-Degueurce, A., Didier, M., and Pujol, J. F. (1981). The viability of transplants of mesencephalic raphe nuclei in the 15th ventricle of adult rat. *Neurosci. Lett.*, 24, 251-4.

McRae-Degueurce, A., Lauder, J. M., and Privat, A. (1983). Adult age destruction versus neonatal age destruction of the serotonin system: two models to investigate the survival of serotonin neurons transplanted in adult rats. *Neurosci. Lett.*, 40, 27-32.

McRae Degueurce, A., Serrano, A., Sandillon, F., Privat, A., and Scatton, B. (1984). *In vivo* voltametric measurement of extra-cellular 5-HIAA in the denervated striatum after transplantation of mesencephalic raphe neurons. *Neurosci. Lett.*, **48**, 97–102.

Mahalik, T. J., Finger, T. E., Stromberg, I., and Olson, L. (1985). Substantia nigra transplants into denervated striatum of the rat: ultrastructure of graft and host interconnections. *J. Comp. Neurol.*, **240**, 60–70.

Nornes, H., Bjorklund, A., and Stenevi, U. (1984). Transplantation strategies in spinal cord regeneration. In Sladek, J. R., and Gash, D. M. (eds.), *Neural Transplants: Development and Function*. Plenum Press, New York, 407–21.

Nygren, L. G., Olson, L., and Seiger, A. (1977). Monoaminergic reinnervation of transected spinal cord by homologous fetal brain grafts. *Brain Res.*, **129**, 227–35.

Privat, A. (1982). *In vitro* cultures of serotonergic neurons from fetal rat brain. *J. Histochem. Cytochem.*, **30**, 185–7.

Privat, A., Mansour, H., Pavy, A., Geffard, M., and Sandillon, F. (1985). Transplantation of foetal 5-HT neurons into the transected spinal cord of adult rats. *Neurosci. Lett.*, **66**, 61–6.

Racine, R. J., and Coscina, D. V. (1979). Effects of midbrain raphe lesions or systemic p-chlorophenylalaline on the development of kindles seizures in rats. *Brain Res. Bull.*, **4**, 1–7.

Steinbusch, H. W. M. (1984). Serotonin-immunoreactive neurons and their projections in the CNS. In Bjorklund, A., Hökfelt, T., and Kuhar, M. J. (eds.), *Handbook of Chemical Neuroanatomy*. Elsevier, Amsterdam, pp. 68–125.

Steinbusch, H. W. M., Verhofstad, A. J., and Joosten, H. W. J. (1978). Localization of serotonin in the central nervous system by immunohistochemistry: desctruction of a specific and sensitive technique and some applications. *Neurosci.*, **3**, 811–19.

Index